Atlas of Lip and Nose Plastic and Cosmetic Surgery

Jianhua Liu • Bing Shi
Editors

Atlas of Lip and Nose Plastic and Cosmetic Surgery

PMPH PEOPLE'S MEDICAL PUBLISHING HOUSE

Springer

Editors
Jianhua Liu
Department of Oral and Maxillo-facial Surgery
First Affiliated Hospital
Zhejiang University School of Medicine
Hangzhou
China

Bing Shi
Department of Cleft Lip and Palate Surgery
Vice Dean, West China Stomatology College
Sichuan University
Chengdu
China

ISBN 978-981-16-1910-6 ISBN 978-981-16-1911-3 (eBook)
https://doi.org/10.1007/978-981-16-1911-3
Jointly published with People's Medical Publishing House, PR of China

This Springer imprint is published by the registered company Springer Nature Singapore Pte Ltd.
The registered company address is: 152 Beach Road, #21-01/04 Gateway East, Singapore 189721, Singapore

Preface

In the recent years, patients' expectation in medical care has shifted from merely being functionally oriented to having the desire to restore both aesthetics and health, in equal weightage. This is especially relevant for maxillofacial surgery. This requires clinicians to have a stronger sense of duty and professionalism. Only by adhering to the principles of form and function, can we meet the growing demands of the patients.

Compared to other parts of the body, the deformities of maxillofacial region have a greater influence on the physical and mental wellbeing of the patients. Even minor deformities deserve special care and attention during treatment.

In the maxillofacial region, nasolabial deformities are the most common. This includes both primary and secondary (acquired) deformities. Previously written plastic or cosmetic surgery books on the nose or lip region focus on management as their key points. The books mostly begin with an introduction to the anatomical structures and discuss a few routine and generic surgical techniques. They generally do not delve into management of specific conditions or deformities. However, in the clinical setting, there are many situations whereby ideal outcome cannot be achieved with these routine methods. If we introduce the different surgical techniques in relation to the different classification of the deformities, it will aid in the conceptualization of customized surgical plans, which will be useful to many clinicians.

For this reason, we compiled a range of knowledge from the normal anatomy of the nasolabial region, cosmetic surgery, to the repair of congenital and acquired malformation of the nasolabial region.

The format of the book is based on the classification of the deformities so as to facilitate referencing and application. Information is relayed in terms of the indications, classic examples of the deformities, points to note, and so on. In the writing of the surgical methods and procedures, we strive to give the reader a clear understanding of the entire operating process with pictures of surgical procedures.

In order to ensure high quality in the academic content of this book, we engaged a team of specialists in China who are experts in this subject. In particular, the team from West China Stomatological Hospital of Sichuan University imparted their knowledge on the management of primary and secondary cleft lip and palate. Although some of these methods have already been published in local or international scientific journals, the format of conveying the information in this book will make comprehension and application easier.

The repair of secondary peri-oral and lip deformities is unique, unlike the repair of the tongue, floor of mouth, cheek and even soft palate. The main objective is to restore function, and it can be achieved with various kinds of skin flaps. It is not uncommon to have residual deformities after cleft lip repair, i.e. microstomia, crooked lips, and deficiency of lip mucosa. The impact of microstomia is greatest on elderly patients as it affects the wearing and removal of removable dentures, whereas younger patients are more affected by appearance of the lip. The lack of strict classifications of the indications and information on the post-operative outcome in many textbooks has created problems for many oral and maxillofacial surgeons.

After hundreds of lip repair surgery for more than 30 years, the oral and maxillofacial surgery team from the First Affiliated Hospital of Zhejiang University has summed up 20 different techniques to manage different types of deformities of various sizes and locations. This allows each patient to get the best treatment possible. With the recommendation of Academician Qiu Wei-Liu (Chinese Academy of Engineering) and Professor Zhang Zhi-Yuan of Oral and Maxillofacial Surgery and Ninth Hospital of Shanghai Jiaotong University, respectively, the seventh edition of Oral and Maxillofacial Surgery Textbook (Chinese edition) has been compiled.

As the leading unit in the field of plastic surgery in China, the plastic surgeons of the Ninth People's Hospital of Shanghai Jiaotong University have also provided strong support for this book. Amongst them, Professor Li Qing-Feng and Professor Liu Kai introduced the method of preparing tissues on the anterior chest into nose or lip-like structures first, and then transferring the structure to the face. This has provided an avenue for surgeons to reconstruct the complete loss of the nasal and upper lip tissues.

Tan Xiao-Yan, president of Hangzhou Plastic Hospital, and Liu Kai, professor of plastic surgery of Shanghai Ninth Hospital contributed the part on the cosmetic surgery of the nose and lip despite given limited time during the editorial process. Here, we express our utmost gratitude for their support.

The case on the repair of a total loss of nose by Professor Choi Chung-yu, Secretary General of the Korean Association of Plastic Surgeons, had given us a visual impact and admirations for the Korean Plastic Surgeons strive for aesthetic excellence. There are many things we can learn from them. In addition, we would also like to express our gratitude to the plastic surgery team of Eshan Hospital, Seoul, Korea.

In the process of translating the Chinese version of the book into English, we have received strong support from Dr. Yong Chee-Weng from National University Centre for Oral Health Singapore (NUCOHS), Dr. Lee Qi-qi and Dr. Sabrina Ng Livia from National Dental Centre Singapore (NDCS) from Singapore. Their hard work has allowed the completion of the English version of this book. We would like to express our deep gratitude for their efforts.

In order to improve the quality of the book, the structure and format of writing was standardized. However, we hope to have the readers' understanding that it is unavoidable for different writers to have a different writing style and characteristics.

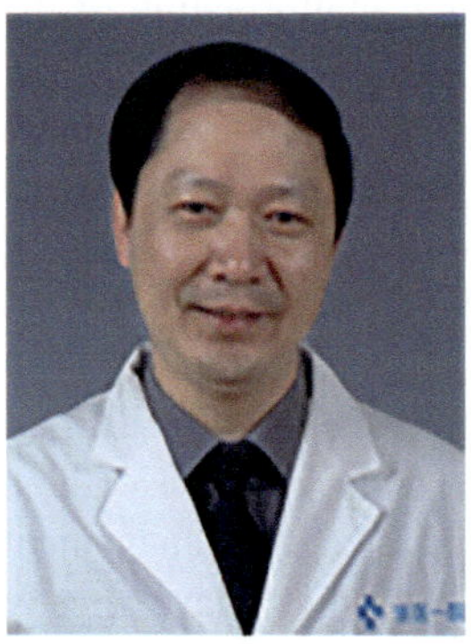

Jianhua Liu
Hangzhou, China

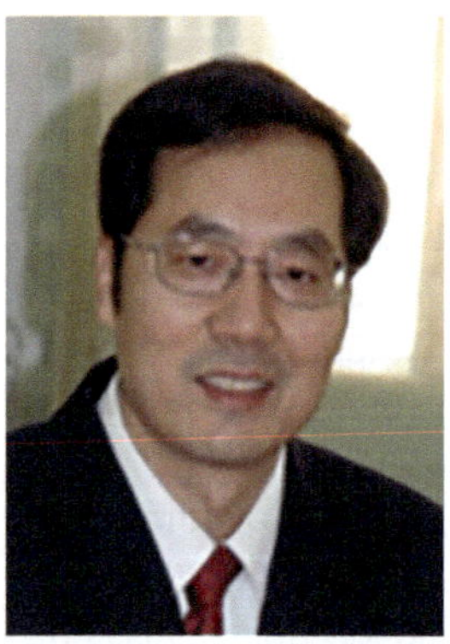

Bing Shi
Chengdu, China

Contents

Part I Anatomy of the Lips and Nose

1 **Applied Anatomy of the Lips and Nose** 3
Zhiyong Li and Jianhua Liu

2 **Embryonic Development of the Lips and Nose** 13
Zhiyong Li and Jianhua Liu

3 **Esthetic Features of Lips and Nose** 17
Zhiyong Li and Jianhua Liu

Part II Esthetic Correction of Lip and Nose Deformities

4 **Esthetic Correction of Lip Deformities** 23
Kai Liu

5 **Cosmetic Surgery of Nose** 29
Xiaoyan Tan

Part III Plastic Surgery of Congenital Nasolabial Deformities

6 **Unilateral Cleft Lip Repair** 57
Bing Shi

7 **Bilateral Cleft Lip Repair** 69
Chenghao Li and Bing Shi

8 **Repair of Secondary Deformities of Unilateral Cleft Lip Surgery** 77
Qian Zheng

9 **Repair of Secondary Deformities of Bilateral Cleft Lip Surgery** 87
Qian Zheng

10 **Correction of Secondary Nasal Deformities of Unilateral Cleft Lip Repair** 103
Wang Zheng and Qian Zheng

11 **Correction of Secondary Nasal Deformities of Bilateral Cleft Lip Repair** 113
Qian Zheng

12 **Plastic Surgery of Facial Cleft** 119
Wang Zheng and Qian Zheng

Part IV Acquired Nasolabial Deformities and Plastic Reconstruction

13 Essentials of Surgical Design for Acquired Lip Defect 129
Jianhua Liu

14 Surgical Methods of Simple Lip Defect 135
Jianhua Liu

15 Modified Bernard's Sliding Flaps for Larger Lower Lip Defect 141
Jianhua Liu

16 Reconstructive Surgery After Total Lower Lip Resection 153
Huiyong Zhu and Jianhua Liu

17 Reconstruction of Upper Lip Defect After Tumor Resection 161
Jianhua Liu

18 Reconstruction of Irregular Lip Defects 177
Xu Huang and Jianhua Liu

19 Reconstruction of Lip Defects with Composite Tissue Flap 191
Jianhua Liu

20 Reconstruction of Total Nasal Defect 197
Kai Liu and Choi Jong-Woo

Contributors

Choi Jong-Woo Department of Plastic Surgery, ASAN Medical Center, University of Ulsan College of Medicine, Seoul, Republic of Korea

Xu Huang, MD, DMD Department of Stomatology, Fourth Affiliated Hospital, Zhejiang University School of Medicine, Yiwu, China

Chenghao Li, MD, PHD, DMD Department of Cleft Lip and Palate Surgery, West China Stomatology Hospital, Sichuan University, Chengdu, China

Jianhua Liu, MD, PHD, DMD Department of Oral and Maxillo-facial Surgery, First Affiliated Hospital, Zhejiang University School of Medicine, Hangzhou, China

Kai Liu, MD, PHD Department of Plastic Surgery, The 9th People's Hospital, Shanghai Jiao Tong University, Shanghai, China

Zhiyong Li, MD, PHD, DMD Department of Oral and Maxillo-facial Surgery, Zhejiang Stomatology Hospital, Hangzhou, China

Bing Shi, MD, PHD, DMD Department of Cleft Lip and Palate Surgery, Vice Dean, West China Stomatology College, Sichuan University, Chengdu, China

Xiaoyan Tan, MD Hangzhou Plastic Surgery Hospital, Hangzhou, China

Wang Zheng Department of Cleft Lip and Palate Surgery, West China Stomatology Hospital, Sichuan University, Chengdu, China

Qian Zheng, MD, PHD, DMD Department of Cleft Lip and Palate Surgery, West China Stomatology Hospital, Sichuan University, Chengdu, China

Huiyong Zhu, MD, PHD, DMD Department of Oral and Maxillo-facial Surgery, First Affiliated Hospital, Zhejiang University School of Medicine, Hangzhou, China

Part I

Anatomy of the Lips and Nose

Applied Anatomy of the Lips and Nose

1

Zhiyong Li and Jianhua Liu

1.1 Position of the Lips and Nose in Relation to the Facial Proportions

The facial region can be divided into multiple anatomical regions based on surface morphology and anatomical characteristics. The lip region is demarcated superiorly from the nose region by the base of the nose, inferiorly from the chin region by the labiomental sulcus, and laterally from the cheek regions by the bilateral labiofacial grooves. The nose region is demarcated from the lip region inferiorly by the base of the nose, laterally from orbital and infraorbital regions by the nasofacial groove traveling from the inner canthus of the eyes to the alar of the nose, and superiorly from the forehead region by the root of the nose. The lip and nose regions are positioned in the center of the face, and in addition to being paramount for respiration, mastication, enunciation, facial expression, and other important bodily functions, are also the most important facial anatomical regions contributing to our perception of facial esthetics. The nose and lips are convex anatomical structures protruding from the surface of the face and are composed primarily of soft tissue and cartilage. As a result, the nose and lips are the most easily traumatized structures in the facial region, resulting in the formation of defects or deformities (Figs. 1.1 and 1.2).

1.2 Normal Anatomical Landmarks of Lips and Nose

1.2.1 Anatomical Landmarks of the Lip

The lip region is located at the lower third of the face and consists of the upper and lower lips, oral fissures, and the adjacent facial structures. These jointly form a valve-like soft tissue structure capable of the largest range of motion in the facial region. The upper and lower lips can be subdivided into three parts: (a) the cutaneous zone (also known as the white lip), which includes the region from the base of the nose to the vermillion border of the upper lip, and the region from the labiomental sulcus to the vermillion border of the lower lip; (b) the vermillion zone (also known as the red lip), from the vermillion border to the interface between the dry and wet vermillion; and (c) oral mucosal zone, posterior to the interface between the dry and wet vermillion (Figs. 1.3 and 1.4).

There are many important anatomical landmarks of the lips:

1. Oral Fissure: The horizontal crevice between the upper and lower lips. The width of the oral fissure is the most important determinant in the diagnosis of macrostomia and microstomia.
2. Angle of Mouth: The point where the vermillion border of the upper and lower lips converge bilaterally. The angle of the mouth is typically located between the upper canines and the upper first premolars. This reference point is an important landmark when determining the width of the oral fissure when performing surgical correction.
3. Vermillion: The transition zone between the cutaneous zone and the oral mucosa of the upper and lower lips. The normal appearance of the vermillion is moist, ruby red, and reflective. Some medical conditions can cause the lower lip to appear cyanosed, pale, or dark purple. The vermillion zone consists of the vermillion border, Cupid's bow, dry vermillion, wet vermillion, prochelion, the peak of Cupid's bow, philtrum, and other morphological landmarks, and is an important anatomical landmark in esthetic corrective surgery.
4. Vermillion Border: The boundary between the cutaneous zone and vermillion. The upper vermillion border forms a flat "M" shape and is also termed the Cupid's

Z. Li (✉)
Department of Oral and Maxillo-facial Surgery, Zhejiang Stomatology Hospital, Hangzhou, China

J. Liu
Department of Oral and Maxillo-facial Surgery, First Affiliated Hospital, Zhejiang University School of Medicine, Hangzhou, China

J. Liu, B. Shi (eds.), *Atlas of Lip and Nose Plastic and Cosmetic Surgery*, https://doi.org/10.1007/978-981-16-1911-3_1

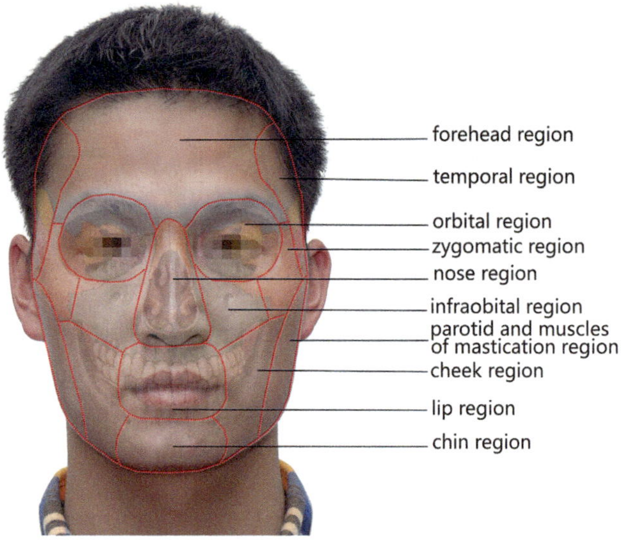

Fig. 1.1 Anatomical regions of the face, frontal view

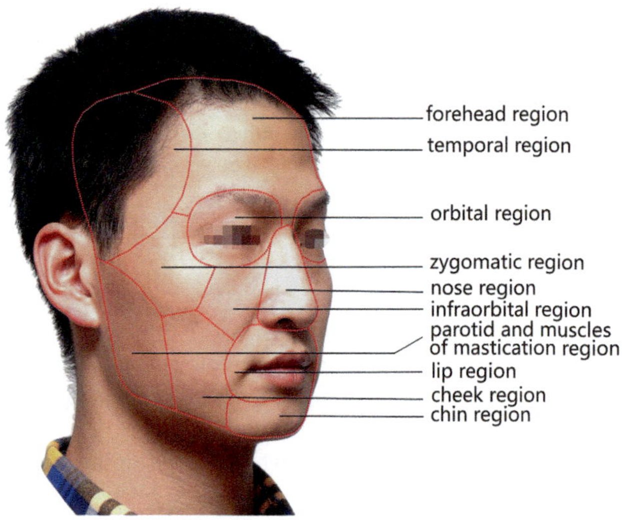

Fig. 1.2 Anatomical regions of the face, side view

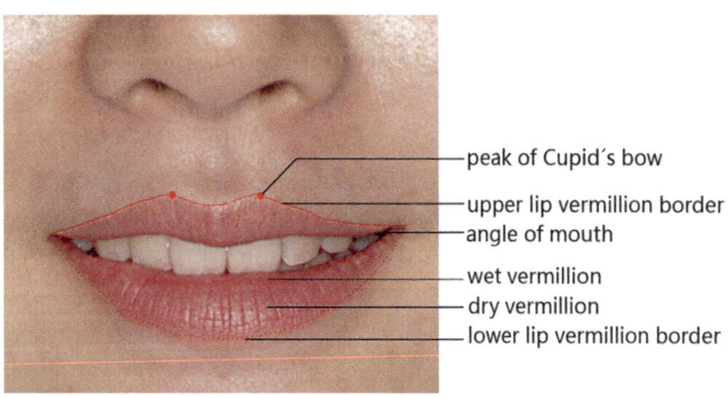

Fig. 1.3 Anatomical landmarks of the lip: Part 1

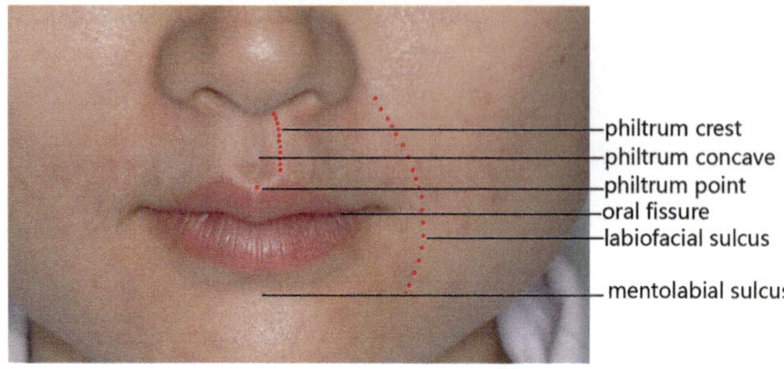

Fig. 1.4 Anatomical landmarks of the lip: Part 2

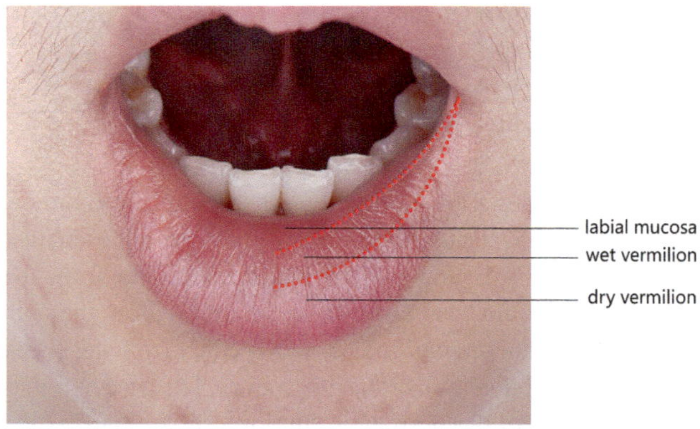

Fig. 1.5 Boundary between the wet and dry vermillion

bow because of its resemblance to a bow. The lower vermillion border forms an indistinct "W" shape and is comparatively simpler in structure.

5. Prochelion: A distinct midline downward protuberance of the upper lip. This is a normal anatomical structure that needs to be reconstructed during cleft lip repair surgery.
6. Peaks of Cupid's bow: The crest formed by the "M" shape on either side of the prochelion. This is the most obvious anatomical landmark that is disrupted in cleft lip patients.
7. Dry Vermillion and Wet Vermillion: The vermillion communicates externally with the skin of the upper and lower lips, and internally with the oral mucosa. The subepithelial layer lacks sebaceous glands and minor salivary glands. The portion of the vermillion adjacent to the skin appears dry and is hence termed the dry vermillion. The portion of the vermillion adjacent to the oral mucosa is moist with saliva and is hence termed the wet vermillion. There is a discernible boundary between the wet and dry vermillion, which is an important anatomical landmark when performing cleft lip surgery or surgical repair of the lips (Fig. 1.5).
8. Philtrum: A midline shallow, vertical depression on the upper lip, between the columella of the nose superiorly to the vermillion border inferiorly.

9. Philtrum Crest: The paired ridges parallel to the philtrum, between the columella of the nose superiorly to the crest of the Cupid's bow inferiorly.
10. Philtrum Point: A point along the line formed between the philtrum and the vermillion border, at the lowest point formed by the "M" shape of the Cupid's bow.
11. Mentolabial Sulcus: The horizontal depression formed between the lower lip and the chin. This is the boundary between the lip region and the chin region. During block resection, this sulcus is often used as the inferior limit of resection to avoid obvious scarring.
12. Labiofacial Sulcus: A diagonal depression between the upper lip and cheek region. An incision along the labiofacial sulcus leaves a surgical scar that is not obvious. This sulcus is also an important anatomical landmark for the preparation and closure of nasolabial flaps.

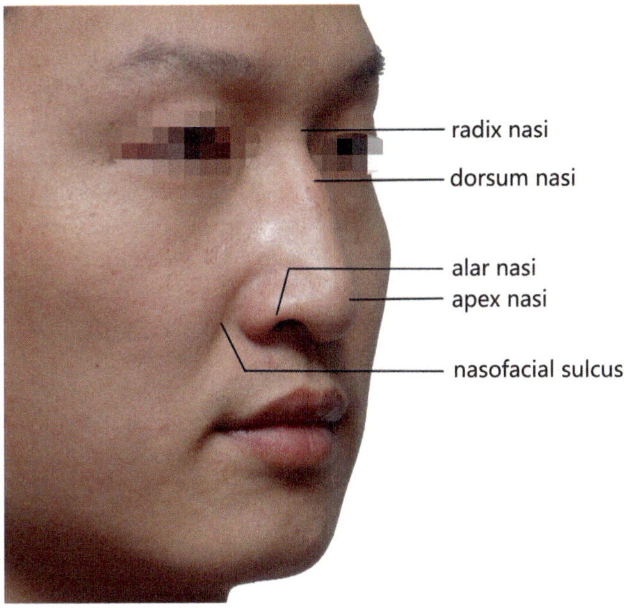

Fig. 1.6 Nose anatomical landmarks

1.2.2 Anatomical Landmarks of the Nose

The nose is consists of three parts, namely the external nose, nasal cavity, and nasal sinus the external nose refers to the part of the nose that projects from the face, consists of bone and cartilaginous support framework, and is covered externally by the skin. The external nose has a three-dimensional, tapering shape, and projects from the center of the face, and is hence easily traumatized. The external anatomical landmarks of the external nose are the radix nasi, apex nasi, dorsum nasi, alar nasi, base of nose, nostrils, and columella nasi.

1. Radix Nasi: The zone between the upper part of the nose and the forehead region.
2. Apex Nasi: The protuberance at the anterioinferior aspect of the nose.
3. Dorsum Nasi: The zone between the radix nasi and apex nasi.
4. Base of Nose: The tapering base of the external nose, which has a triangular outline. The oval openings at the base of the nose form the paired nostrils.
5. Columella Nasi: The soft tissue strut between the paired nostrils.
6. Alar Nasi: The bilateral protuberances on the external aspect of the nostrils.
7. Nasofacial Sulcus: The longitudinal depression formed between the lateral border of the nose and the infraorbital region. The collective term for the nasofacial sulcus and the labiofacial sulcus is the nasolabial sulcus. Incisions oriented along the nasolabial sulcus leave less visible scars. The obliteration of the nasolabial sulcus is an important clinical sign of potential damage to the buccal branch of the facial nerve (Figs. 1.6 and 1.7).

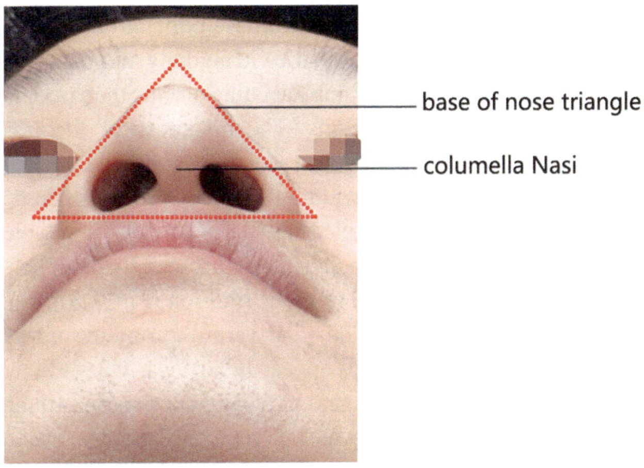

Fig. 1.7 Base of nose anatomical landmarks

1.3 Structural Characteristics of Lips and Nose

I. Structural Characteristics of the Lips [1]
   (1) The morphology and structure of the lips.
      1. The color of the lips: The color exhibited by the vermillion is primarily due to the capillary loops in the submucosal layer. It is usually ruby red in color. An anemic individual may exhibit pallor of the lips, whereas a hypoxic individual may exhibit cyanosis of the lips. In order to objectively assess the color of the lips, any lipstick or lubricants applied to the lips must be removed.

2. The thickness of lips: The thickness of the upper and lower vermillion when the lips are generally closed. The thickness of the vermillion is different between the upper and lower lips, and at different regions of each lip. There are two key points: firstly the thickness between the upper and lower lips is not uniform, and secondly, the thickness of each lip varies from the midline to the angle of the mouth.
   (A) The thickness: The thickness of the lips can be classified into four types, based on the average thickness at the midline. (a) Thin Type: with a thickness of less than 4 mm; (b) Moderately Thick Type: with a thickness of approximately 5 mm; (c) Thick Type: with a thickness of 9 to 12 mm; (d) Thick and Protrusive Type: with a thickness of more than 12 mm. The upper and lower lips are not uniform in thickness, with the lower lip usually being thicker than the upper lip. There are also racial differences in the thickness of the lips—Afro-Americans have thicker lips than the Caucasian or Chinese population. People originating from the Guangdong and Guangxi regions of China have thicker lips than people of other regions. The thickness of the lips needs to be in harmony with the facial shape, height, and width of the patient in order to be esthetically pleasing. In a portion of people with thin lips, it can be attributed to the underdevelopment of the vermillion (Fig. 1.8).
   (B) The vermillion: The vermillion of the upper and lower lips appear fullest near the midline, and the thickness gradually decreases until the upper and lower lips meet at the angle of the mouth. The structural anatomy of the upper lip is especially complicated, of which the vermillion border forms a bow shape, and is also referred to in literature as the Cupid's bow. In the middle portion, the philtrum lies superiorly, and the prochelion forms a downward protuberance. These anatomical landmarks are visually obvious and have a pronounced effect on the external appearance. Hence, when performing lip surgery, utmost care must be taken in order not to disrupt the appearance of these important landmarks. When performing esthetic repair of the lip in cleft lip and palate patients, restoration of these landmarks is both important and challenging. As the intrinsic muscles of the lip have a large degree of activity, the shape varies depending on whether the lip is in the active or passive state. Hence, in patients with progressive degenerative disease of the lips or in patients with loss of lip tissue (such as in cleft lip and palate patients), complete restoration back to normal anatomy is particularly challenging.

(2) Muscles of the Lip Region

The muscles around the lip can be classified into four groups based on position, namely the upper group, lower group, the orbicularis oris, and buccinator, of which the orbicularis oris is the primary muscle. The upper and lower groups radiate from and are oriented circumferentially around the orbicularis oris. In isolation, the action of the orbicularis oris muscle is the closure of the oral fissure. The wide range of motion of the upper and lower lips is due to contribution from the other perioral musculature (Fig. 1.9).

1. Muscles around the lip (upper group) include: risorius, zygomaticus major, zygomaticus minor, levator labii superioris, levator labii superioris alaeque nasi, and levator anguli oris muscles.

Upper Group Muscles	Origin	Insertion	Action
Risorius	Parotid Fascia	Skin at the angle of the mouth and lips	Pulls the angle of the mouth posteriorly and laterally
Zygomaticus Major	Posterior to the zygomaticotemporal suture of the zygoma	Skin at the angle of the mouth and lips	Pulls the angle of the mouth superiorly and laterally
Zygomaticus Minor	Posterior to the zygomaticomaxillary suture of the zygoma	Skin at the medial aspect of the angle of the mouth and lateral aspect of the upper lip	Pulls the angle of the mouth superiorly and laterally
Levator Labii Superioris	Infraorbital margin of the maxilla and the tubercle of the zygoma	Merges with the orbicularis oris muscle	Pulls the upper lip superiorly
Levator Labii Superioris Alaeque Nasi Muscle	Infraorbital margin and frontal process of the maxilla	Terminates medially at the cartilaginous portion of the alar of the nose, laterally merges with the orbicularis oris muscle	Pulls the alar of the nose superiorly
Levator Anguli Oris	Canine fossa	Skin of the angle of the mouth	Pulls the angle of the mouth superiorly

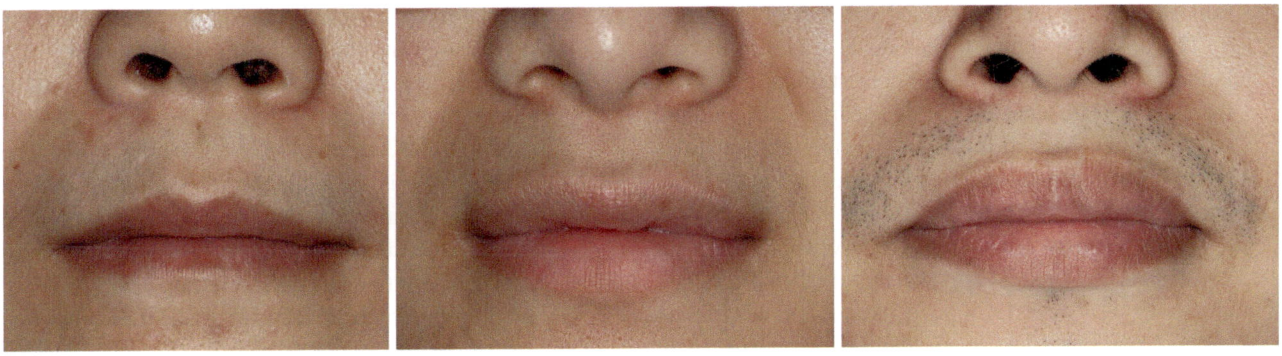

Fig. 1.8 Comparison of different lip thickness

Fig. 1.9 Muscles of the lip and nose region

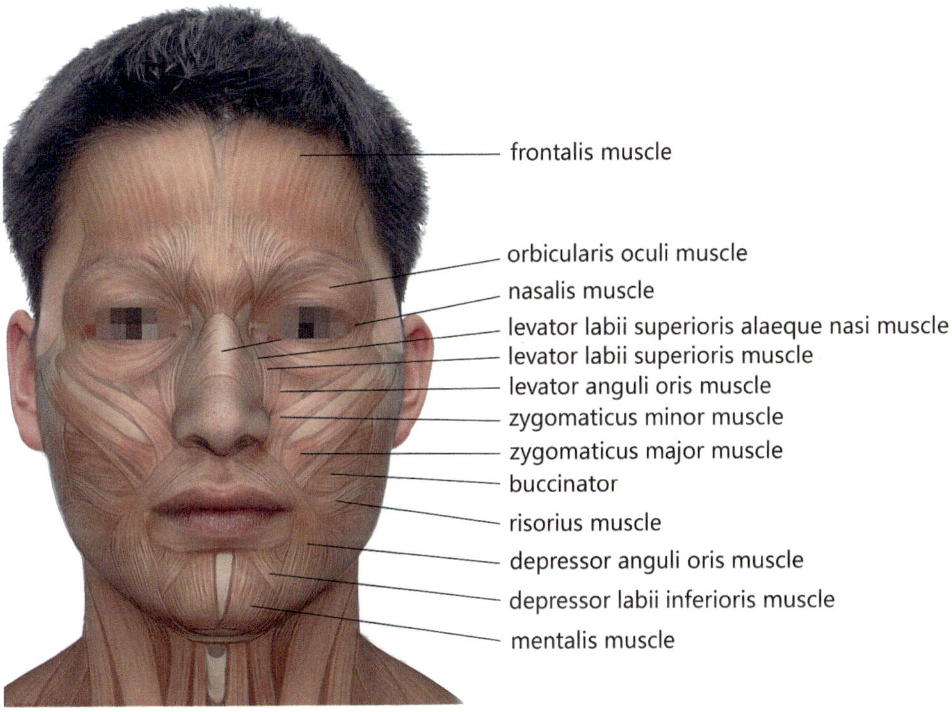

2. Muscles around the lip (lower group): from superficial to deep consists of the depressor anguli oris muscle, depressor labii inferioris, and mentalis muscles.

Lower Group Muscles	Origin	Insertion	Action
Depressor Anguli Oris (or Triangularis)	Oblique line of the mandible	Skin at the angle of the mouth	Pulls the angle of the mouth inferiorly
Depressor Labii Inferioris (or Quadratus Labii Inferioris)	Oblique line of the mandible	Skin of the lower lips and chin	Pulls the lower lip inferiorly
Mentalis	Prominence between the lower incisors and canine	Skin of the chin	Extends the lower lip

3. Orbicularis Oris: A flat, circular-shaped muscle around the oral fissure that is innervated by the buccal branch of the facial nerve. The main functions are to maintain the natural form of the face, and the upper and lower lips, closure of the oral commissure, and allows for a range of other motion such as eversion of the lips, pouting, whistling, and aids in sucking, swallowing, mastication, speech, and other important functions.
4. Buccinator: A quadrilateral shaped muscle, which originates posteriorly from the pterygomandibular raphe, lying between the perioral muscles and buccal mucosa and inserts into the angle of mouth and skin of the cheeks. It is innervated by the marginal mandibular and buccal branches of the facial nerve, and its action is to pull the angle of the mouth posteriorly, and aids in mastication, sucking, and blowing actions.

(3) Fundamentals of the function and esthetics of the lip

The lips are a common anatomical structure of both humans and mammals. The lips consist primarily of soft tissue. They are capable of a large range of motion, which allows them to fulfill many important functions including ingestion, phonation, speech, and facial expression.

The lips are the only part of the face with an obvious pigmentation. Regardless of whether the lips are tightly closed or gently parted and regardless of whether to express happiness or anger, the lips are capable of expressing an individual's personality and mood. The lips are capable of a wide range of expression, and hence are an important visual point of interest on the face. The lips are also one of the most sensitive parts of the human body, and stimulation of the lips can lead to sexual arousal.

Ideally, the shape of the lip must be harmonious with the eyes, nose, and face, with a well-defined structure and outline, gently upturned at the angles of the mouth, with the upper lip slightly thicker than the lower lip, and full of depth and dimension. Our assessment of esthetics is based on the eyes, lips, facial outline, nose, chin, and lastly ears, in the sequence of importance. Hence, the importance of the lips in facial esthetics is secondary only to the eyes. In some circumstances, the esthetic importance of the lips may even exceed that of the eyes.

(4)Layers of the Lip

The lip can be divided into five layers, namely (from superficial to deep): skin, subcutaneous tissue, muscular layer, submucosa, and mucosa. The labial artery is usually located deep to the boundary between the wet and dry vermillion, superficial to the orbicularis orisoris muscle. When performing lip surgery, the labial artery must be identified and protected if possible (Fig. 1.10).

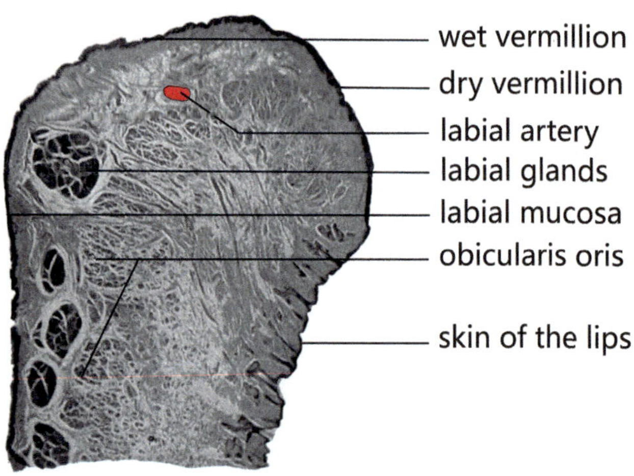

Fig. 1.10 Sectional view of the lip

II. Special anatomical characteristics of the external nose

(1) Morphology and structure of the external nose:

The nose is situated in the midline of the face, of which the part that is of greatest significance to our perception of esthetics is the external nose. The external nose is the focus of this section. Based on anatomical characteristics, the external nose can be divided into three parts: the bony framework, supporting structure, and covering structures.

(1) Bony Framework: refers to the nasal bone and nasal cartilage.

(1) Nasal Bone: The nasal bone is paired structures meeting in the midline, and articulates superiorly with the frontal bone, laterally on both sides with the frontal processes of the maxilla, and posteriorly with the nasal bone crest and the perpendicular plate of the ethmoid bone and inferiorly with the soft tissues and the paired upper lateral cartilages. The superior portion of the nasal bones is thick and narrow, while the inferior portion of the nasal bones is thin and wide. The nasal bones are easily fractured, giving rise to a saddle nose deformity. The nasal bone has a good vascular supply and hence heals well after fracture reduction.

(2) Nasal Cartilage: The nasal cartilages include the paired upper lateral cartilages, accessory cartilages, and the greater alar cartilages (also known as the lower lateral cartilages), lesser alar cartilages, and the single septal cartilage. Aside from the nasal septal cartilage, the rest of the nasal cartilages are all paired (Figs. 1.11, 1.12, 1.13).

(2) Supporting Framework: consists of the connective tissue and ligaments that attach the nasal bones to the nasal cartilages.

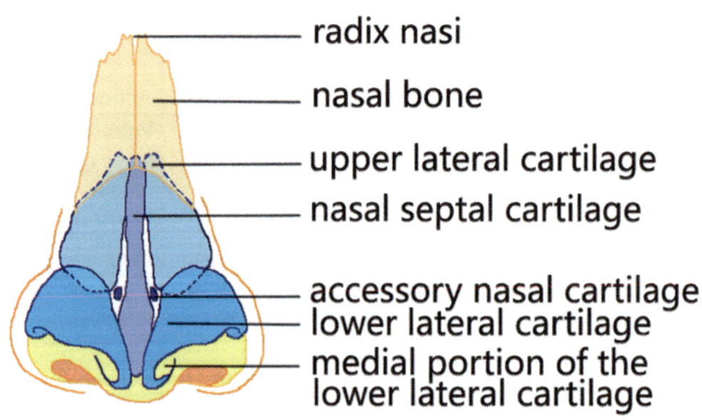

Fig. 1.11 Anatomical structure of the nasal cartilages: frontal view

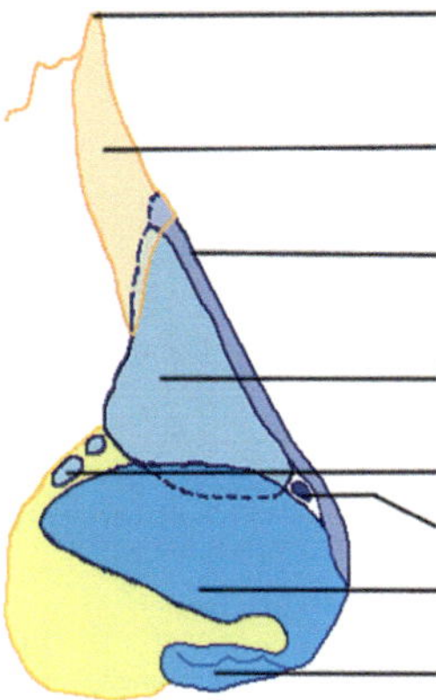

Fig. 1.12 Anatomical structure of the nasal cartilages: side view

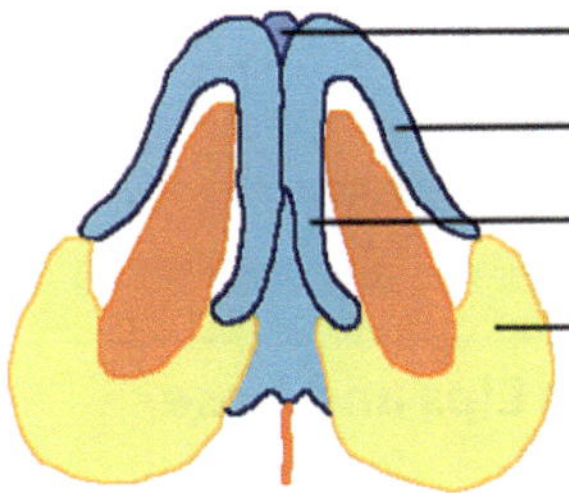

Fig. 1.13 Anatomical structure of the nasal cartilages: inferior view

(3) Covering Structures: consists of the external skin, and the respiratory mucosa of the nasal cavity. The skin overlying the nasal bone is thin and relatively mobile, while the skin over the apex of the nose is thicker, and rich with sebaceous glands, and relatively immobile and fixed to the underlying structures. The nasal lining consists of epithelium and mucosa. The nasal vestibule and nasal septum surface is lined primarily with epithelial cells and dries easily.

(2) Peri-nasal musculature (refer to Fig. 1.3)

The musculature of the nose can be divided into two groups based on their function. The first group is muscles responsible for enlarging the aperture of the nostrils, while the second group is muscles responsible for reducing the aperture of the nostrils. The muscles responsible for the enlargement of the aperture of the nostrils include procerus muscle, levator labii superioris alaeque nasi muscle, and alar portion of the nasalis muscle. The muscles responsible for reducing the aperture of the nostrils are the transverse portion of the nasalis muscle and depressor septa nasi muscle. Additionally, some fibers of the orbicularisoris muscle also attach to the alar of the nose and skin of this region and serves the function of depressing the alar of the nose and closure of the nostrils.

Of all the peri-nasal musculature of the nose, the one with the most clinical significance is the levator labii superioris alaeque nasi muscle and depressor septa nasi muscle. The levator labii superioris alaeque nasi muscle is thin and broad, with the medial head arising from the superior aspect of the frontal process of the maxilla. The muscle travels inferiorly and laterally in an oblique direction, dividing into two bundles. The first bundle terminates at the lower lateral nasal cartilages and the deep part of the skin of the alar of the nose, while the second bundle terminates at the upper lip. The main function is to enlarge the aperture of the nostrils and to elevate and evert the upper lip, which results in deepening and lengthening of the nasolabial groove. Injury to the levator labii superioris alaeque nasi muscle can lead to functional nasal obstruction, and obliteration of the nasolabial groove. The depressor septi nasi muscle originates from the canine fossa of the maxilla, and its fibers terminate at the alar of the nose and nasal septum. Contraction of these muscles causes depression of the nasal septum and shortening of the upper lip. Hence, in corrective surgery for deformities of the nose, the function of the levator labii superioris alaeque nasi muscle should be preserved intact, in order not to affect the attached structures. If the depressor septi nasi muscle is more obvious, it will present clinically as a shortened upper lip. In these patients, contraction of this muscle can cause significant depression of the apex of the nose. In such situations, the origin of the depressor septi nasi can be detached from its underlying attachments, and the free ends of the muscles sutured to each other, in other to preserve the fullness of the upper lip and to prevent the apex of the nose from depressing too significantly during facial expression.

(3) Nasal Subunits

The morphology of the external nose is determined primarily by the underlying bony framework and the overlying skin. There are areas of prominence and areas of depression, which under lighting presents as areas of highlight and areas of shadow. Burget et al. first presented the concept of nasal subunits based on the different visual effects of different regions of the nose and the specific anatomical characteristics of each region. The nasal subunits include the dorsal subunit, the lateral wall subunits, nasal tip subunit, alar subunits, columella, and the soft tissue triangles. Burget proposed that incisions placed along the boundaries of these subunits produced the best esthetic outcomes, partly because these lie within areas of shadow on the external nose (Figs. 1.14 and 1.15).

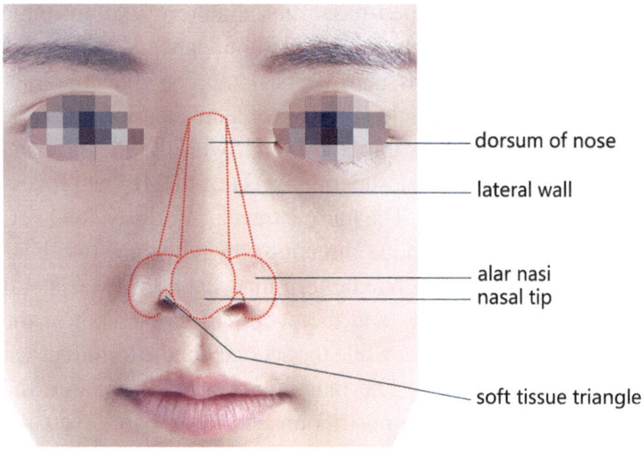

Fig. 1.14 Nasal subunits: frontal view

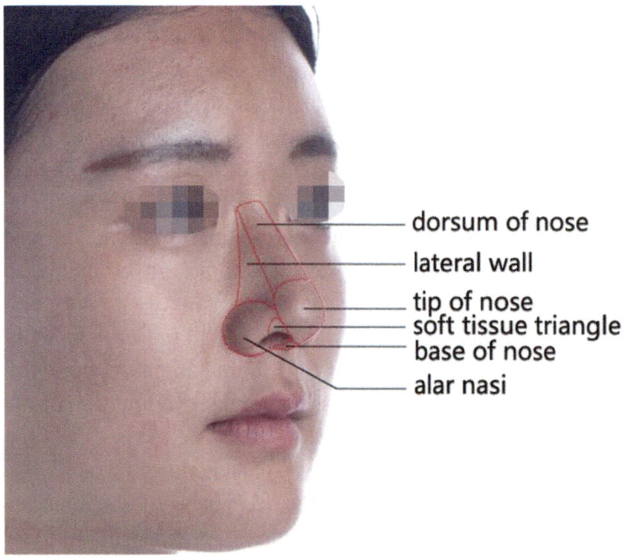

Fig. 1.15 Nasal subunit: side view

(4) Anatomical Structures of the Nose and its Effect on Form and Function

The normal bony framework of the nose gives the external nose its basic morphology and shape. The nasal bone articulates with both the frontal bone and maxilla and provides the radix of the nose with a hard foundation. The nasal cartilages are connected to each other via dense connective tissue and ligament, and have a certain degree of elasticity and mobility, and are an important support structure at the entrance to the respiratory tract. Therefore, during the reconstruction of nasal defects and deformities, it is important to consider restoration of this hard support framework, to provide the soft tissue structures with a stable foundation. The material used for reconstruction should be similar to the nasal cartilages, such as autogenous cartilage grafts, silicone, and other similar materials.

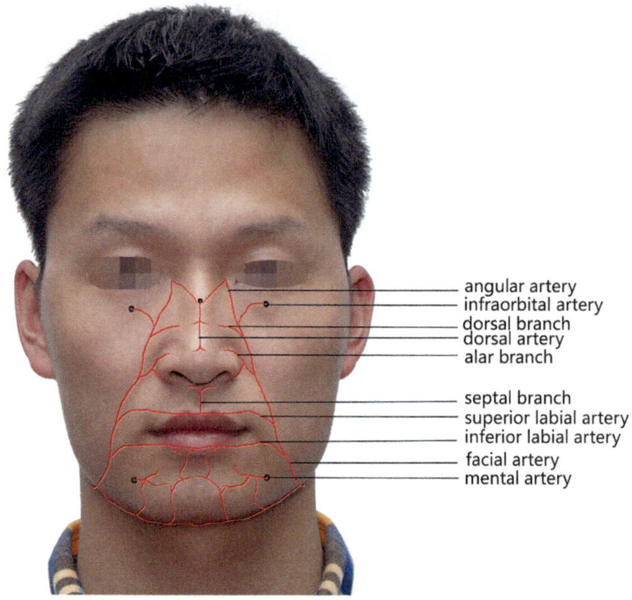

Fig. 1.16 Facial artery and its communicating branches

1.4 Blood Supply of the Lips and Nose

The lips and nose regions are well vascularized (Fig. 1.16). Aside from a small portion of the dorsum of the nose which is supplied by branches of the internal carotid artery, the rest of the lips and nose regions are supplied by branches of the facial artery and maxillary artery. In particular, the lips and external nose are supplied by branches of the facial artery, while the nasal cavity and the maxillary sinuses are primarily supplied by the maxillary artery. The lip and nose region is well vascularized by branches of the facial artery, maxillary artery, and internal carotid artery, which anastomose freely and extensively. This is a significant advantage in surgical repair of lip and nose defects because it allows larger, longer, and wider sliding flaps to be designed.

1. Characteristics of the Vascular Supply of the Lip: The main arterial supply of the upper and lower lips is the facial artery. The facial artery branches into the superior labial artery and the inferior labial artery at the angle of the mouth [2].
   1. Labial Arteries
      1. Inferior Labial Artery: branches from the facial artery near the angle of the mouth, enters deep to the depressor anguli oris muscle, pierces the orbicularis oris, and travels medially in the submucosal layer to the midline to anastomoses with the contralateral inferior labial artery. The inferior labial artery, mental artery, and sub mental artery can sometimes have minor branches that anastomose with each other.
      2. Superior Labial Artery: after giving off the inferior labial artery branch, the facial artery contin-

ues traveling superoanteriorly. The facial artery gives off the superior labial artery branch slightly superior to the angle of the mouth, which enters the upper lip and travels medially between the orbicularis oris and intraoral mucosa toward the midline, where it anastomoses with the contralateral superior labial artery. The caliber of the superior labial artery is slightly greater than the inferior labial artery. Blood flow in the superior and inferior labial arteries can be stopped with digital pressure to the upper or lower lips. The upper and lower lips are all supplied by branches of the facial artery. These branches anastomose at the midline with the contralateral branches, forming a vascular ring supplying the perioral region.

2. Applied anatomy of Labial Arteries:

   The arterial ring formed by upper and lower lip arteries creates many advantages in making various kinds of local soft tissue flap that is often used in repairing perioral defects. For example, when preparing the Abbe flap, even if one side of the upper lip artery is cut off, the other side of the upper lip artery can still ensure enough blood supply. As a matter of fact, the soft tissue flap in the blood supply of the arterial ring can be harvested in different shapes, as long as one side of the blood supply to the flap is reserved.

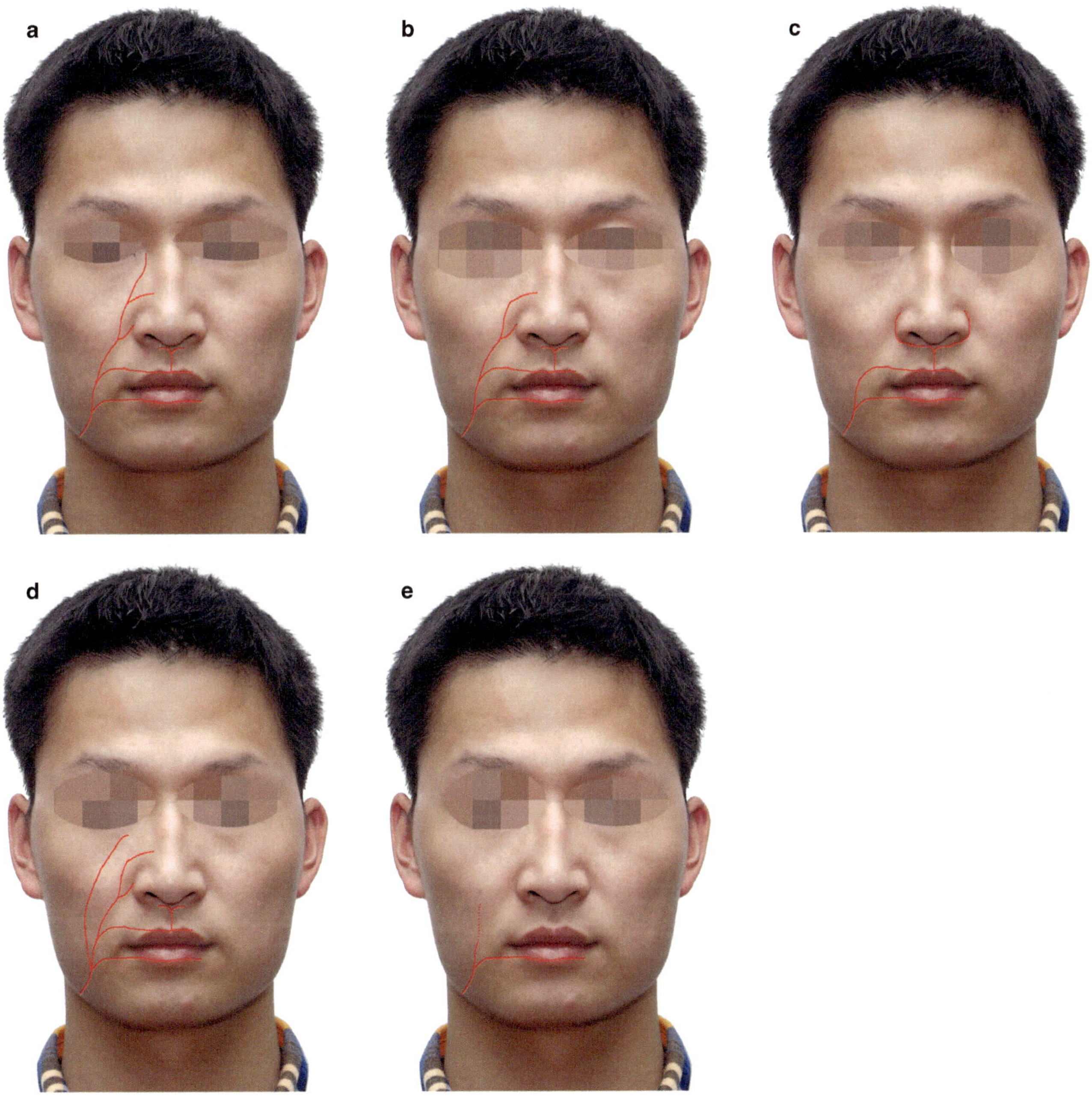

Fig. 1.17 (**a**–**e**) Common variations of branches of the labial artery

3. Variation of Labial Arteries:

Depending on specimen anatomy, Loucas classified branches of the facial artery into five types (type A; B; C; D; E), some of which include subtypes (Fig. 1.17) [3].

Type A is the most common vascular distribution pattern, accounting for 47.5% of cases. In Type A, the nasolabial artery runs parallel deep to the nasolabial groove and travels superiorly and medially, giving rise to the inferior and superior labial arteries, lateral nasal artery, of which the latter gives rise to the inferior and superior alar arteries before terminating as the angular artery. Type B pattern accounts for 38.7% of cases and differs primarily from Type A in that the lateral nasal artery terminates as the superior alar artery. Type C pattern accounts for 8.4% of cases and is characterized by the lack of the lateral nasal branch, with the facial artery instead terminating as the superior labial artery. In Type C pattern, the superior and inferior alar arteries arise from the nasal septal artery. Type D pattern accounts for 3.8% of cases and is characterized by the angular artery arising directly from the main facial artery branch. Type E pattern is the rarest, and only accounts for 1.4% of cases, and is characterized by a lack of branches, with the inferior labial artery being the only discernible branch from the main facial artery branch. Cumulatively, Types A, B, and D account for up to 90% of cases. In these cases, the extensive vascular distribution allows for greater freedom in the design of local flaps. In Types C and E cases, identification of an obvious and reliable arterial supply when designing nasolabial flaps may be particularly challenging. In these cases, it is more appropriate to place an initial incision to identify the arterial supply first before raising the whole flap.

2. Characteristics of the Vascular Supply of the Nose:

The structure of the nose and its arterial supply is more complicated, with a specific supply to the external nose, nasal cavity, and maxillary sinus

1. Vascular Supply to the External Nose:

The external nose, nasal dorsum, and alar of the nose are primarily supplied by the angular artery. Different parts of the external nose are supplied by different sources. The dorsum of the nose is primarily supplied by the ophthalmic artery and the angular artery, while the tip of the nose is primarily supplied by branches of the facial artery. The branches of the facial artery supplying the tip of the nose typically arise from the deep portion of the base of the nose and terminate in the vascular network in the subcutaneous layer of the tip of the nose. Excessive removal of the subcutaneous structures of the tip of the nose can result in ischemia of overlying skin, resulting in skin necrosis. Hence, when performing corrective surgery of the tip of the nose, changing the morphology of the nose is achieved by reconstruction of the deep structural framework of the nose, and not by removal of the subcutaneous structures (Fig. 1.18).

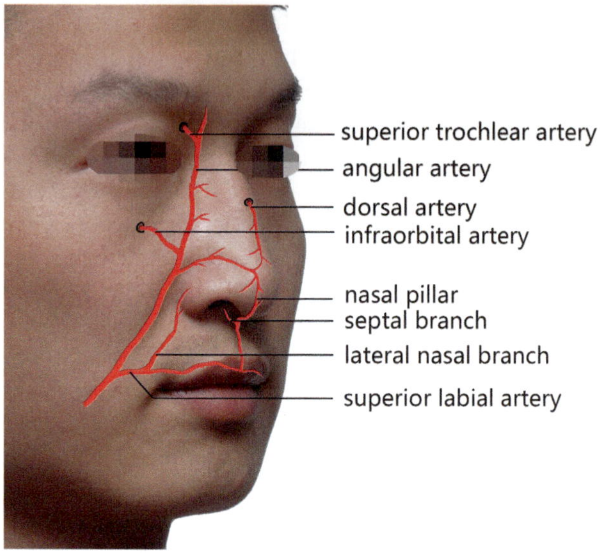

Fig. 1.18 Arterial branches of the nose region

2. The arterial supply of the nasal cavity and maxillary sinus is derived primarily from the ophthalmic artery (which is a branch of the internal carotid artery), and the internal maxillary artery (which is a branch of the external carotid artery). The anterior ethmoid artery, posterior ethmoid artery septal branch, superior labial artery, descending palatine artery, and nasopalatine artery form a rich vascular network at the anterior inferior portion of the nasal septum. This is the reason why there is usually profound bleeding from this region.

References

1. Wang M-Q, He S-G. Oral anatomical physiology. 7th ed. Beijing: People's Medical Publishing House (in Chinese); 2013.
2. Jian-Hua L, Ming Z, Wu Q-L. Facial artery casting mould and its significance in selecting labial and buccal flaps (in Chinese). J Stomatol Progress. 2001;6(3):8–10.
3. Marios L, Joel H, Robert G, et al. A detailed observation of variations of the facial artery, with emphasis on the superior labial artery. Surg Radiol Anat. 2006;28:316–24.

Embryonic Development of the Lips and Nose

2

Zhiyong Li and Jianhua Liu

The lips and nose are derived primarily from the frontonasal process and the first pharyngeal arch and are an important part of the development of the face. This region is also the most prone to developmental deformities or defects [1].

2.1 Developmental Process of the Lips and Nose

In the third week of development of the fetus, a frontonasal prominence develops at the inferior part of the forebrain. On the 28th day of gestation, it is divided by the cribriform plate into the medial nasal process and lateral nasal process, which eventually develops into the medial and lateral structures of the nose, respectively. On the inferior portion of both sides of the frontonasal prominence, the neural crest cells migrate and hypertrophy to form the first pharyngeal arch. On the 24th day of gestation, the maxillary process appears, eventually forming the upper lip. The mandibular processes at the inferior part of the first pharyngeal arch develop into the lower lip (Figs. 2.1 and 2.2).

Developmental origins of the lips and nose and the structures derived from the facial processes

Origin	Facial Process	Derived Soft Tissue Structures	Derived Hard Tissues Structures
Frontonasal Prominence	Medial Nasal Process	Dorsum of Nose、Apex of Nose、Nasal Septum	Ethmoid, Vomer, Nasal Bone
	Globular Process	Middle segment of the upper lip	Maxillary Incisor, Premaxilla
	Lateral Nasal Process	Lateral aspect of the nose, Alar of the nose	Frontal Process of the Maxilla、Lacrimal Bone
1st Pharyngeal Arch	Maxillary Process	Outer 2/3 of the Upper Lip	Maxilla
	Mandibular Process	Lower Lip	Mandible, Mandibular Teeth

2.2 Development Deformities of Lips and Nose

In the development of the face, the various facial processes unite and fuse together, gradually forming the lips, nose, maxilla and mandible, and other soft tissue structures. The development of the facial processes can be affected by various mutagenic factors, causing developmental delays or disruption, causing the facial processes to fail to unite and fuse, resulting in developmental defects such as lip and facial clefts [2] (Fig. 2.3).

1. Cleft Lip: results from failure of union or partial union of the globular processes with the maxillary processes. In most patients, the cleft lies along the philtrum crest, and unilateral clefts are more common than bilateral clefts. Failure of bilateral globular processes to fuse on the other hand results in a midline cleft of the upper lip. Failure of the mandibular processes to meet and fuse results in a midline cleft of the mandible. Midline clefts of the upper and lower lips are rarer (Fig. 2.4).

Z. Li (✉)
Department of Oral and Maxillo-facial Surgery, Zhejiang Stomatology Hospital, Hangzhou, China

J. Liu
Department of Oral and Maxillo-facial Surgery, First Affiliated Hospital, Zhejiang University School of Medicine, Hangzhou, China

J. Liu, B. Shi (eds.), *Atlas of Lip and Nose Plastic and Cosmetic Surgery*, https://doi.org/10.1007/978-981-16-1911-3_2

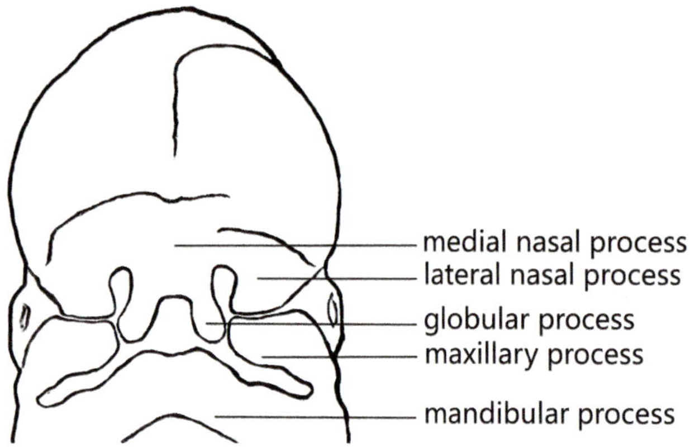

Fig. 2.1 Development of the various processes at sixth in utero

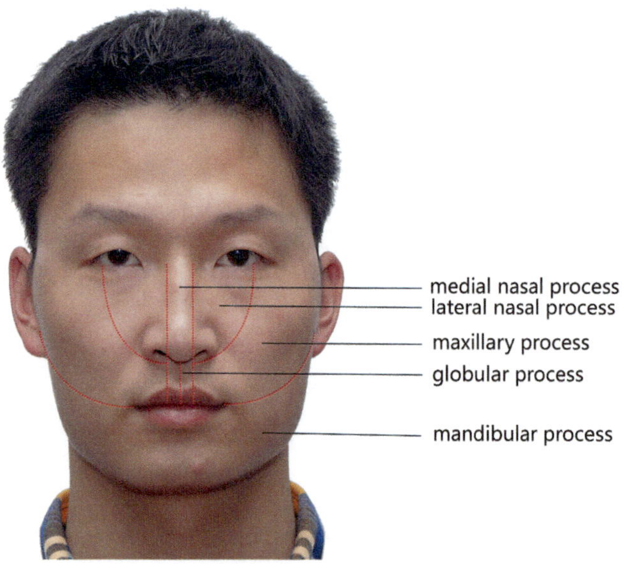

Fig. 2.2 The lines of fusion of the processes that form the face

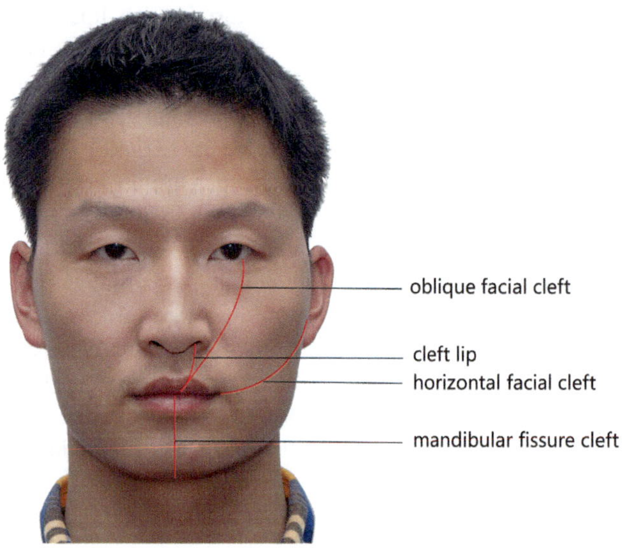

Fig. 2.3 Location of facial clefts

2. Facial Cleft: Failure of fusion of the maxillary and mandibular processes can result in horizontal clefts of the face, which presents clinically as macrostomia. Over-fusion of these processes on the other hand results in microstomia. Failure of the maxillary process and lateral nasal process results in oblique facial clefts, with the cleft traveling from the upper lip, past the alar base, toward the inferior margin of the eyes. Failure of fusion of the lateral nasal process and the medial nasal process can result in lateral nasal clefts. Facial clefts are relatively rarer compared to clefts of the lips (Figs. 2.5 and 2.6).

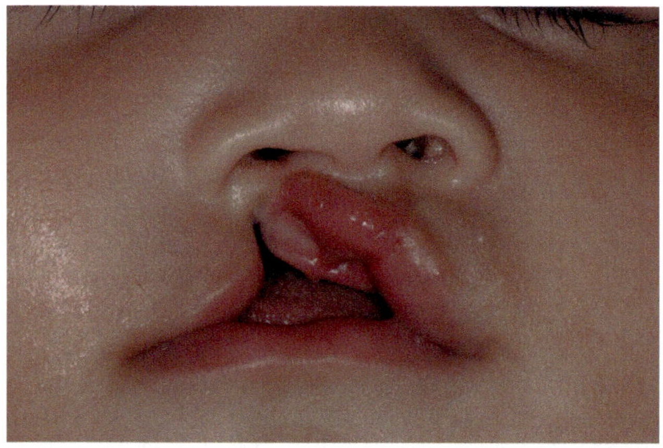

Fig. 2.4 Cleft lip

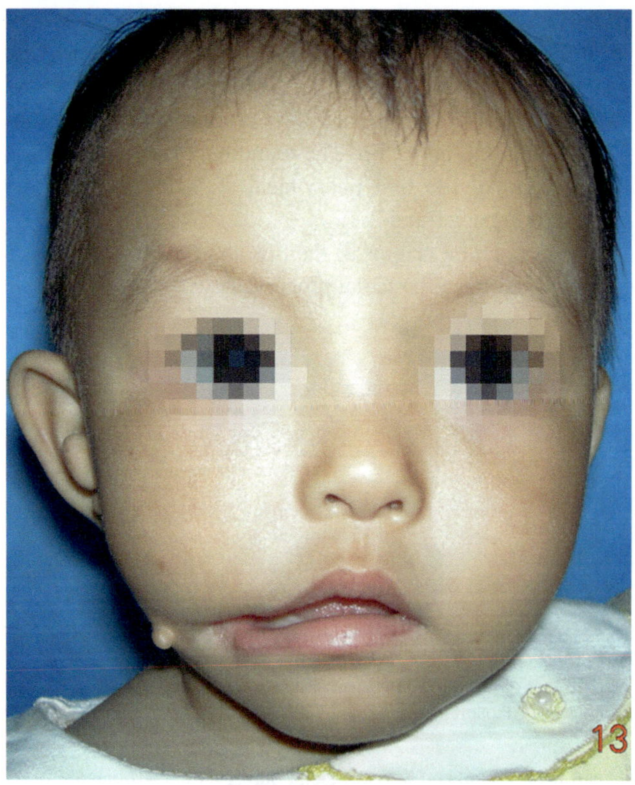

Fig. 2.5 Horizontal facial cleft

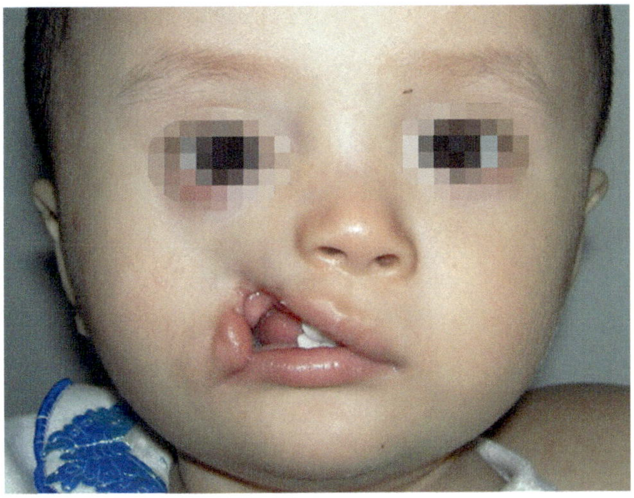

Fig. 2.6 Oblique facial cleft

3. Bilateral Nasal Deformities: Partial or complete separation of the nasal tip is due to failure of fusion of the medial nasal processes.
4. Button Nose: disturbance of the growth of the external nose, and incomplete growth results in the nose presenting with a button shape.
5. Saddle Nose: Obstruction to the normal development of the dorsum of the nose results in depression of the bridge of the nose, forming a saddle shape. These types of deformities can also be acquired.

References

1. Wang M-Q, He S-G. Oral anatomical physiology (in Chinese). 7th ed. Beijing: People's Medical Publishing House; 2013.
2. Sudler MT. The development of the nose, and of the pharynx and its derivatives in man. Am J Anat. 2005;1(4):391–416.

3 Esthetic Features of Lips and Nose

Zhiyong Li and Jianhua Liu

3.1 Common Reference Points of the Lips and Nose

The face is paramount as the assessment of one's beauty. Facial reference points serve as consistent, repeatable landmarks for the assessment of the face [1].

1. Glabella: the midpoint between the bilateral eyebrows.
2. Nasion: the intersection between the frontonasal suture and median sagittal plane, located slightly superior to the most depressed point on the dorsum of the nose.
3. Pronasale: the most anterior point of the tip of the nose.
4. Subnasale: the point where the columella meets the upper lip.
5. Alare: the most protuberant on the lateral border of the alar.
6. Supramental (Soft Tissue B Point): the intersection between the labiomental fold and the median sagittal plane.
7. Pogonion: the most anterior point of the chin in the midline.
8. Menton: the most inferior point of the chin in the midline (Figs. 3.1 and 3.2).

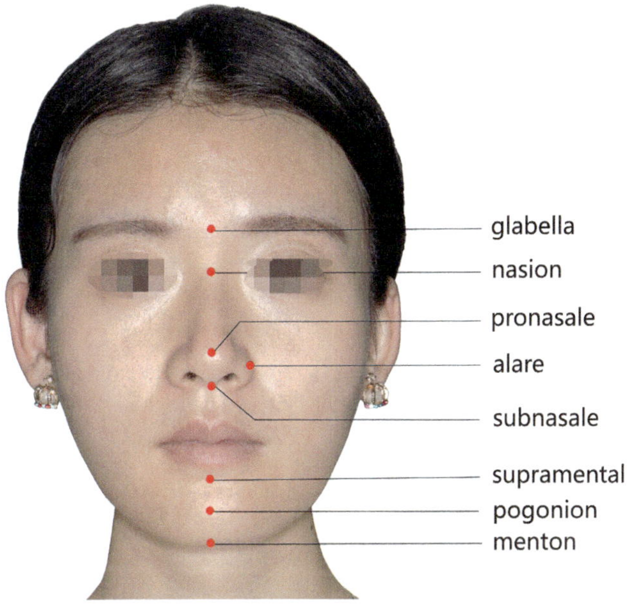

Fig. 3.1 Common cephalometric landmarks of the face: frontal view

3.2 The Esthetics of Important Angles of the Face

Many esthetically important angles are formed by the various structures of the face. These angles are termed esthetic angles. The important angles in the lip and nose region are:

1. Nasofrontal Angle: the angle between the line formed between the glabella and nasion, and the line formed between the nasion and pronasale. The normal nasofrontal angle is between 125 and 135°. The angle is determined primarily by the morphology of the frontal region and the projection of the tip of the nose.
2. Nasomental Angle: the angle between the line between the nasion and pronasale, and the line between the pronasale and pogonion. The normal nasomental angle is 120–132°. Orthognathic surgery involving movement of the maxilla can significantly affect this angle.
3. Nasolabial Angle: the angle between the columella and the upper lip. The normal nasolabial angle is 90–100°. Orthognathic surgery involving movement of the maxilla can significantly affect this angle.
4. Nasofacial Angle: the angle formed by the line between the nasion and pogonion, and the line between the nasion and the pronasale. The normal nasofacial angle is 36–40°.

Z. Li (✉)
Department of Oral and Maxillo-facial Surgery, Zhejiang Stomatology Hospital, Hangzhou, China

J. Liu
Department of Oral and Maxillo-facial Surgery, First Affiliated Hospital, Zhejiang University School of Medicine, Hangzhou, China

J. Liu, B. Shi (eds.), *Atlas of Lip and Nose Plastic and Cosmetic Surgery*, https://doi.org/10.1007/978-981-16-1911-3_3

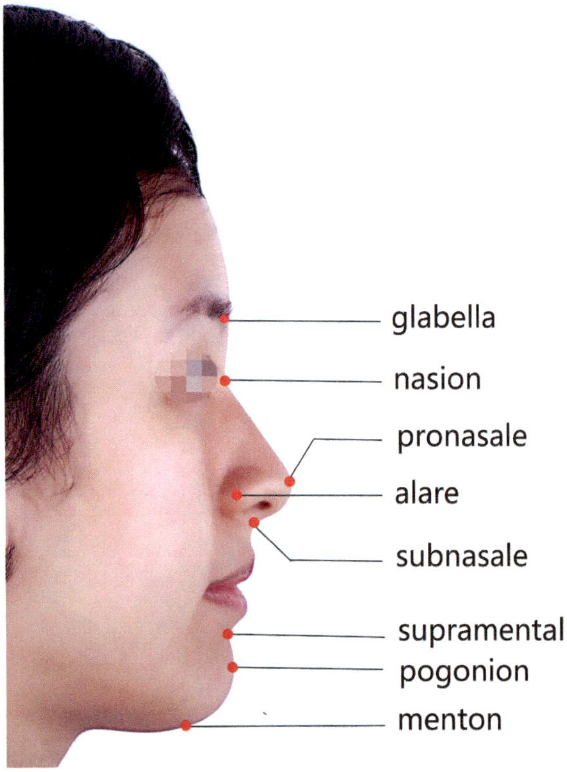

Fig. 3.2 Common cephalometric landmarks of the face: profile view (Soft Tissue B Point: Supramental point)

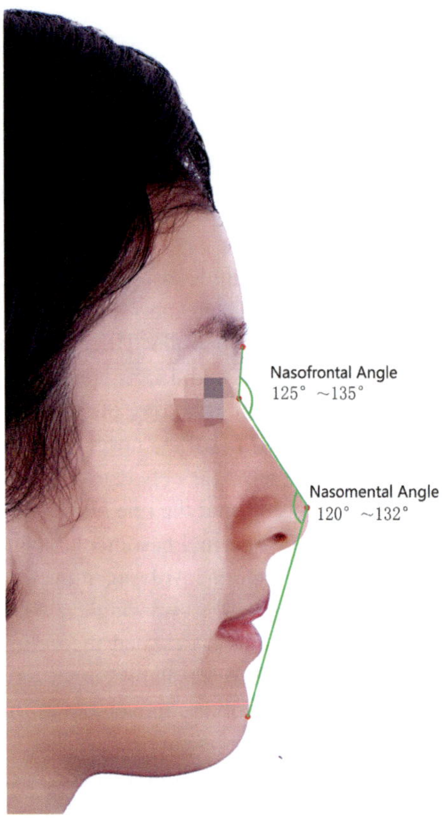

Fig. 3.3 Common esthetic angles of the face: nasofrontal and nasomental angles

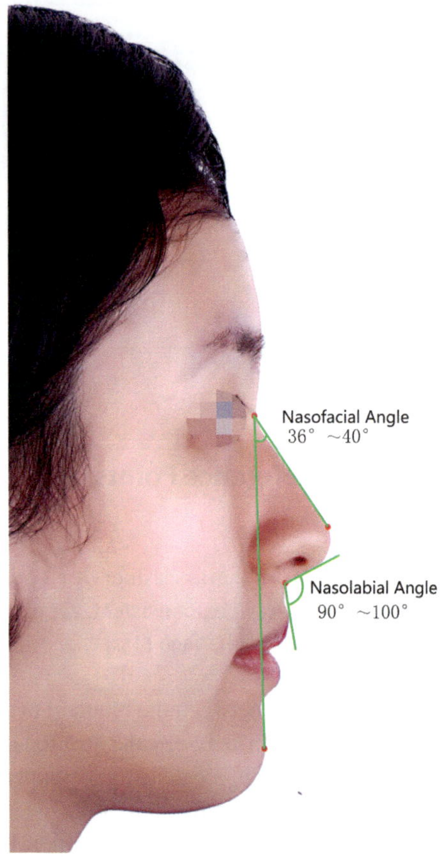

Fig. 3.4 Common esthetic angles of the face: nasolabial and nasofacial angles

Orthognathic surgery involving movement of the mandible, as well as genioplasty can significantly affect this angle (Figs. 3.3 and 3.4).

3.3 Esthetic Proportions of the Face, and Lip and Nose Region

The proportion of the face is a primary determinant of our perception of facial esthetics. This concept of facial proportions has been described both in Chinese and Western literature. Concepts such as the golden proportion are attempts at quantifying the analysis of facial esthetics, to achieve symmetry and harmony of the face. In facial esthetic surgery, in particular correction of deformities in the lip and nose region, these analyses need to be conducted both pre-operatively and post-operatively [2].

1. The "Three Stops and Five Eyes"

   The concept of three stops and five eyes is a concept created by ancient Chinese artists based on average proprotions of the adult face. This concept determines the ideal facial proportions and relationships from the frontal view using horizontal and vertical lines. It is important

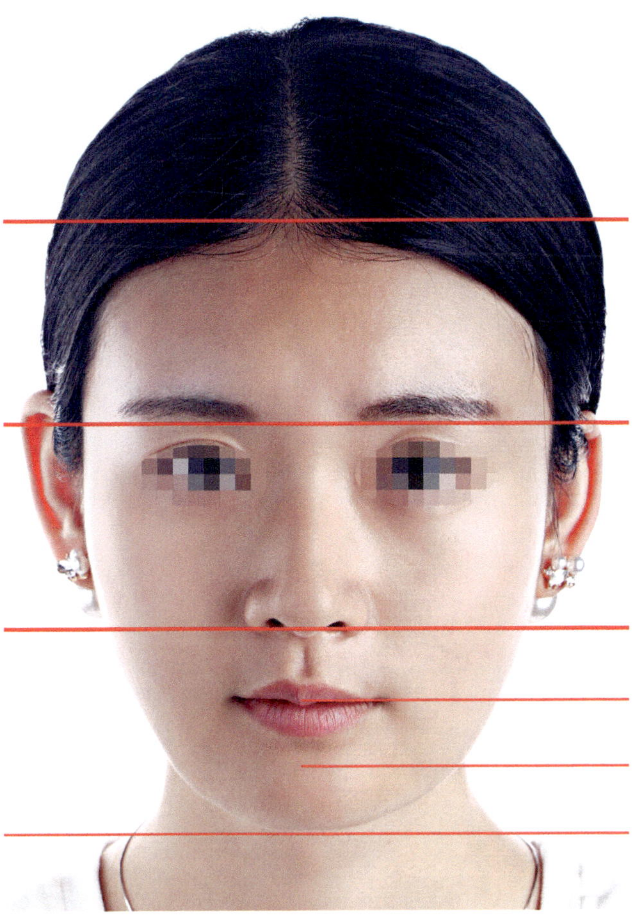

Fig. 3.5 Three stops and three minor stops

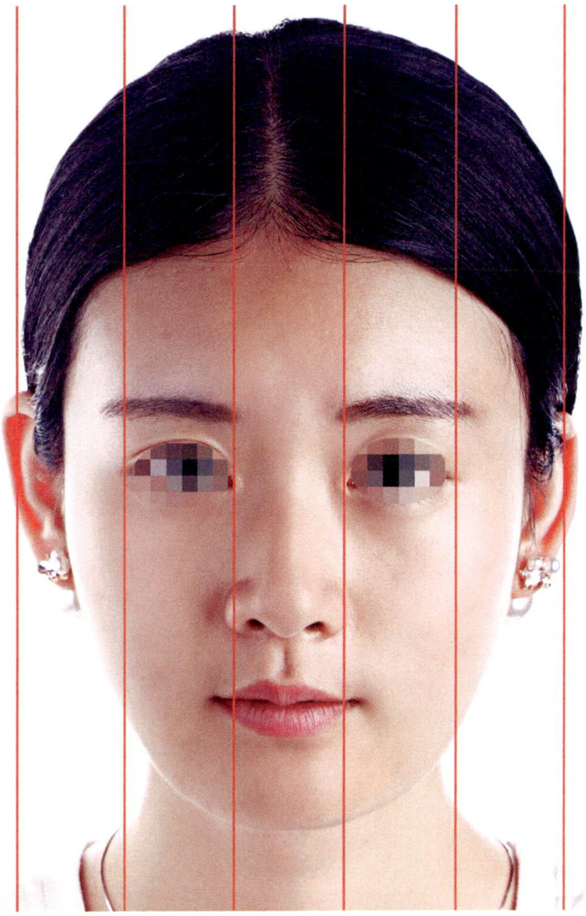

Fig. 3.6 The Five Eyes

that these proportions are not absolute, as there may be variations depending on the gender, race, and skin color, or how fat or thin an individual is. There are also slight differences between the Asian perception of beauty compared to other parts of the world.

1. Three Stops: The face can be divided into three equal horizontal thirds. The upper third lies between the hairline and the glabella. The middle third lies between the glabella and the base of the nose. The lower third lies between the base of the nose and menton.
2. Three Minor Stops: The lower third can be further divided into three additional equal minor thirds, using the oral commisure and menton as reference points. The upper minor third determines the height of the upper lip. This is an important reference in surgical repair of deformities of the oral commissure and in planning for genioplasty procedures.
3. The Five Eyes: The face can be divided into five equal vertical fifths, with each fifth being the width of the eyes. The distance from the external ear to the outer canthus of each eye, the distance between the inner and outer canthus of each eye, and the distance between both inner canthus should be equal, the width of each fifth being the width of one eye.

2. The Golden Ratio

   In the sixth century B.C., the Greek mathematician Pythagoras discovered that if a straight line is divided in such a way that the ratio of the longer segment to the shorter segment equal to the ratio of the entire length to the longer segment, which is 0.618, there is profound proportionality, esthetic, and harmony. This ratio is of great importance in facial esthetics. For example, facial harmony is achieved if the ratio between the vertical distance from the hairline to the menton and the horizontal distance of both ears are in the ratio of 1:0.618 (Figs. 3.5 and 3.6).

References

1. Wang M-Q, He S-G. Oral anatomical physiology (in Chinese). 7th ed. Beijing: People's Medical Publishing House; 2013.
2. Ru-Yao S, Zhang-Lin F. Cosmetic and plastic surgery (in Chinese). 2nd ed. Beijing: Beijing Publish House; 1992. p. 132–9.

Part II

Esthetic Correction of Lip and Nose Deformities

4 Esthetic Correction of Lip Deformities

Kai Liu

The lips form the most important esthetic and functional structure of the lower third of the face [1]. They are complex and delicate organs that require special mention. The most notable feature of the upper lip is the Cupid's bow, which is formed by the harmonious union of the philtrum, philtrum crest, and the upper vermillion border. Both the upper and lower lips have a cutaneous zone, a vermilion zone, and an oral mucosal zone. The vermillion zones of the upper lip to the lower lip are normally in the ratio of 1:2. The thickness of the lips is not uniform, with the middle being the thickest and thereafter slowly tapering toward the lip commissures. These features must be understood and adhered to for the success of any esthetic surgery involving the lips.

4.1 Surgical Correction of the Hypertrophic Lip

Lip thickness varies between individuals, and this variation is known to occur between genders and races. Males tend to have thinner lips than females, whereas individuals of African heritage tend to have the thickest lips, as opposed to Asians and Caucasians. Although significant deviation from normal lip thickness and proportions should be corrected, the surgeon must take note of a growing number of patients who wish to correct the non-obvious deviation in lip proportion. When dealing with such patients, great care in communication must be taken to ensure that the patient is given a realistic post-surgical expectation and the operator understands the esthetic demands of the patient.

In the surgical correction of the hypertrophic lip, a full-thickness wedge is removed from the wet vermillion zone at the interface between the dry and wet vermillion zones. The thickness of the wedge should be according to the amount of reduction required, whereas the length should be greater than the inter-commissure distance (Figs. 4.1 and 4.2).

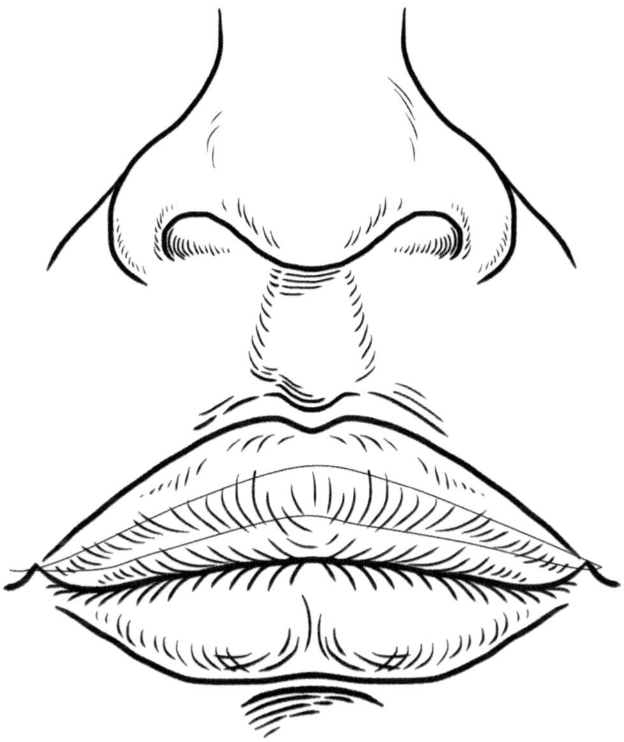

Fig. 4.1 Pre-correction of the hypertrophic upper lip

After removal of the full-thickness wedge as planned, the thickness of the upper lip should be less than that of the lower lip or achieve the ideal 1:2 ratio as compared to the lower lip (Figs. 4.3 and 4.4).

K. Liu (✉)
Department of Plastic Surgery, The 9th People's Hospital,
Shanghai Jiao Tong University, Shanghai, China

J. Liu, B. Shi (eds.), *Atlas of Lip and Nose Plastic and Cosmetic Surgery*, https://doi.org/10.1007/978-981-16-1911-3_4

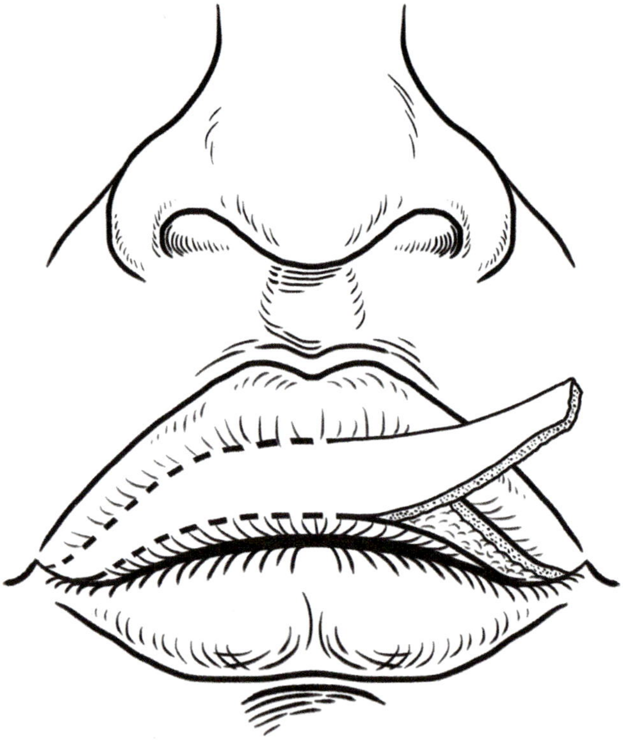

Fig. 4.2 A full-thickness wedge is removed from the vermillion zone at the interface between the dry and wet vermillion zones

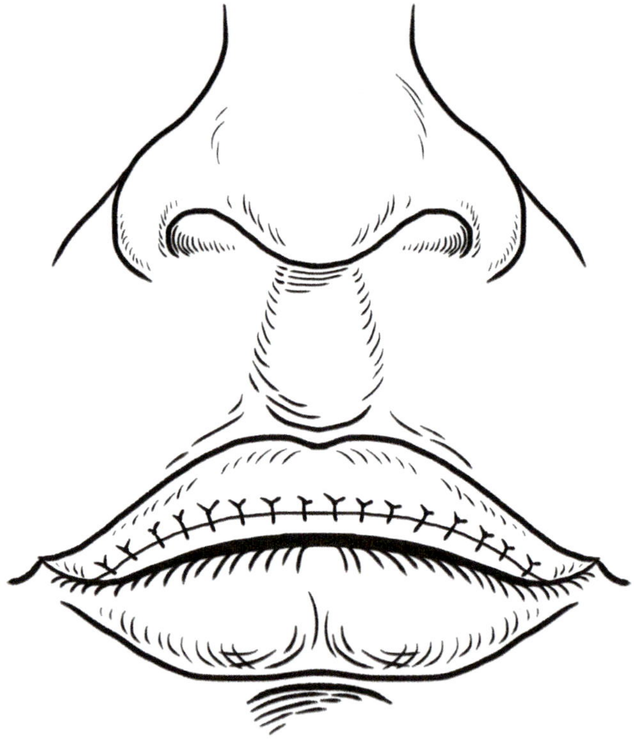

Fig. 4.3 Post-surgical closure

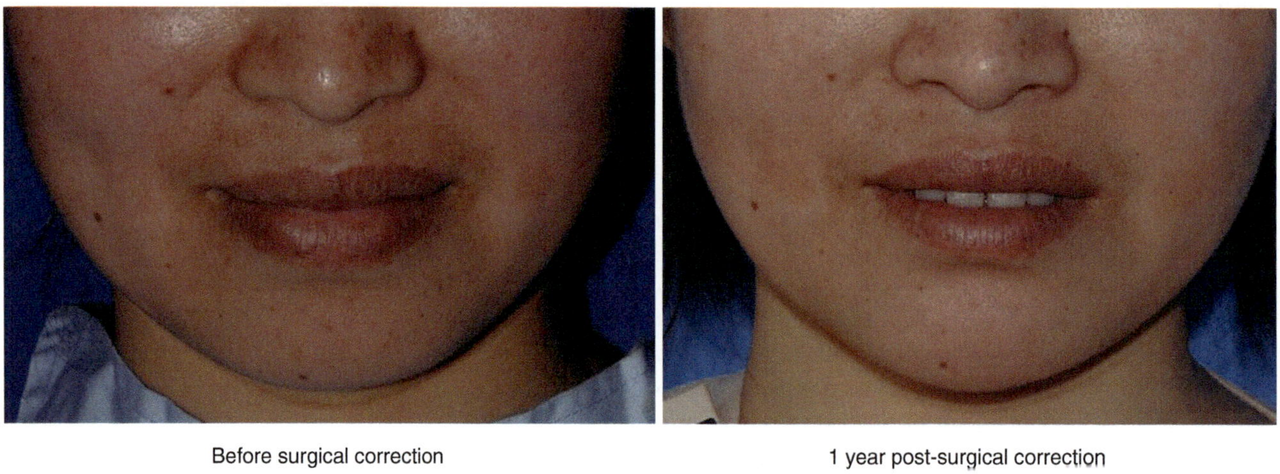

Fig. 4.4 Before and after surgical correction

4.2 Depressed Deformity Correction of Nasolabial Groove

The nasolabial groove is formed from the confluence of the alar nasi and the lateral commissure of the lip. Superficially, it appears to be a triangular depression, with the base of the triangle at the lateral border of the upper lip. An excessively depressed nasolabial groove could be due to three reasons:

1. Under-development of the midface
2. Excessively low piriform rim
3. Excessively wide piriform rim

Several corrective techniques are known—local injection of filler material, insertion of implants such as e-PTFE and Medpore implants, etc. Of course, the use of rib grafts in the correction of the depression deformity of the nasolabial groove is the most predictable and therefore most ideal

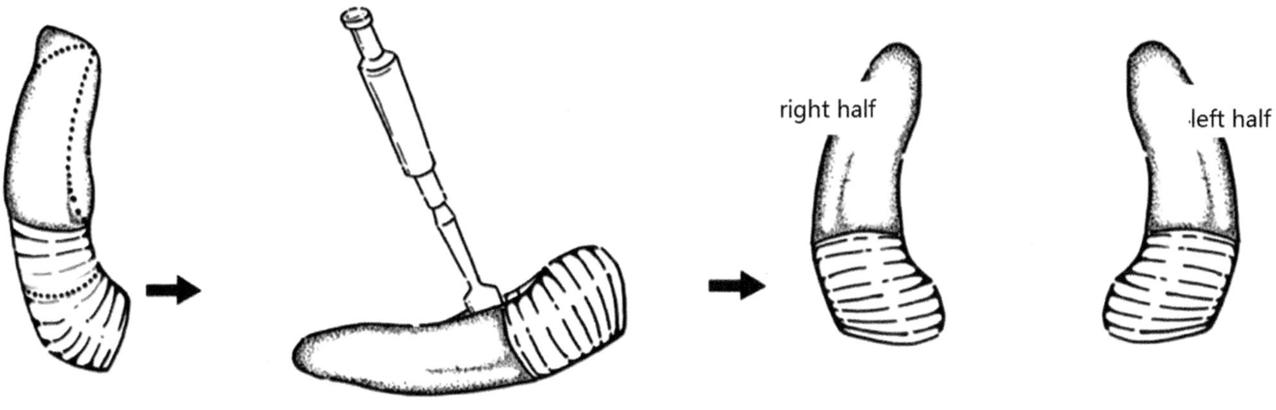

Fig. 4.5 Preparation of autogenous rib osteocartilaginous graft

treatment option. Usually, the sixth or seventh rib with attached cartilage is used. After harvest, it is split lengthwise, to form left and right halves. The bone grafts are then shaped and prepared for insertion. A small incision is made in the buccal sulcus and extended sub-periosteal to expose the lateral nose bilaterally. The prepared bone graft is then inserted. Usually, if the preparation of the graft is adequate, it will stay firmly in place and will not require further fixation (Figs. 4.5, 4.6, 4.7).

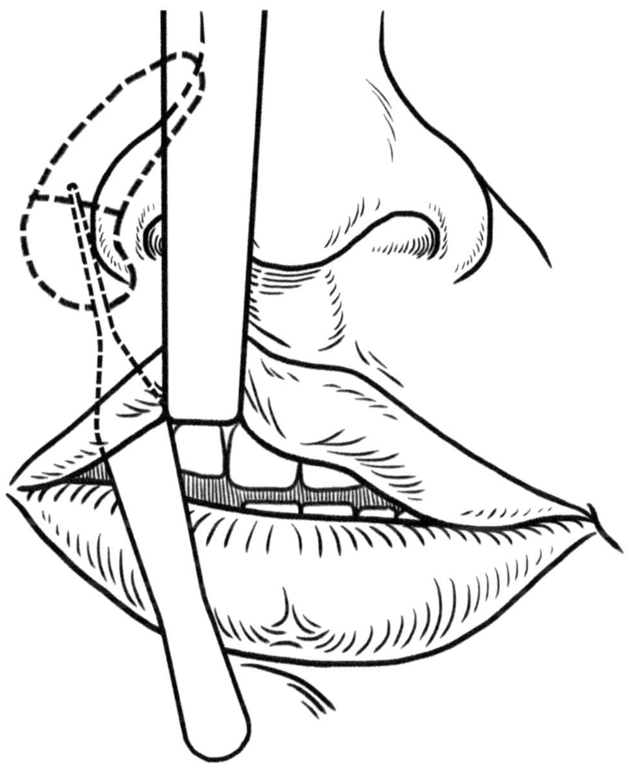

Fig. 4.6 Insertion of autogenous rib osteocartilaginous graft

4.3 Lip Augmentation

Injection of absorbable fillers, such as hyaluronic acid, or autogenous fat, may be used in the treatment of the patient with excessively thin lips [2]. The point of injection is at the junction between the dry and wet lips and to the depth of the submucosa. The decision for injection of such fillers into the upper or lower lip, or both upper and lower lips, depends greatly on the patient's esthetic demands.

Injection to the upper lip is at three points, with each point receiving 0.1–0.3 ml of filler. Injection to the lower lip is at two points, with each point receiving 01–0.5 ml of filler. It is of paramount importance to ensure that the filler material is distributed evenly throughout the lip. It is also important to ensure that only absorbable fillers are injected. The lips are the most active organs in the face, and non-absorbable material will move during lip movement, eventually aggregating to form a mass that will compromise the shape and esthetics of the lips. The operator must make all attempts to ensure that fillers are not injected directly into any vessels in the lips (Figs. 4.8 and 4.9).

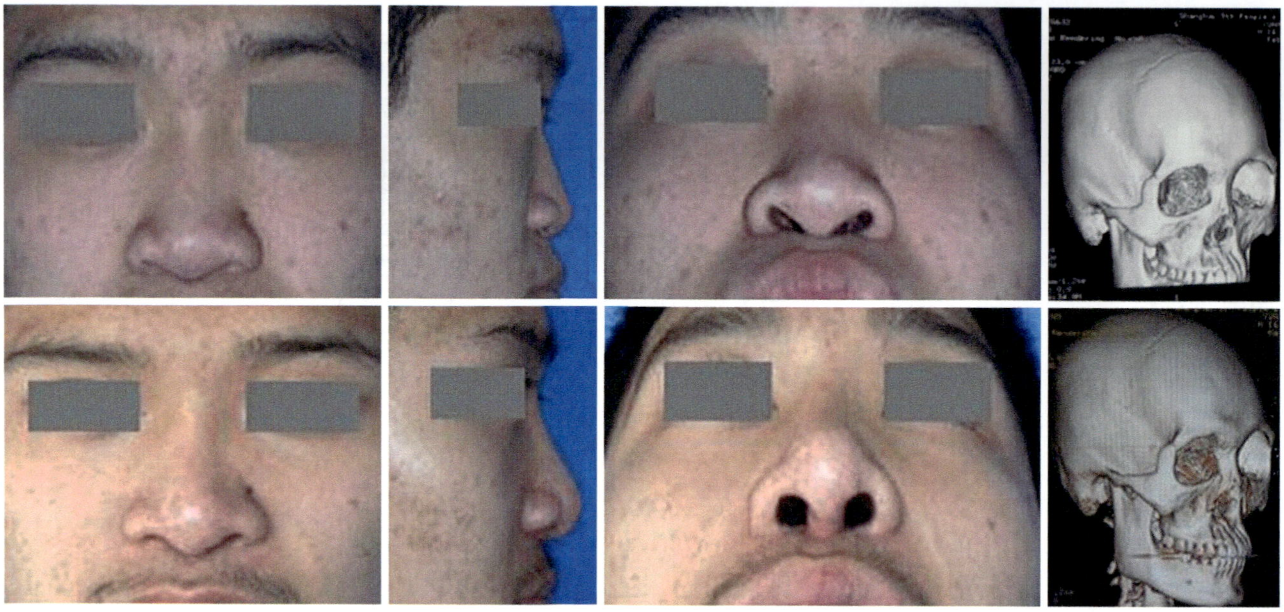

Fig. 4.7 Augmentation of depressed nasolabial groove with autogenous rib osteocartilaginous graft

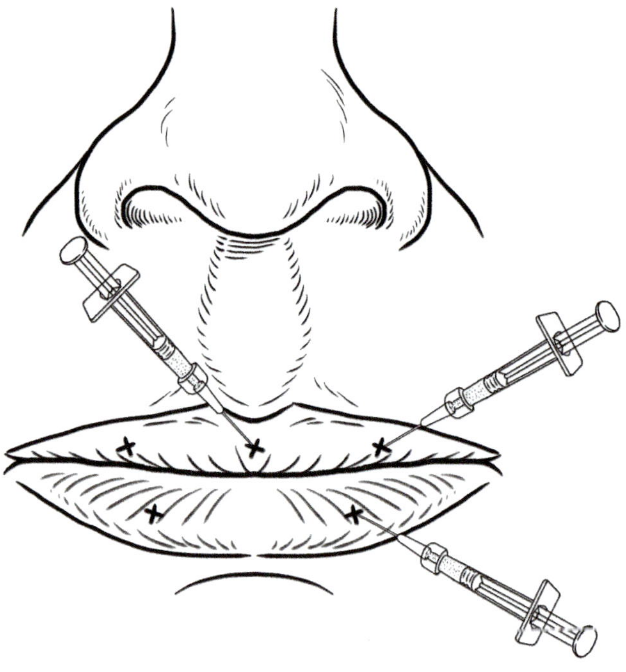

Fig. 4.8 Injection of fillers into the upper lips are at three points and at two points into the lower lip

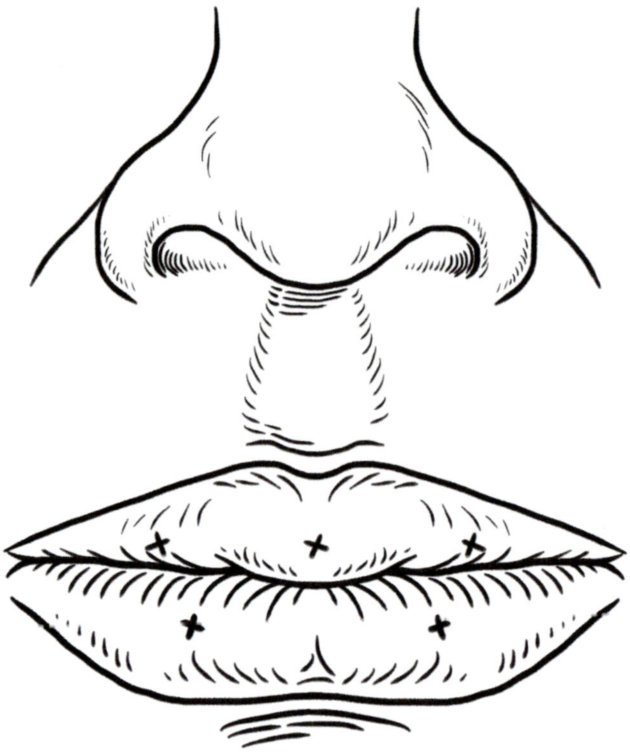

Fig. 4.9 Illustrating the change of lips after injection of fillers

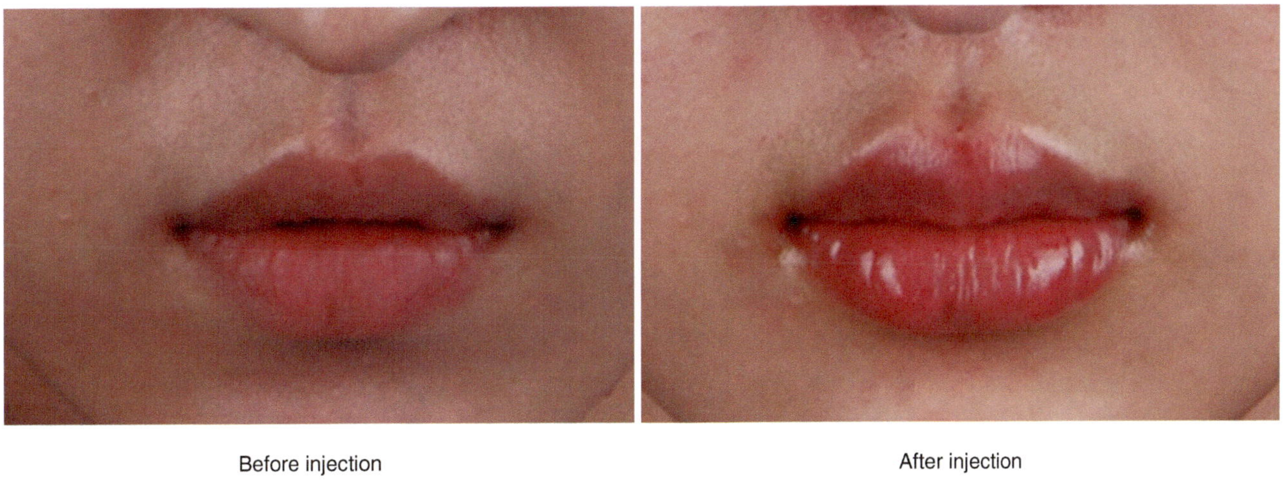

Fig. 4.10 Pre- and post-injection of fillers to augment the thin lips

Take note of the change in the external appearance of the lips after injection of fillers (Fig. 4.10).

References

1. Ru-Yao S, Zhang-Lin F. Cosmetic and plastic surgery (in Chinese). 2nd ed. Beijing: Beijing Publish House; 1992. p. 132–9.
2. Peng J, Peng HP. Classifications and injection strategy for lip reshaping in Asians. J Cosmet Dermatol. 2020;19(2):21–3.

5 Cosmetic Surgery of Nose

Xiaoyan Tan

5.1 Plastic Surgery of Saddle Nose and Augmentation Rhinoplasty

1. Indication
   (i) Flat radix and nasal bridge, an acute nasofacial angle less than 30° (see Fig. 5.1), note: at profile view, connect a line from glabella to pogonion, connect another line from radix to the nasal tip, the angle formed by the intersection of both lines is the nasofacial angle.
   (ii) Pre-operatively, assess for the presence of abnormalities in olfaction and nasal air passage.
2. Surgical methods and procedures
   Anesthesia: Local infiltration or general anesthesia.
   Surgical methods:
   (i) Radix position: level of the upper eyelid with eyes open.
   (ii) Incision: Place skin incision at the inferior border of left or right lower lateral cartilage, or trans-columellar flying-bird incision (as shown in Fig. 5.2).
   (iii) Material: Silicon, expanded polytetrafluoroethylene (ePTFE), autogenous rib, or fascial graft.
   (iv) Carving of grafts or cartilage: carve the graft according to the individual patient's facial characteristics, pay particular attention to the width and curvature of the dorsum of the nose. Immerse the carved graft in antibiotics (see Fig. 5.3).
   (v) Dissection: Incise along the planned incision line, dissect superiorly between the lateral nasal cartilage subcutaneous fats of the nasal tip until the keystone area (the connection between the nasal bone and cartilage), continue subperiosteal dissection superiorly until radix, and create a subperiosteal pouch of about 10–12 mm wide to receive the graft (see Fig. 5.4). Care must be taken to ensure an intact dorsal periosteum, avoid elevating beyond radix, the asymmetrical or inadequate elevation of the subperiosteal pocket, as well as excessively large pocket resulting in movement and inadequate stability of the graft.
   (vi) Graft insertion: After removal of accumulated blood, insert and carefully position the graft into the subperiosteal pocket with a clamp, avoid folding, distortion, and displacement of the graft. Close the incision with interrupted sutures.

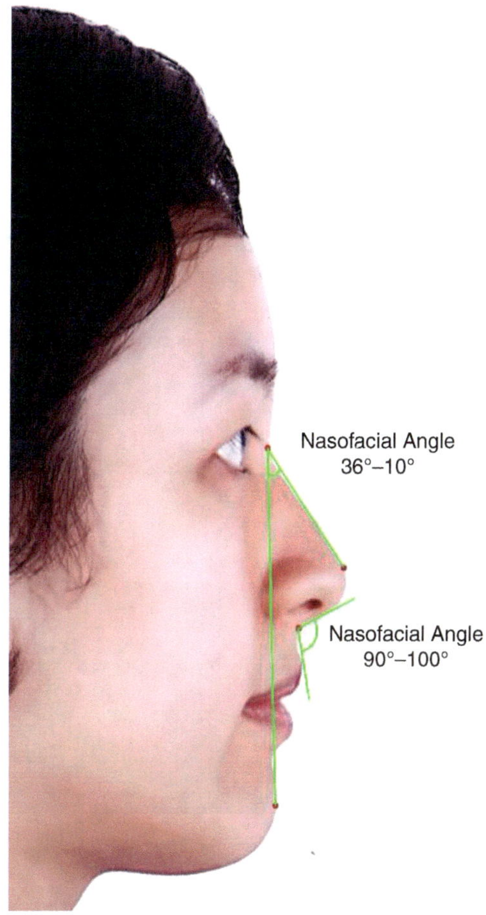

Fig. 5.1 Nasofacial Angle

X. Tan (✉)
Hangzhou Plastic Surgery Hospital, Hangzhou, China

J. Liu, B. Shi (eds.), *Atlas of Lip and Nose Plastic and Cosmetic Surgery*, https://doi.org/10.1007/978-981-16-1911-3_5

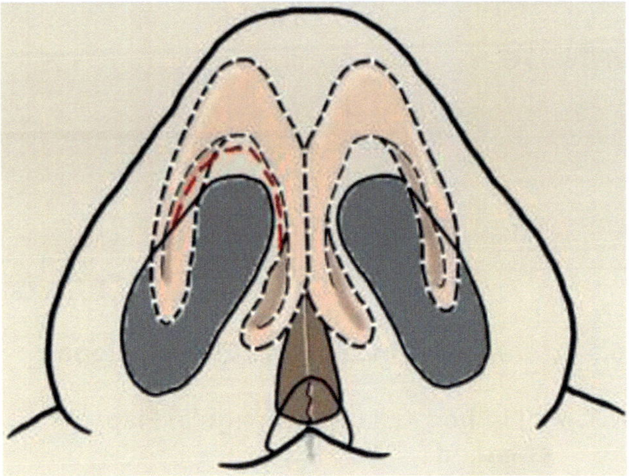

Fig. 5.2 Schematic designs of surgical incisions

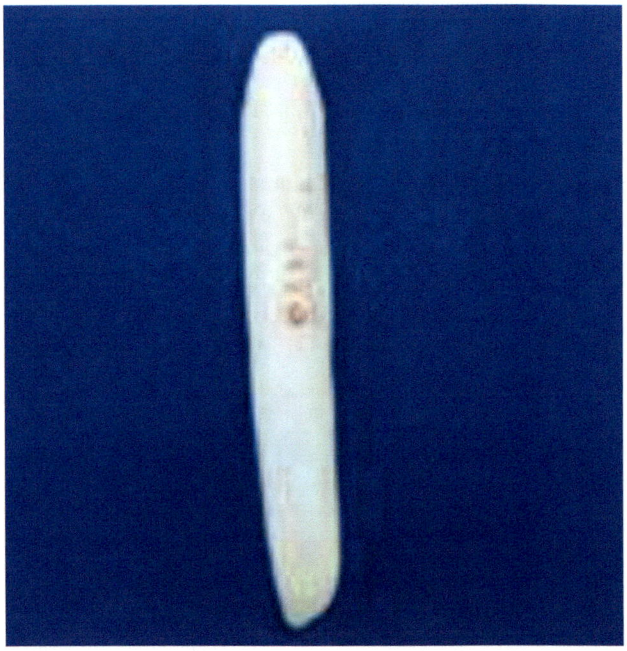

Fig. 5.3 The carved graft

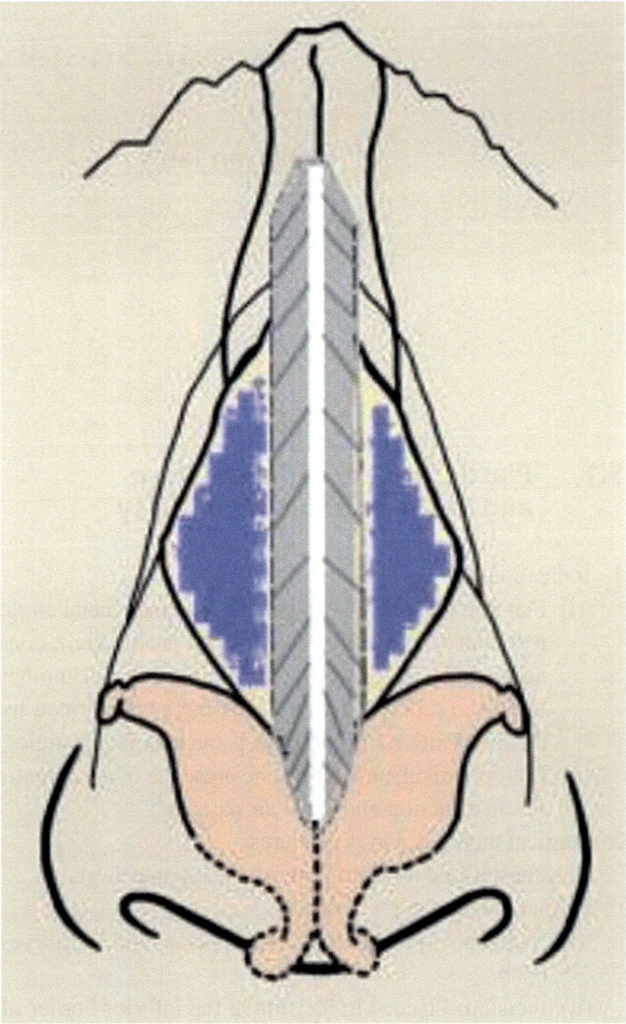

Fig. 5.4 Illustration showing the extent of dorsal dissection

Classic Case 1 (Fig. 5.5)

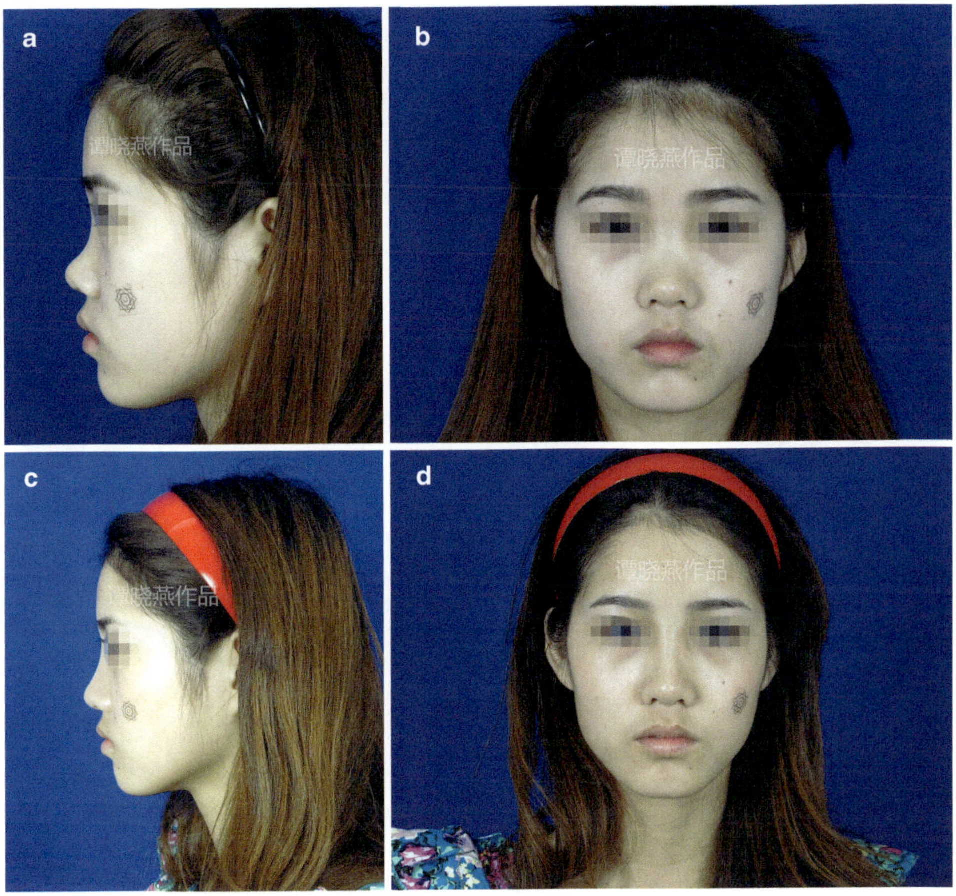

Fig. 5.5 (**a**–**d**) Classic case 1 (augmentation rhinoplasty with silicon). **a**: lateral view, pre-op; **b**: frontal view, pre-op; **c**: lateral view, post-op; **d**: frontal view, post-op

Classic Case 2 (Fig. 5.6)

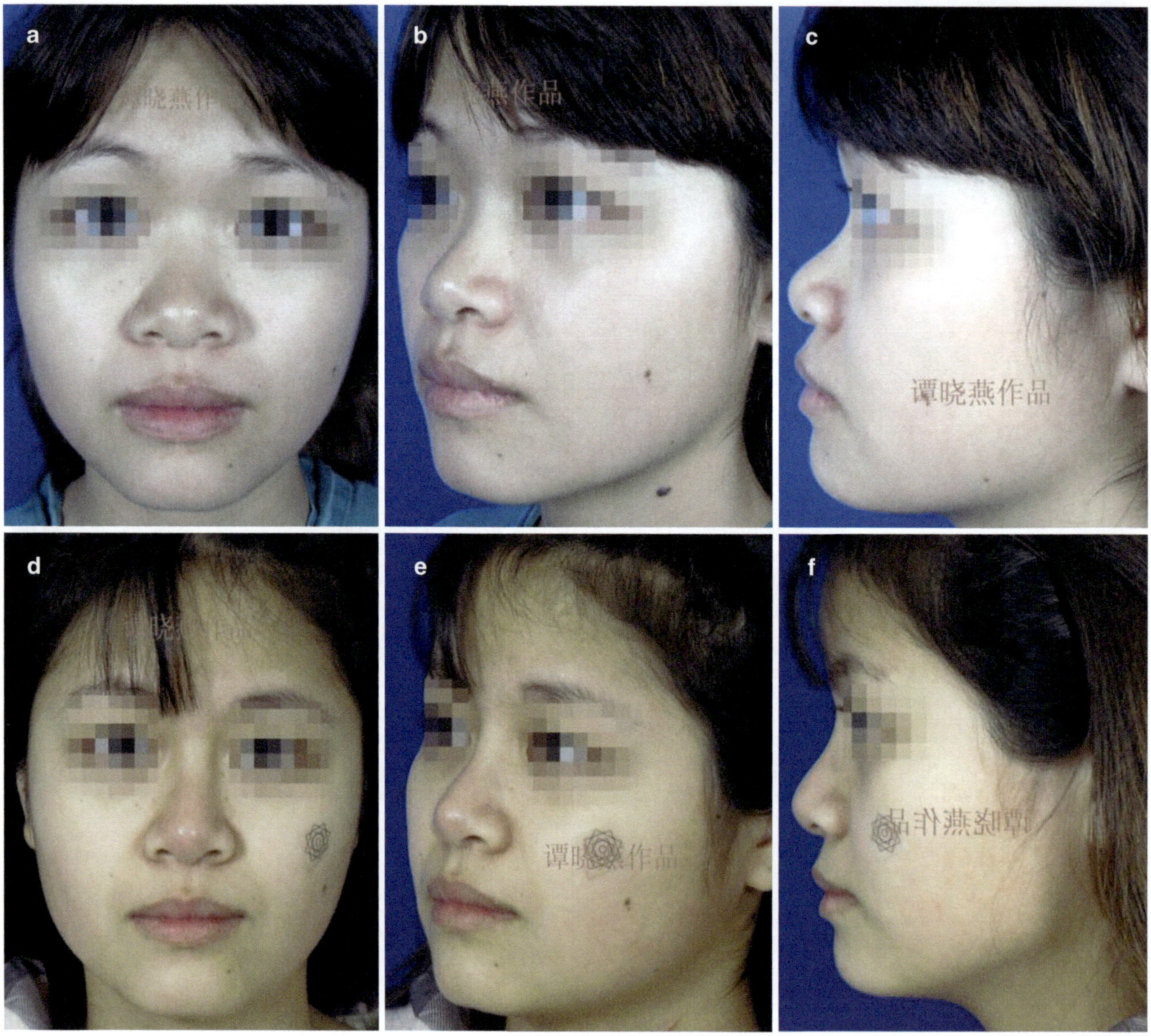

Fig. 5.6 (**a–f**) Classic Case 2 (augmentation rhinoplasty with PTFE). **a–c**: frontal; oblique lateral; and lateral view, Pre-op; **d–f**: frontal; oblique lateral; and lateral view, Post-op

3. Points to note:
   (i) Radix is at the level of the upper eyelid with eyes open. With significantly depressed radix, the graft can be placed slightly superior to radix to allow for a natural transition and avoid a stairstep appearance.
   (ii) The height of the dorsum should be in harmony with that of the nasal tip. With a low-hanging nasal tip, consider augmentation rhinoplasty with simultaneous autogenous cartilage grafting of the nasal tip. Refer to the section on nasal tip correction for details [1–3].
   (iii) Severe cases of saddle nose deformities are frequently accompanied by a short nose, flat tip, and upturned nostrils. The degree of correction with simple augmentation rhinoplasty is limited. A simultaneous nasal tip reconstruction with autogenous rib graft should be considered for better clinical outcomes [4, 5].
   (iv) Reasons for post-operative asymmetry include asymmetry of graft carving, asymmetry of the graft chamber dissection, and incomplete severance of subperiosteal fibrotic bands. One easily overlooked

factor is pre-existing asymmetry or deviation of the nasal bone and/or nasal septal cartilage. A thorough pre-operative clinical examination is necessary, including CT imaging when indicated.

5.2 Correction of Deviated Nose Deformity

1. Indications
   Nasal deviation due to congenital deformities, trauma, previous surgeries, or pathologies, including a deviation of the nasal tip, deviation and rotation of nasal bridge [6–8].
2. Surgical methods and procedures
   Anesthesia: general anesthesia with intro-oral endotracheal intubation
   Surgical methods:
   (i) Design: mark out the dorsal midline and bilateral base of the nose.
   (ii) Incision: standard open rhinoplasty incision.
   (iii) Exposure and dissection: adequate exposure of abnormally positioned nasal bone, lateral nasal cartilages, and nasal septum.
   (iv) Osteotomy: (1) Post-traumatic asymmetry: osteotomize previous fracture site and reposition. (2) Congenital asymmetry: Perform midline and lateral osteotomies of the nasal bone, manipulate and reposition accordingly to correct asymmetry. Midline osteotomy is done with the osteotome placed superficial to upper lateral nasal cartilages, splitting the roof of nasal bone; lateral osteotomies are done at the junction between nasal bone and maxilla on each side. See Fig. 5.7.

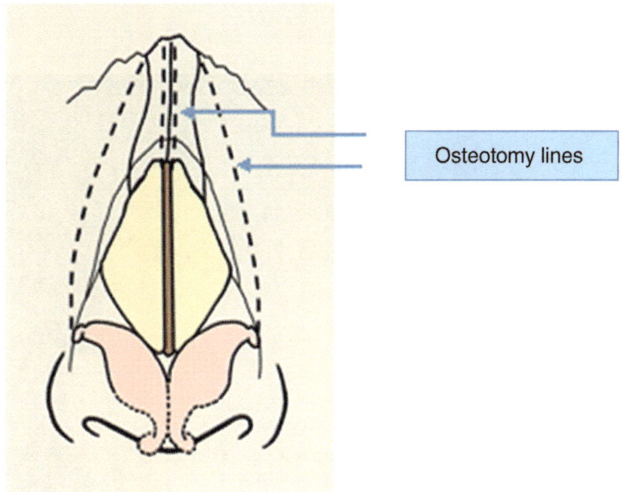

Fig. 5.7 Midline and lateral osteotomy lines

   (v) Correction of the deviated nasal septum: Patients with concurrent nasal septal deviation, reconstruction is often inadequate without simultaneous septal correction. Refer to Sect. 5.3 for surgical correction of the deviated nasal septum.
   (vi) Post-op fixation: After osteotomy, in order to ensure symmetrical positioning and healing of the detached bilateral nasal bones and maintain the repositioned nasal septal cartilage, both internal and external nasal splints are required. Bilateral nostrils are packed with BIPP gauze, ensuring a symmetrical appearance of the external nose and central position of the nasal bones and septum. External splinting can be achieved with tapes or rigid splints.

Classic Case 1 (Fig. 5.8)

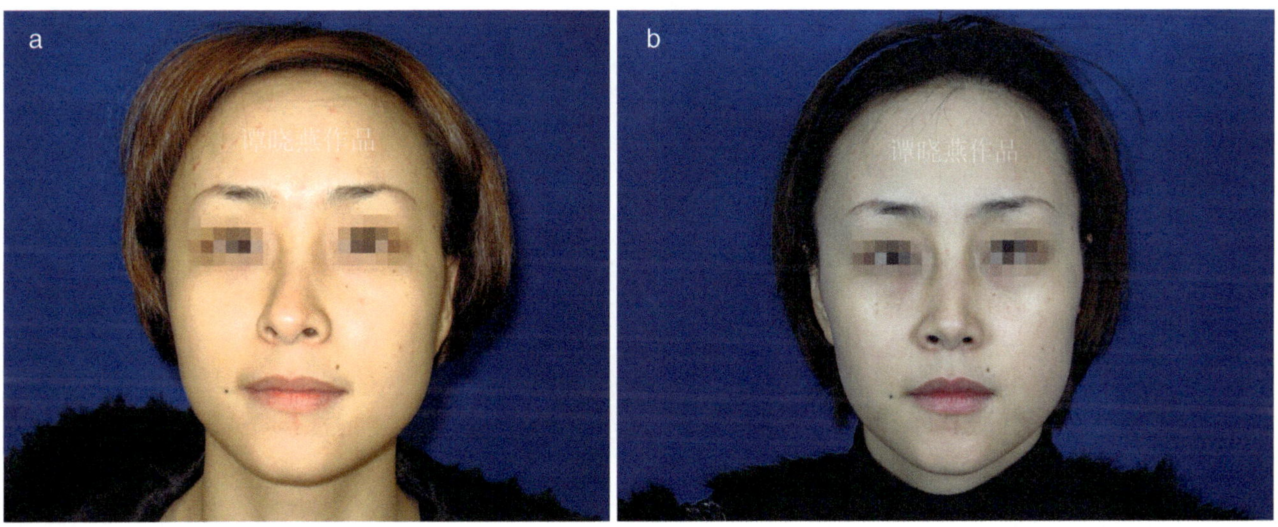

Fig. 5.8 (**a** and **b**) Surgical correction of deviated nose, pre- and post-operative appearances. **a**: Pre-operative; **b**: 1.5 months post-operative

Classic Case 2 (Fig. 5.9)

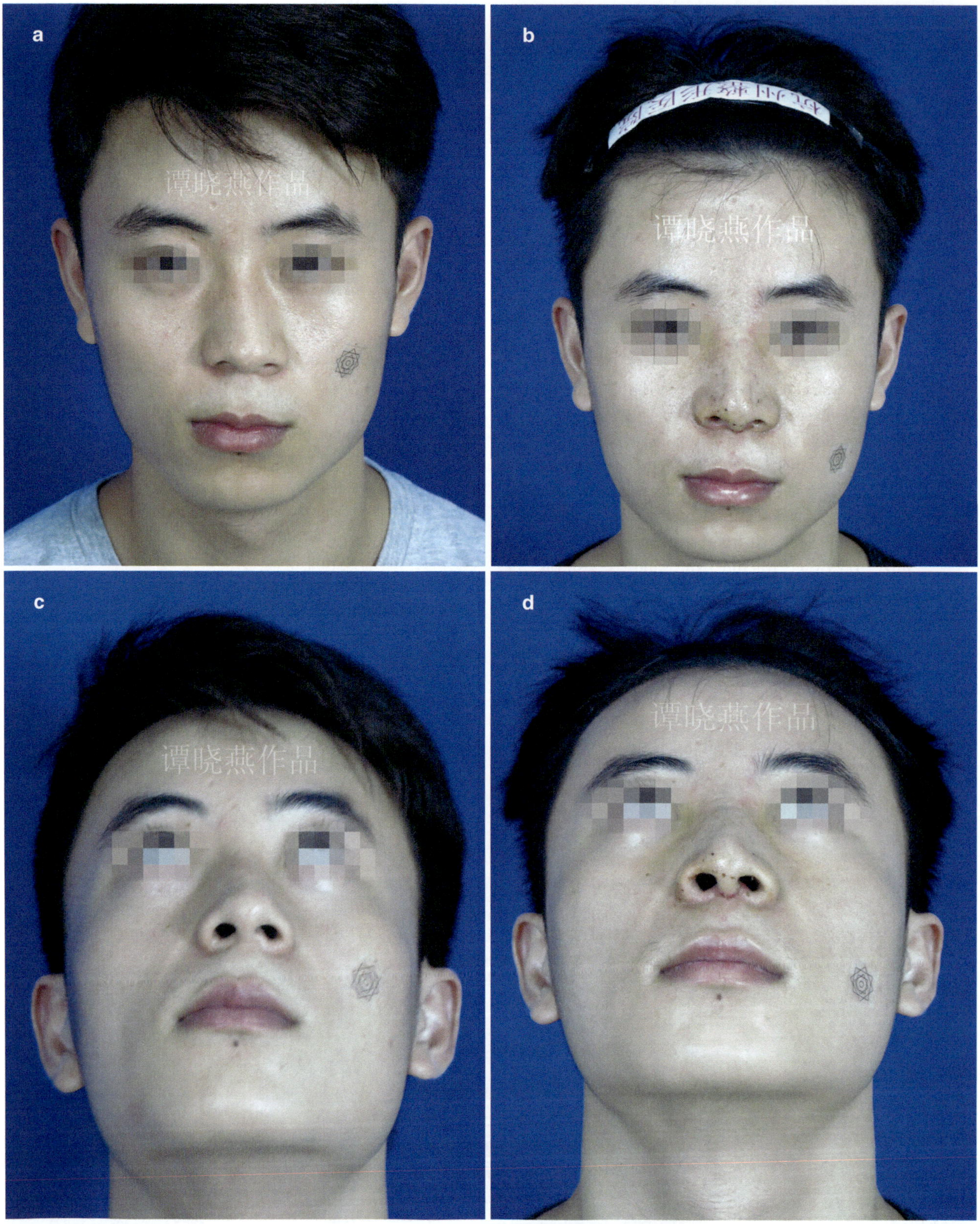

Fig. 5.9 (**a**–**d**) Surgical correction of deviated nose, pre- and post-operative appearances. **a**: Frontal view pre-op; **b**: Frontal view post-op; **c**: Worm's eye view, pre-op; **d**: Worm's eye view, post-op

3. Points to note
   (i) Common expectations of patients seeking surgical correction of nasal deviation include correction of nasal asymmetry, improvement of nasal obstruction and esthetic improvement of the external nose. Patients should be well informed before treatment; these three outcomes may be completely or only partially achievable with surgery, especially those with pre-existing nasal obstruction with which a complete resolution can be difficult. Clear patient understanding should be obtained with appropriate signed clinical documentation [3, 8].
   (ii) For post-traumatic nasal deformities, the first 20 days after the initial injury is deemed optimal for relatively straightforward and fast surgical correction. There is a small risk for residual or relapse of asymmetry with tissue healing.
   (iii) Nasal osteotomy often leaves the dorsal nasal bone irregular and/or asymmetrical, which is more apparent in patients with thin overlying skin. In such situations, this can be masked by overlying the dorsal bonny surface with grafts such as silicon, ePTFE, or autogenous soft tissue fascia.
   (iv) Correction of nasal deviation is deemed the most complex of all nasal surgeries owing to the multifactorial etiology. This requires a tailored treatment plan for each patient, and a high risk for relapse exists.
   (v) Common surgical complications include: (1) incomplete correction; (2) relapse of asymmetry; (3) loss of nasal tip support due to weakening of cartilage; (4) incomplete correction of nasal obstruction, or creation of nasal obstruction.

5.3 Correction of Nasal Septum Deviation

1. Indications
   Nasal asymmetry accompanied by nasal septal deviation (bony and/or cartilaginous) due to congenital deformities, trauma, previous surgeries, or pathologies. This includes midline deviation and rotation, or with significant nasal obstructions.
2. Surgical methods and procedures
   Anesthesia: local infiltration or general anesthesia with oral intubation
   Surgical methods:
   (i) Design: mark out facial midline, the deviated nasal midline, area of deviation and asymmetry, bilateral alar cartilage, and trans-columellar incision line.
   (ii) Incision: standard open rhinoplasty incisions (bilateral anterior cartilaginous incision with a trans-columellar incision).
   (iii) Exposure and dissection: dissection between a bilateral medial portion of the lower lateral cartilages, exposing the distal end of the nasal septum. With a periosteal elevator, staying close to the septal cartilage, elevate the perichondrium bilaterally at distal and dorsal aspects of the septal cartilage fully avoiding tear, thereby releasing any tension causing the deviation. Severe fibrous connection between the dorsal surface of the nasal bone and lateral nasal cartilage create a greenstick fracture at the vertical plate of the ethmoid bone and reposition accordingly.
   (iv) Correction of gross septal asymmetry: after the release of tension, excess septal cartilage can be excised, leaving a 1.5 cm strut in the shape of a "7" at the dorsal and distal end (as shown in Fig. 5.10a, b); the repositioned septum is then secured and sutured at the midline. Adjust the alar position and deviated columella and close the incision with interrupted sutures (The excised portion of septal cartilage can be used as grafts for nasal tip adjustment, details refer to subsequent section).
   (v) Insert expandable sponges to bilateral nostrils, secure with externally sutured plastic sheets (Fig. 5.11).

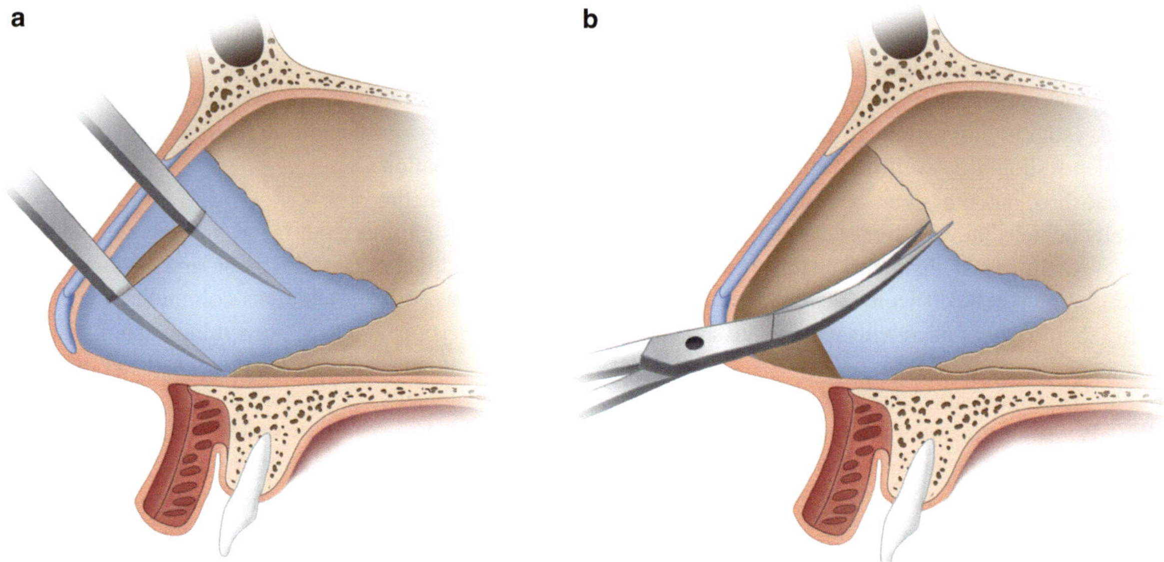

Fig. 5.10 (**a** and **b**) Schematic illustration of the surgical procedures. **a**: Left:elevation of bilateral septal periosteum; **b**: Right: selective excision of septal cartilage, leaving a 1.5 cm "7"-shaped strut at the dorsal and distal end as shaded

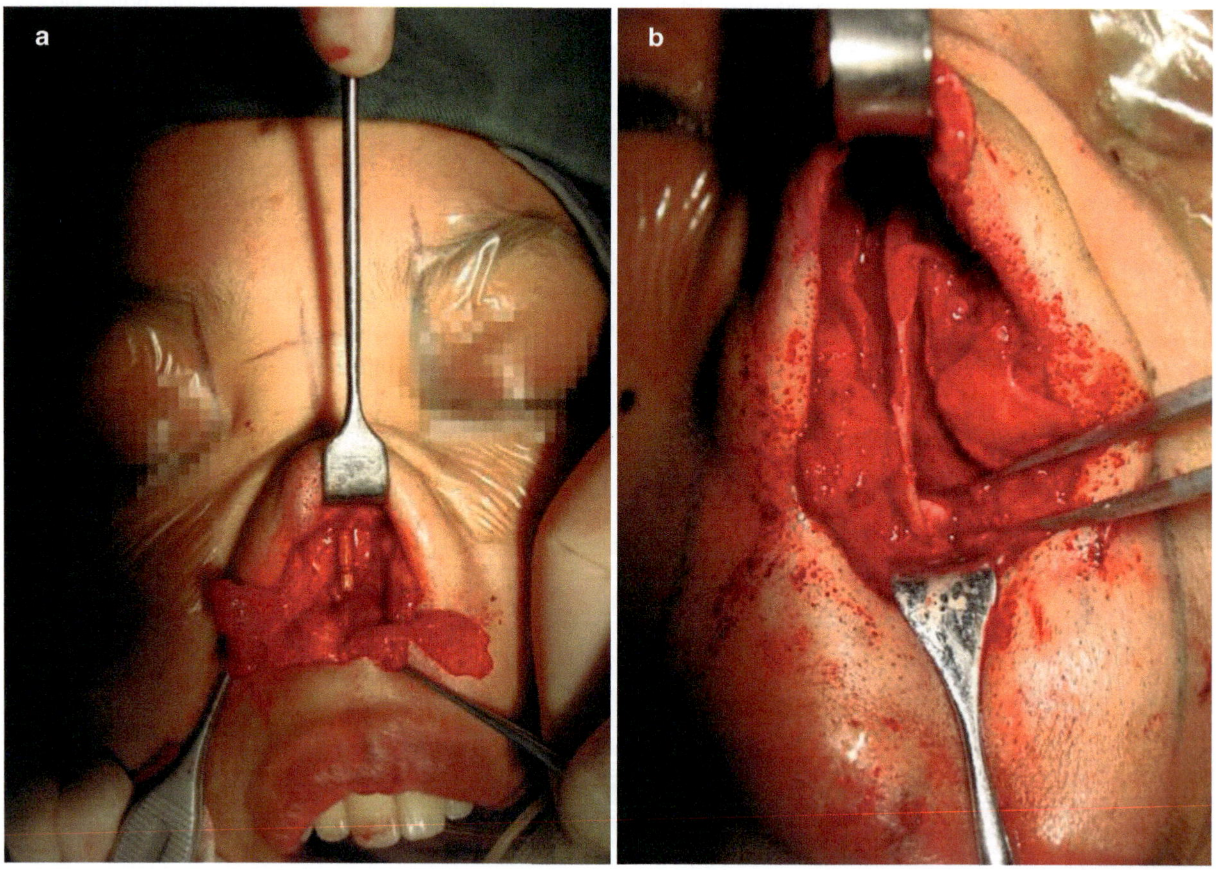

Fig. 5.11 (**a** and **b**) Illustration showing the exposure of septal cartilage. **a**: Left: exposure of distal end of the septal cartilage; **b**: Right: the deviated septal cartilage

Classic Case 1 (Fig. 5.12)

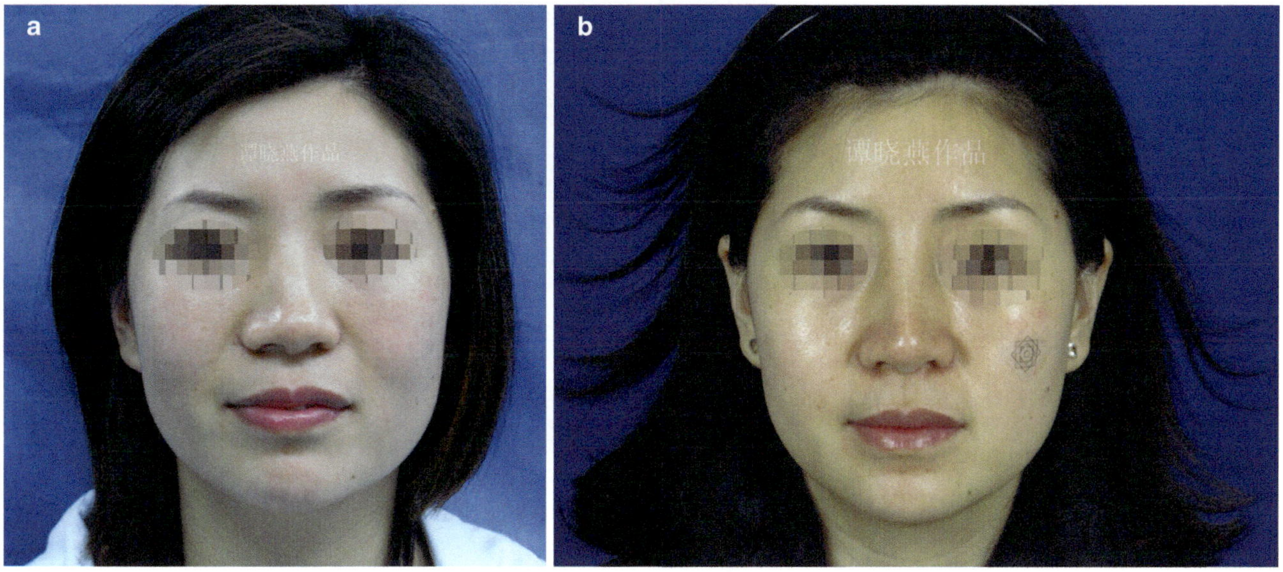

Fig. 5.12 (**a** and **b**) Deviated nasal septum, classic case 1. **a**: pre-operative (deviated nasal midline); **b**: 3-month post-operative

Classic Case 2 (Fig. 5.13)

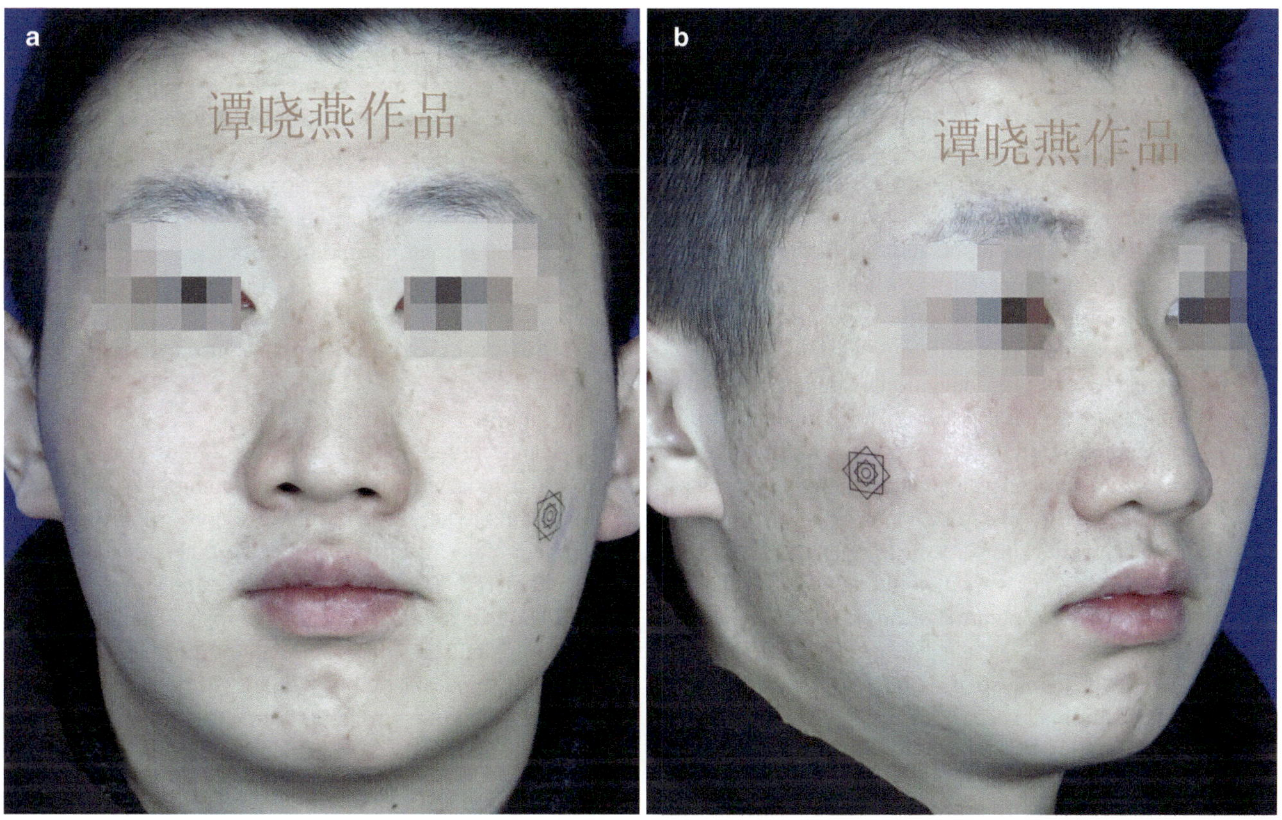

Fig. 5.13 (**a**–**d**) Deviated nasal septum, classic case 2. **a**, **b**: Pre-operative (deviated nasal midline accompanied by dorsal hump; **c**, **d**: 1-month post-operative

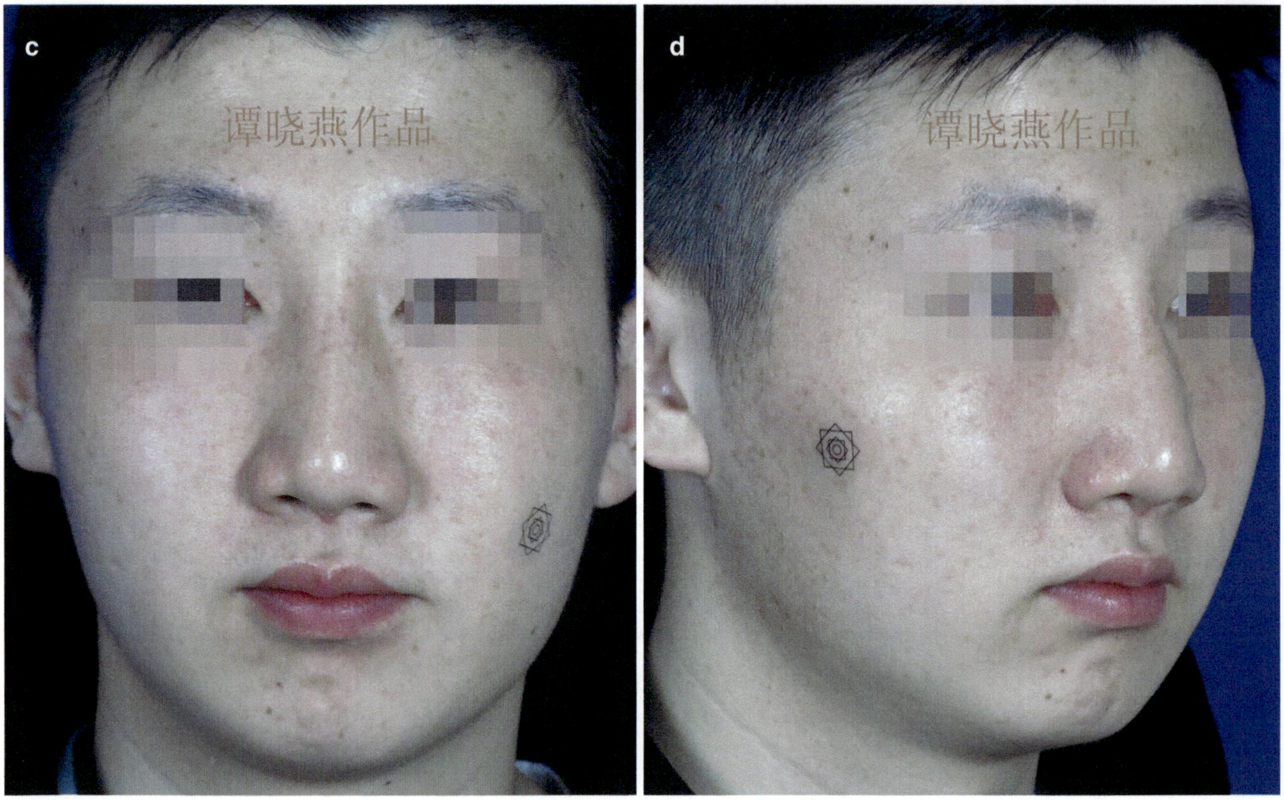

Fig. 5.13 (continued)

3. Points to note:
   (i) For proper pre-operative preparation, patient communication, and documentation, refer to Sect. 5.2 (Correction of deviated nose deformity) in this chapter.
   (ii) For post-traumatic nasal septal deviation, early correction should be performed within 20 days from the initial injury. Delayed correction can be done 6 months after injury.
   (iii) Correction of nasal deviation is deemed the most complex of all nasal surgeries owing to the multifactorial etiology [8, 9]. This requires a tailored treatment plan for each patient, and a high risk for relapse exists. For cases of nasal asymmetry with concurrent nasal septal deviation, reconstruction of symmetry is often inadequate without simultaneous surgical correction of the septum. Post-op fixation: Both external and internal nasal stabilizations are required. Insert expandable sponges into bilateral nasal cavities, position and secure the nasal bone and septum at facial midline, and ensure symmetry. Additional external stabilization with tapes or plastic splint for 7–10 days.
   (iv) Common surgical complications include (1) incomplete correction; (2) relapse of asymmetry; (3) loss of nasal tip support due to weakening of distal end of septal cartilage; (4) incomplete correction of nasal obstruction, or creation of nasal obstruction; and (5) septal hematoma and infection.

5.4 Correction of Hump Nose Deformity

1. Indications

   Spinal projections at the dorsum of the nose are referred to as hump nose, most commonly caused by congenital hyperplasia of the nasal bone, septal cartilage, and lateral nasal cartilages. When septal and lateral cartilage hyperplasia is accompanied by a down-turned nasal tip, it is referred to as an aquiline nose. Traumatic deformation usually results from malunion of fractured nasal bone for hyperplastic bony repair forming a spinal projection at the dorsum and is frequently seen with a concurrent nasal asymmetry. Incidence of a hump nose is much less frequent in Asian populations compared to Caucasians.

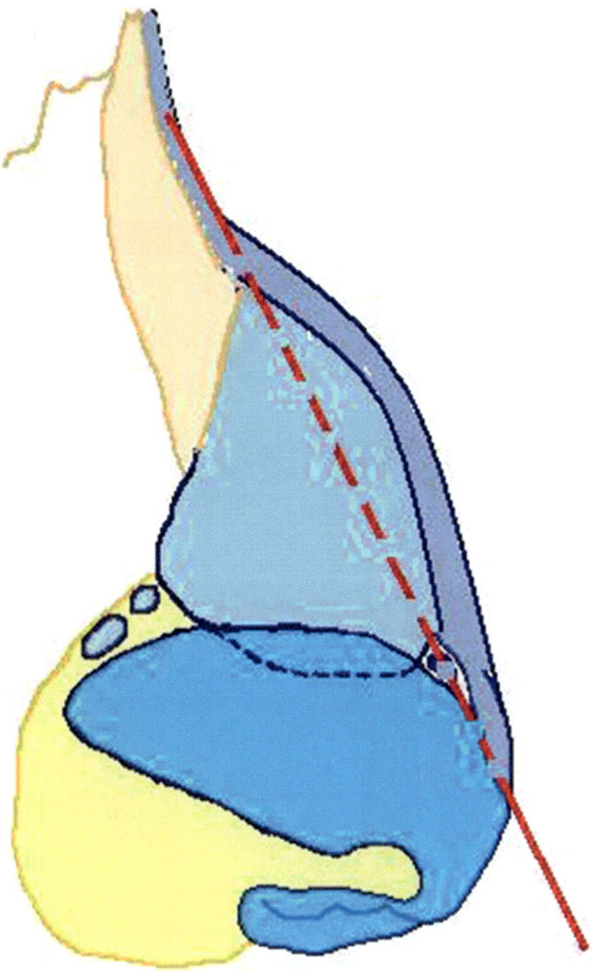

Fig. 5.14 Schematic illustration of surgical incision for dorsal hump reduction

Congenital hump noses rarely present with any functional deficits. However, post-traumatic hump noses can exhibit respiratory impairments due to excessive septal deviation blocking one side of the nostril [10, 11].

2. Surgical methods and procedures

The basic techniques of surgical correction follow Joseph's rhinoplasty method via endonasal approach (suitable for Caucasians and patients with high and prominent noses), or Anderson & Ries' external nasal approach (suitable for the Asian population). Surgical principles include reduction osteotomy of the bony hump, narrowing of the nasal dorsum, and reconstruction of the caudal nose. In the presence of excessive septal deviation, a corrective septoplasty should be performed first.

(i) Mark the intended bony hump osteotomy line. Connect a line sagittally from nasion to the tip of the nose, the portion above this line should be osteotomized and removed (see Fig. 5.14).

(ii) Incision: Bilateral marginal incisions; for more prominent humps, bilateral marginal incisions combined with trans-columellar incision can be used for sufficient surgical exposure and easier manipulation.

(iii) Dissection: Using scissors and periosteal elevator, perform wide subcutaneous dissection superficial to nasal bone and cartilages, elevate the periosteum around the intended osteotomy area.

(iv) Reduction of bony hump: Using a nasal saw, cut and remove the bony hump in a left-to-right and then right-to-left manner. Residual bony irregularities can be smoothened with an osteotome or a rasp. The hump can also be removed directly with an osteotome.

(v) Narrowing of nasal dorsum: Incisions are made via endonasal or flying-bird nasal tip incision, or at the piriform rim. Insert the periosteal elevator and bluntly dissect the periosteum, muscle and skin off the frontomaxillary process, and osteotomized the connection between nasal bone and maxilla. During osteotomy, care must be taken to protect the integrity of the endonasal periosteum and mucosa to ensure the stability of the bony segment. While holding gauze, exert inward pressure on the osteotomized bilateral nasal bones to cause a fracture, therefore reducing the width of the nasal dorsum.

(vi) Tip adjustments: For cases with excessive nasal tip length, pull the lower lateral cartilage through the incision, excise unwanted portion of lateral or distal septal cartilage according to pre-operative measurements; with down-turned nasal tips, excise a portion of caudal nasal septal cartilage posterior to medial crura, suture the alar cartilages with septal cartilage to increase the nasal tip projection; For excessive alar base width, a small wedge of alar cartilage at lateral and superior aspects can be removed by pulling the alar cartilages through the incisions.

(vii) Post-operative management: Insert BIPP packing or expandable sponges into bilateral nasal cavities for internal stabilization. External nasal splints are achieved with thermoplastic or titanium splints. Internal nasal packings are removed 3–7 days post-operatively, and external splints are removed after 2 weeks. Patients should avoid trauma to the nose for several months after surgery.

Classic case 1 (Fig. 5.15)

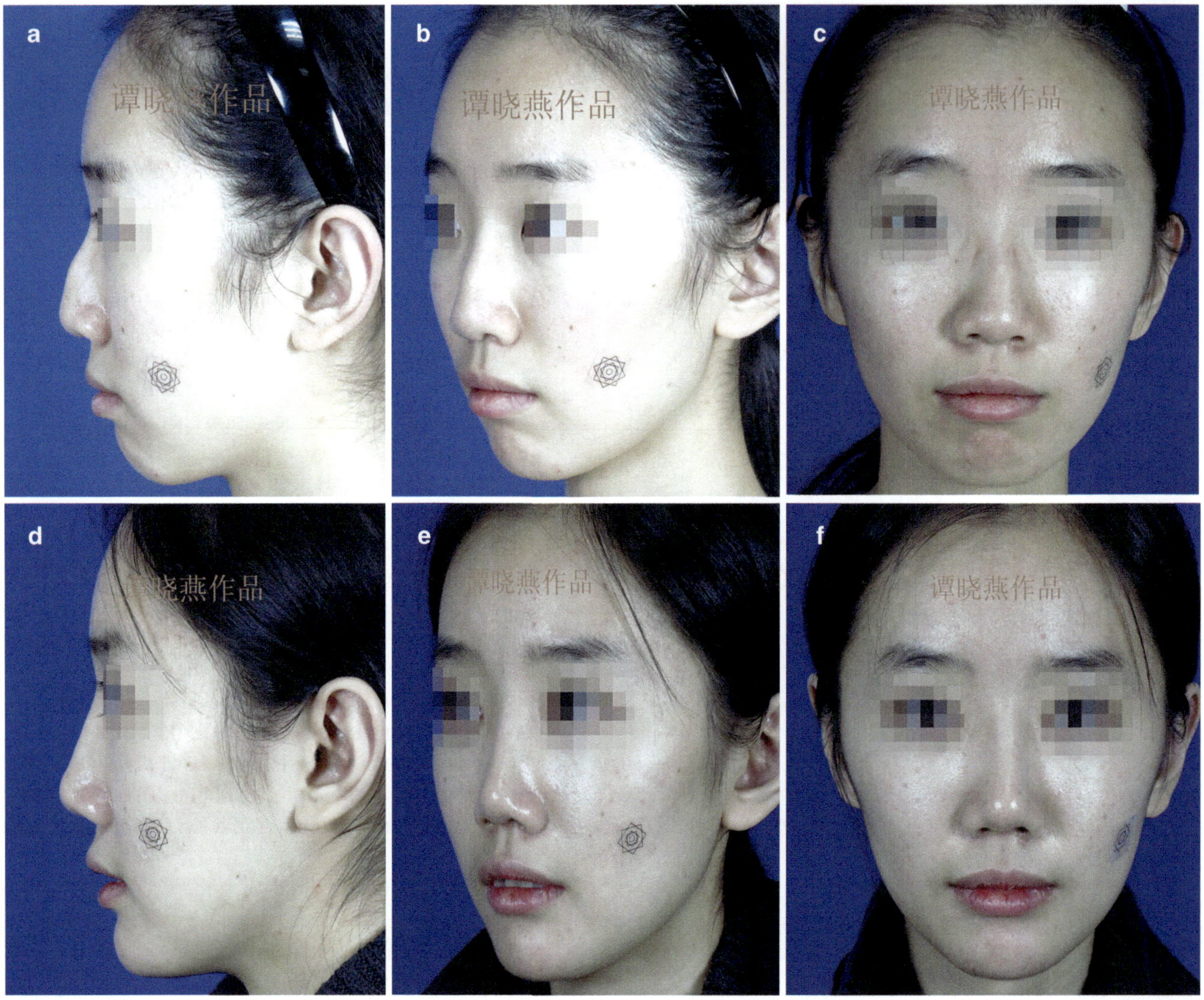

Fig. 5.15 (**a**–**f**) Hump nose classic case 1. **a**, **b**, **c**: lateral; oblique lateral; and frontal view, Pre-op; **d**, **e**, **f**: lateral; oblique lateral; and frontal view, 3 months Post-op

Classic case 2 (Fig. 5.16)

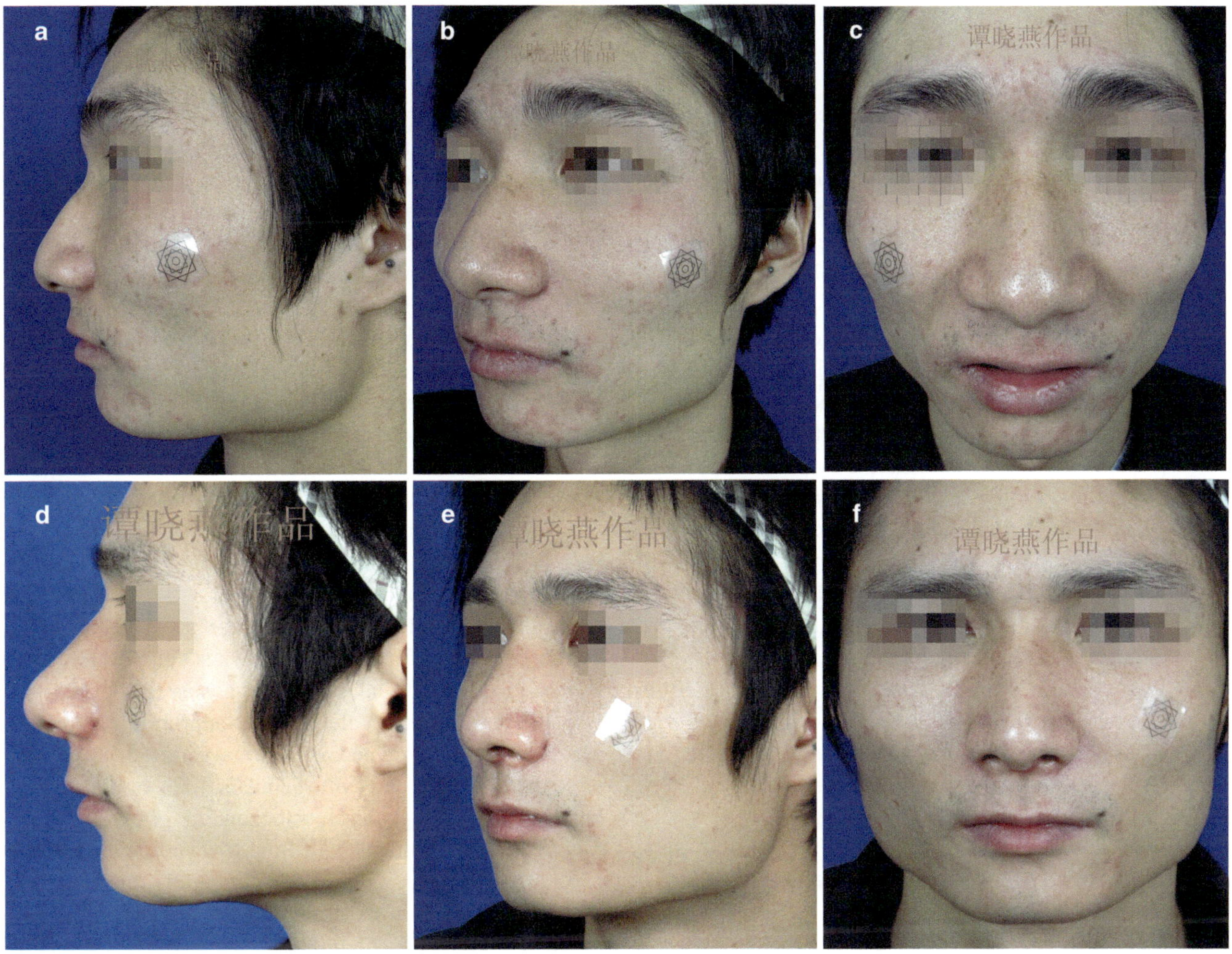

Fig. 5.16 (**a**–**f**) Hump nose classic case 2. **a**, **b**, **c**: lateral; oblique lateral; and frontal view, Pre-op; **d**, **e**, **f**: lateral; oblique lateral; and frontal view, 1 month Post-op

3. Points to note
   (i) Bleeding and infection: can be caused by intra-operative bleeding, drainage, inadequate aseptic preparation, and inadequate post-operative infection control. Manage by appropriate use of hemostatic medications and antibiotics, and ensure unobstructed drainage from the nasal cavity.
   (ii) Inadequate correction: Inadequate removal of boney segments and cartilage is the main cause of this issue. Careful intra-operative assessment and prompt management are the key points. Young patients are prone to bony hyperplasia, and patients should be warned pre-operatively. Slight over-reduction can be considered to compensate for this; otherwise, pressure dressing can be applied to the dorsal hump area to prevent excessive bone regrowth.
   (iii) Step-deformity: This is caused by placing the lateral nasal osteotomy too dorsal. Lateral osteotomies should be carried out at the base of bilateral nasal bones.
   (iv) Saddle nose deformity: This is caused by excessive removal of nasal bone and cartilage. It can be corrected with augmentation rhinoplasty.
   (v) Asymmetrical nasal dorsum: This is caused by unequal inward fracture and reposition of bilateral nasal bones after lateral osteotomy. It can be corrected with local tissue or alloplastic grafts.

5.5 Correction of Brachyrhinia Deformity

1. Indications
   (i) Short mid-facial third; length of the nose measuring from radix to infra-tip point (midpoint between tip of the nose and columella) shorter than 4.5 cm; and those accompanied by a nasolabial angle greater than 100°.
   (ii) Special brachyrhinia deformities: Patients with Binder's syndrome present with midface hypoplasia or deficiency, severe nasal dorsum depression, short nasal tip with a dished-in facial appearance.
   (iii) Pre-surgical assessment should include the presence of any functional deficiencies such as olfactory impairment, septal deviation, turbinal hypertrophy, and nasal airflow obstruction.
2. Surgical methods and procedures
   Anesthesia: General anesthesia or regional blocks.
   Surgical methods:
   (i) For patients requiring simultaneous augmentation rhinoplasty, refer to the subsection on augmentation rhinoplasty for surgical steps to elevate the dorsum.
   (ii) Extra-nasal incision to raise the nasal tip flap: bilateral marginal incisions combined with a flying-bird incision at columella, step trans-columella incision, v-shaped trans-columella incision, or w-shaped trans-columella incision.
   (iii) Tip and surrounding soft tissue release:
      (1) Dorsum: Following the nasal cartilage to nasal bony periosteum and release muscular attachments between nasal bone and cartilages.
      (2) Tip: Release the inter-domal ligaments while preserving the subcutaneous vascular network at the nasal tip.
      (3) Release ligaments between left and right alar cartilages and fibrous connection between alar and lateral nasal cartilages.
      (4) Separate the cephalad septal cartilage at the dorsal aspect from the lateral nasal cartilage in preparation for subsequent insertion of the septal extension cartilage graft.
   (iv) Tip extension:

Selection of cartilage grafts:

Commonly used sources of cartilage grafts include septal cartilage, conchal cartilage from cavitas conchae or cymba conchae (harvested via anterior or posterior conchal incision and perichondrium elevation, an appropriate amount of cartilage can be obtained with preservation of shape and structure of cavitas and cymba conchae); for severe cases of brachyrhinia, autogenous costochondral grafts are commonly used; For patients with Binder's syndrome, source of cartilage is limited to costochondral graft due to innate underdevelopment of nasal cartilages. Acellular allogeneic cartilage grafts are available overseas; however, their clinical application has not been approved in China.

Method of assembly for cartilage graft:

Methods to extend the nasal septal cartilage is largely divided into septal advancement graft and septal strut graft:

(1) Septal advancement: Preserving 1–1.5 cm of cartilage at superior and caudal aspect to ensure adequate support, harvest a portion of septal cartilage (or autogenous costochondral graft), reposition the graft anteriorly to, and partially overlap with caudal septal cartilage and secure with sutures. This will function as an anterior extension of the nasal septum.
(2) Septal strut: two long pieces of cartilage (harvesting method same as described above) are placed lateral to the dorsal aspect of septal cartilage, with partial extension into pre-septal space. Cartilage grafts are sutured to the septal cartilage at areas of overlap and function as a septal extension.

(3) For patients with septal cartilage deficiency related to Binder's syndrome or other conditions, reconstruction of nasal septal with autogenous costochondral graft is necessary (Figs. 5.17 and 5.18).

Elevation of nasal tip cartilage framework can be achieved either by advancement or strut as well:

(1) A single piece of transparent cartilage is inserted between bilateral medial crura of lower lateral cartilage (the graft can be of a harvested septal cartilage with adequate length or a costochondral graft) and secured with sutures. If two-piece septal extension grafts do not provide adequate support, the three cartilages can be further secured with additional sutures at the nasal tip. Transparent cartilages are relatively rigid; therefore, the resultant grafted nasal tip lacks flexibility but exhibits good structural support.

(2) Alternatively, two pieces of long conchal cartilages can be sandwiched between and sutured to bilateral medial crura. Conchal cartilages are more flexible, therefore the resultant nasal tip exhibit better flexibility but relatively poorer support.

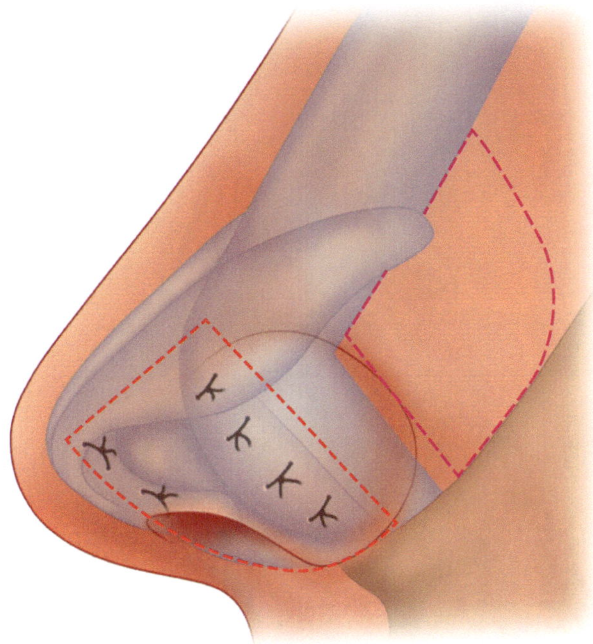

Fig. 5.17 Schematic illustration of septal cartilage harvesting and reposition. The red dotted lines demonstrate the repositioned septal cartilage at pre-septal space

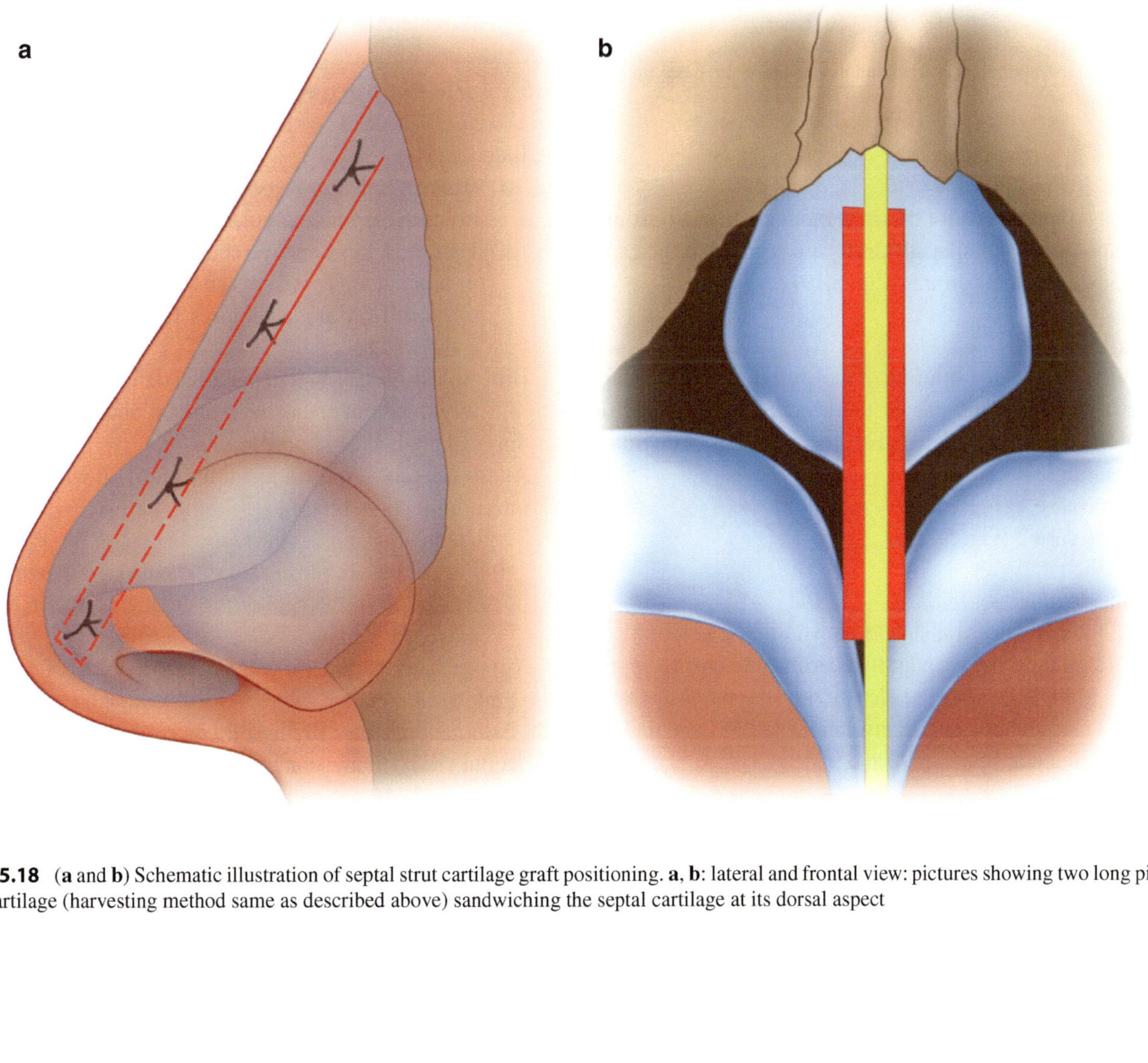

Fig. 5.18 (**a** and **b**) Schematic illustration of septal strut cartilage graft positioning. **a**, **b**: lateral and frontal view: pictures showing two long pieces of cartilage (harvesting method same as described above) sandwiching the septal cartilage at its dorsal aspect

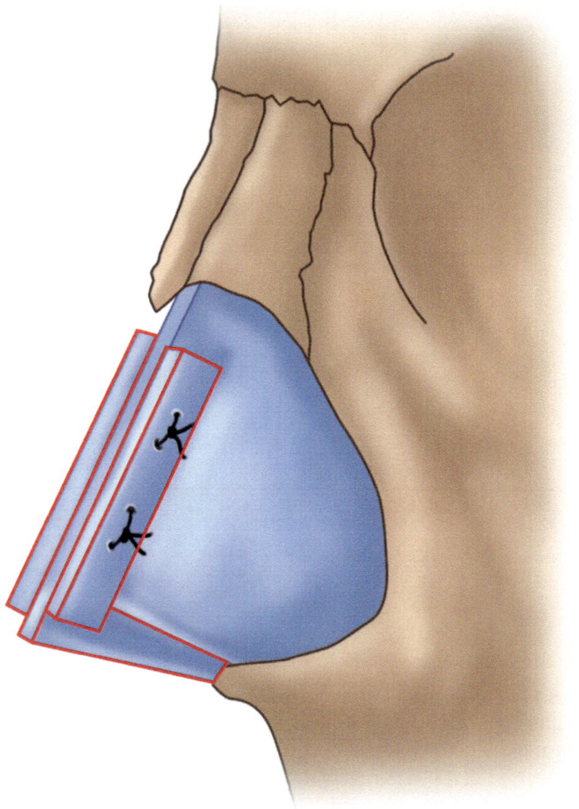

Fig. 5.19 Illustration of elevation and extension of the nasal tip with cartilage grafts

Cartilaginous grafts for the tip defining point can be round cap-shaped or shield-shaped. Grafts are secured to the cartilage framework with sutures (Fig. 5.19).

(v)Graft position:

After insertion and suturing of the graft to the tip cartilage framework, assess and ensure the absence of dorsal or tip deviation, then proceed to close the incisions with interrupted sutures.

Classic case 1 (Fig. 5.20)

Classic case 2 (Fig. 5.21)

3. Points to note
   (i) Special attention should be paid to the position and angulation of each grafted cartilage to ensure appropriate extension and elevation of the nasal tip; keep the nasofacial angle between 30 and 35° and nasolabial angle between 90 and 95°.
   (ii) Ensure adequate overlap between extension graft and septal cartilage for suturing to achieve adequate structural stability.
   (iii) The width between the nasal tip defining points should be within 4–8 mm to avoid excessively narrow or wide nasal tip.
   (iv) When harvesting the septal cartilage, ensure adequate struts are preserved at caudal and dorsal aspects to maintain nasal support. Pre-operative assessment of septal cartilage is necessary. For patients with a poorly developed septum, an alternative source from autologous rib cartilage should be adopted.
   (v) Due to the high incidence of septal deviation, a pre-operative thorough discussion with patients is necessary. Deviation can be corrected intra-operatively during the harvesting of septal cartilage. If the harvested cartilage is curved, it should be trimmed appropriately before insertion and checked for any tip deviation afterward.
   (vi) Surgical extension of brachyrhinia is limited to the volume and stretchability of nasal skin and soft tissue, and the patient should be informed of this limitation before surgeries. If pre-existing dorsal deviation or alar asymmetries are noted during the pre-operative assessment, CT scans and other tests are indicated as appropriate.

5.6 Plastic Surgery of Nasal Tip

1. Indications
   (i) Blunt nasal tip: Hypertrophic and blunt nasal tip, excessive tip-alar angulation.
   (ii) Upturned or down-turned nasal tip: the average nasolabial angle is between 90 and 95°. Too large or too small an angle requires tip rotation for better esthetics.
   (iii) Assess for any functional nasal deficits such as olfactory impairment and nasal airflow obstructions.
2. Surgical methods and procedures

   Anesthesia: local infiltration at the nasal tip with bilateral infraorbital nerve blocks

   Surgical methods:
   (i) For patients requiring simultaneous nasal augmentation, refer to the subsection on augmentation rhinoplasty for details.
   (ii) Incision: endonasal and external nasal incisions.

(1) Endonasal incision: bilateral nasal vestibular incisions

(2) External incisions: Flying-bird incision at the base of the columella, step incision at mid-columella level, v-shaped

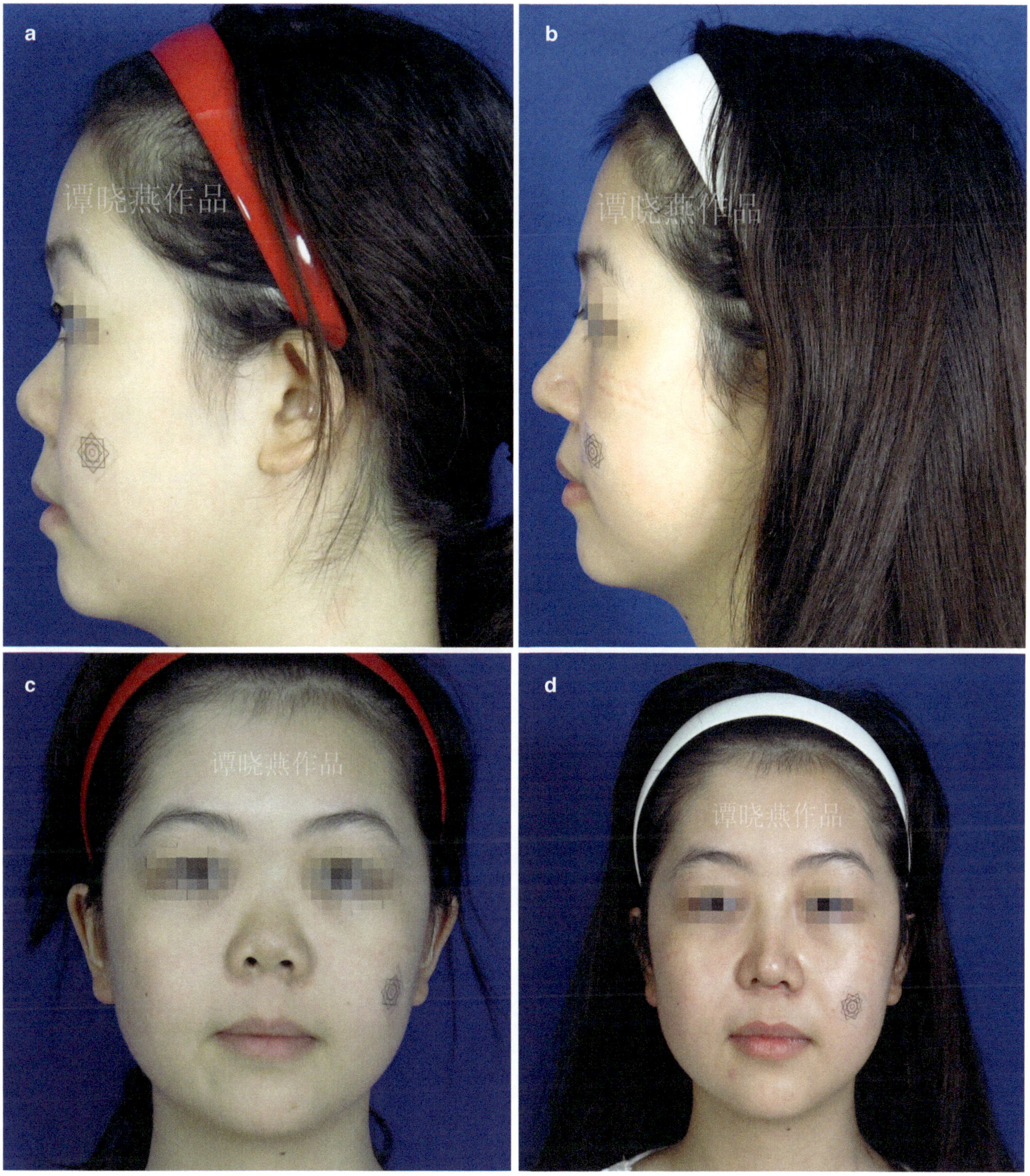

Fig. 5.20 (**a**–**d**) Brachyrhinia classic case 1. **a**: Pre-operative profile view; **b**: 1-month post-operative profile view. **c**: Pre-operative frontal view; **d**: 1-month post-operative frontal view

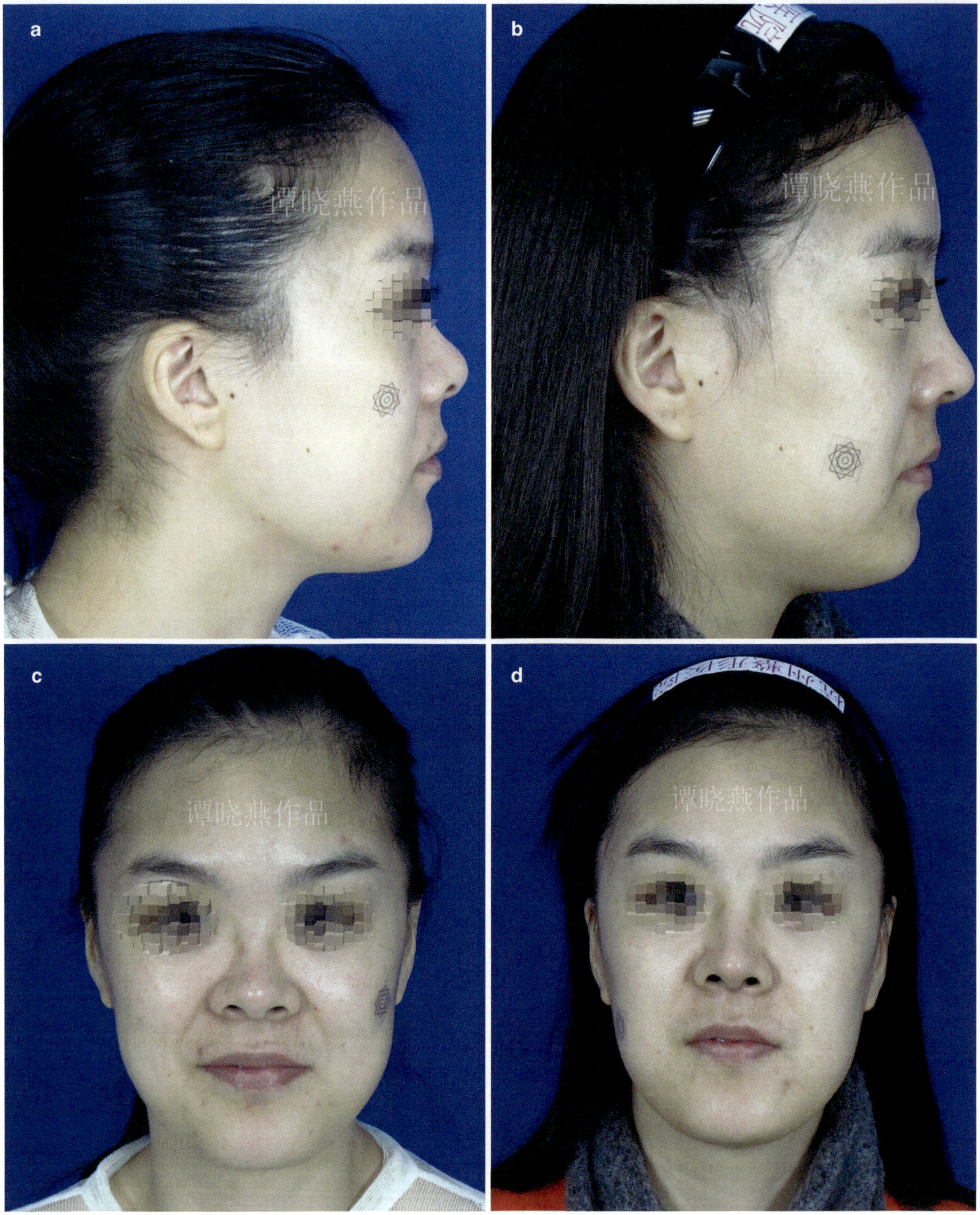

Fig. 5.21 (**a**–**d**) Brachyrhinia classic case 2. **a**: Pre-operative profile view; **b**: 2-month post-operative profile view; **c**: Pre-operative frontal view; **d**: 2-month post-operative frontal view

trans-columella incision, w-shaped trans-columella incisions; extended with bilateral vestibular incisions.

(iii) The extent of dissection: after planned incision, staying superficial to lower lateral cartilages and underneath nasal tip fat, dissect superiorly until keystone area (joint between nasal cartilage and bone), exposure the borders of bilateral upper and lower lateral cartilages and dorsal septal cartilage. Dissect and expose the caudal septal cartilage from bilateral medial crura. Carefully separate out bilateral lower lateral cartilage domes until medial surfaces of lateral crura.

(iv) Tip fibrofatty tissues: To resect for patients with a hypertrophic blunt tip (soft tissue type) (Fig. 5.22).

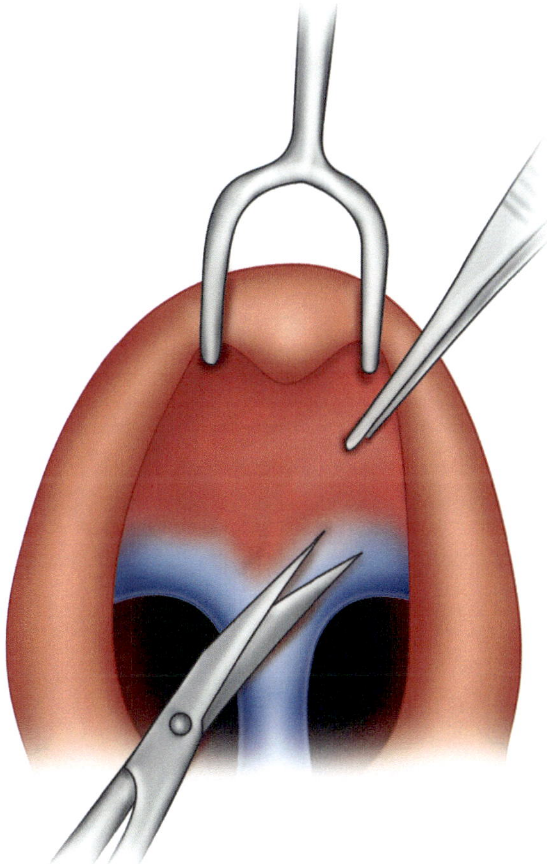

Fig. 5.22 Schematic illustration of surgical incision and dissection

(v) Management of nasal tip crura cartilages.

(1) Crural suturing techniques (Figs. 5.23, 5.24, 5.25):

(2) By adjusting the angulation of crural-septal suturing, minor sagittal adjustment of tip projection can be achieved.

(3) To reduce excessively wide lateral crura, the shaded portion of cartilages can be resected, followed by an inward rotation of lateral crura and secure with mattress sutures (Fig. 5.26).

(vi) Nasal tip graft:

(1) Nasal tip cartilage shield graft (Fig. 5.27).

(2) Nasal tip cartilage cap graft (Fig. 5.28).

(3) Nasal tip cartilage umbrella graft, with insertion of cartilage grafts from columella to nasal tip in a shape resembling an umbrella (Fig. 5.29).

(vii) After wound closure, leave negative-pressure drainage and secure with tape or plastic splints at the nasal tip for 3–7 days.

(viii) Post-operative management: Suture removal at seventh post-operative day. Maintain nasal cavity cleanliness and oral antibiotics for 3 days.

Classic case (Fig. 5.30)

3. Points to note

Including: Pre-operative surgical design, intra-operative and post-operative considerations.

(i) Tip surgery is the most difficult and variable procedure of all nasal surgeries. Depending on an individual case, a combination of the abovementioned techniques should be adopted as required for better clinical outcomes compared to a singular method [1, 12].

(ii) Excised nasal tip fibrofatty tissues can be repurposed as needed, such as wrapping of the tip graft or overlying cartilage graft surfaces to mask any irregularities or to increase overlying tissue thickness.

(iii) Considerations during trimming, rotation, and closure of nasal tip: preserve the natural physiological structures of the nasal tip as well as normal nasal functions such as olfaction and airflow; at the same time ensure the stability of the nasal tripod framework.

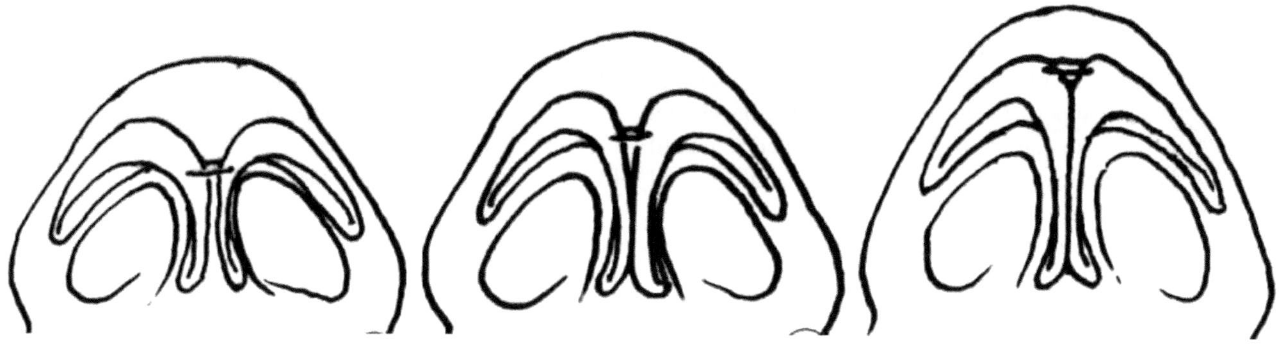

Fig. 5.23 Schematic illustration of crural suturing. Left: medial crural suturing; Center: intermediate crural suturing; Right: interdomal suturing

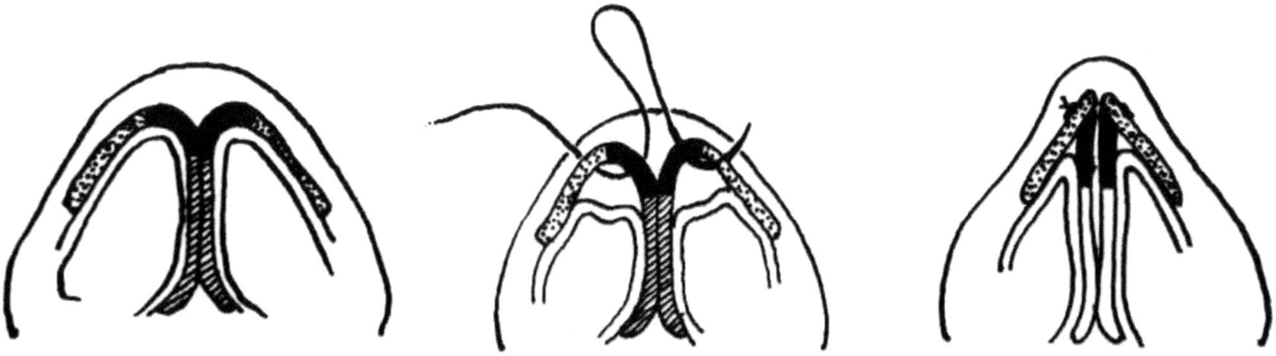

Fig. 5.24 Lateral crural steal

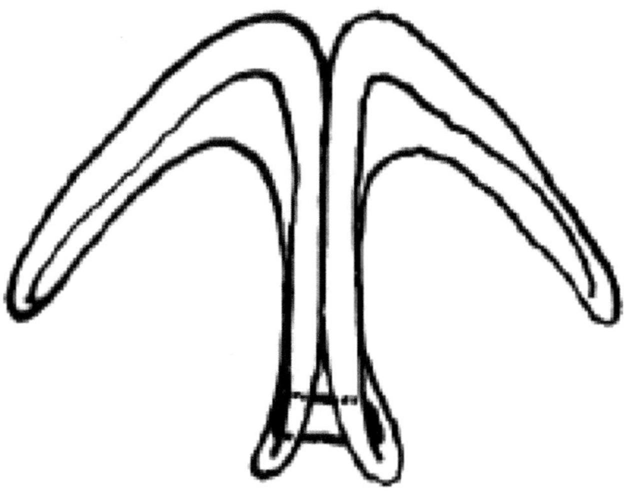

Fig. 5.25 Medial crural footplate suturing

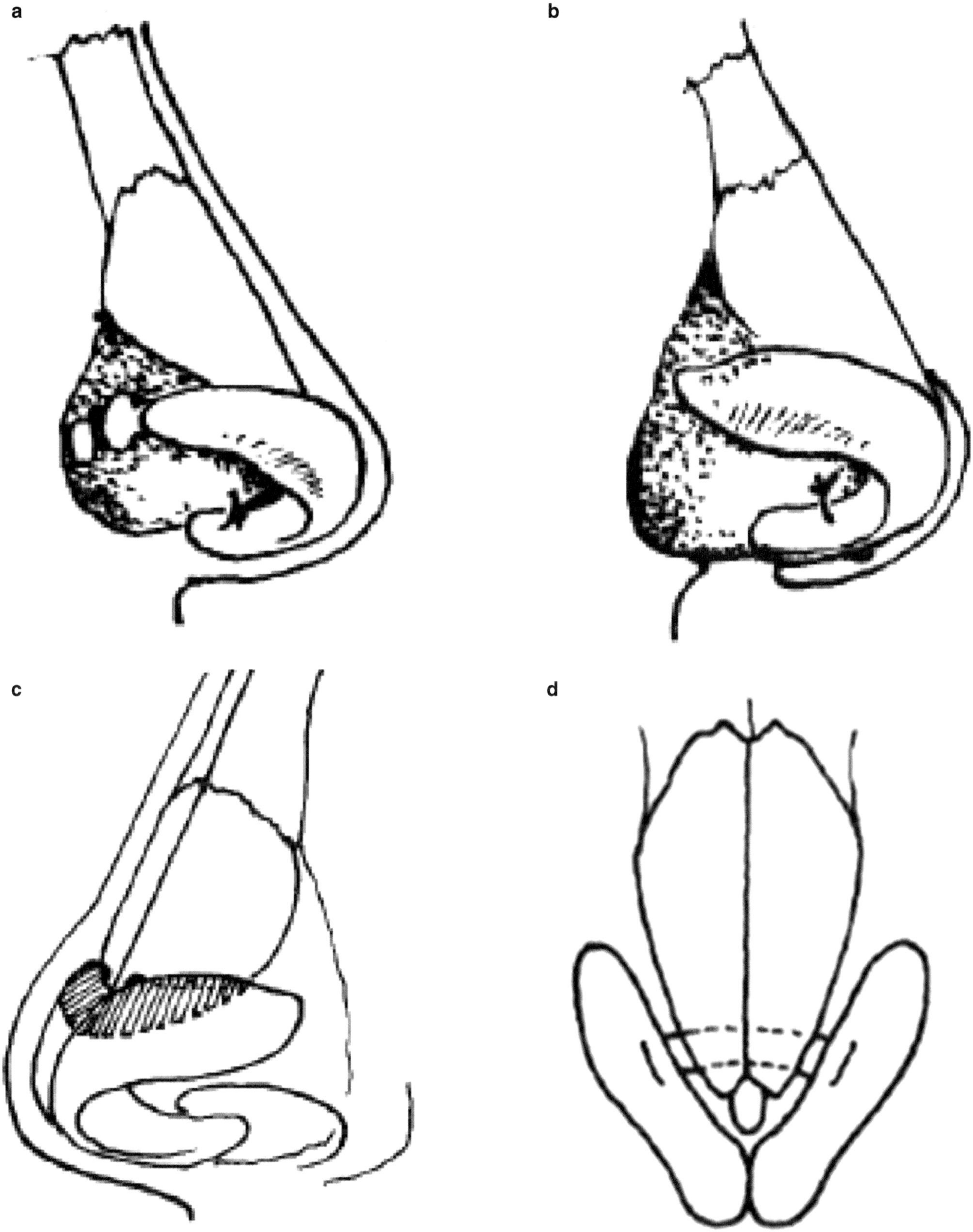

Fig. 5.26 (**a**–**d**) Correction of broad lateral crura

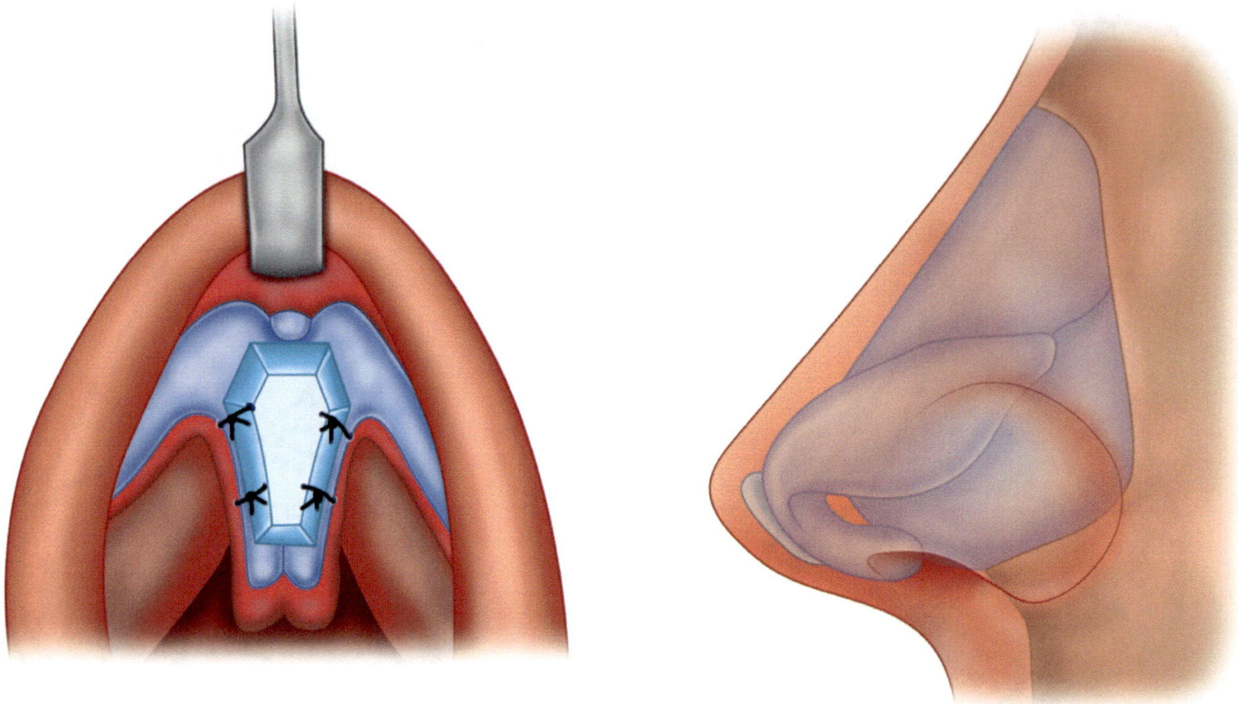

Fig. 5.27 Nasal tip cartilage shield graft

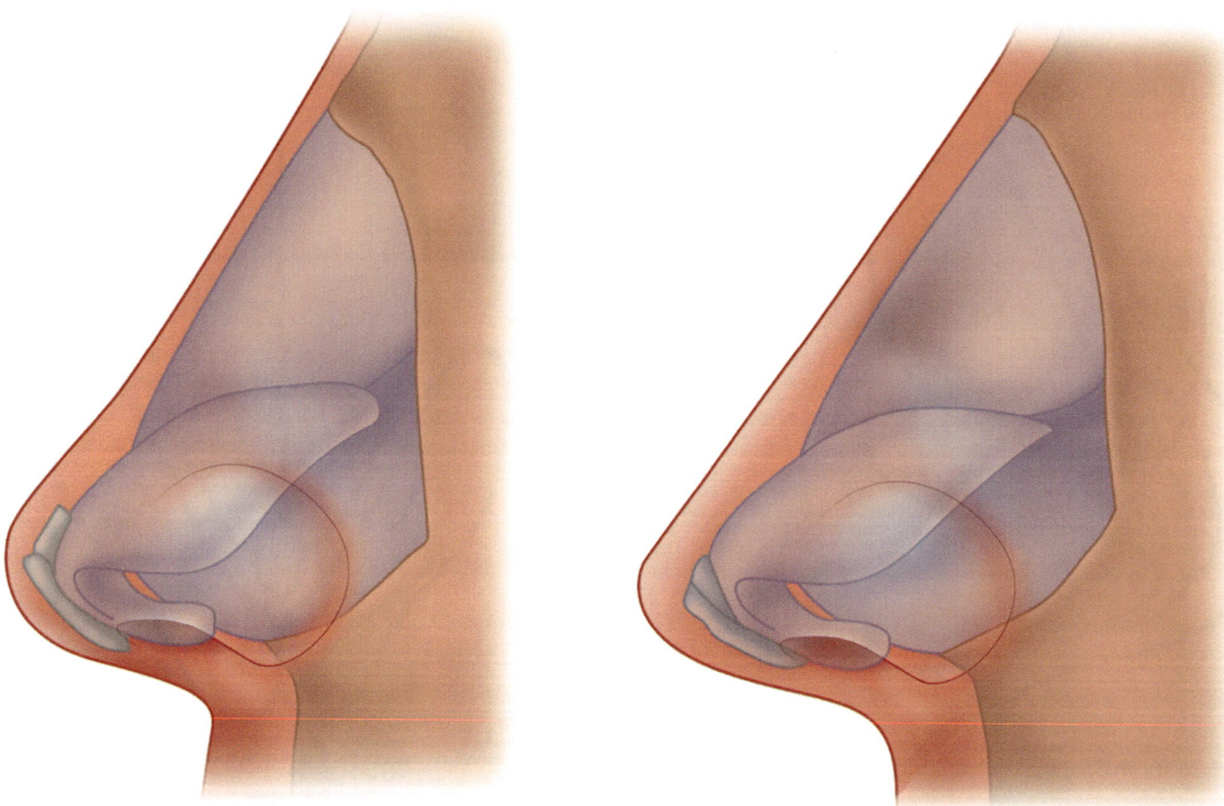

Fig. 5.28 Nasal tip cartilage cap graft

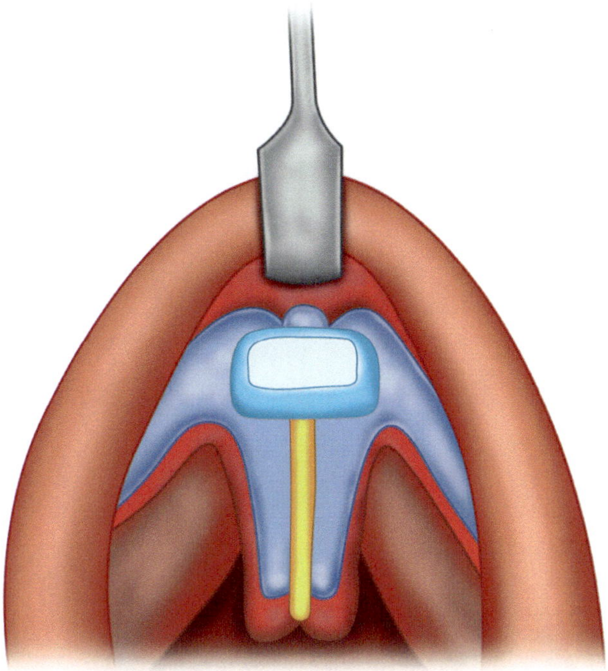

Fig. 5.29 Nasal tip cartilage umbrella graft

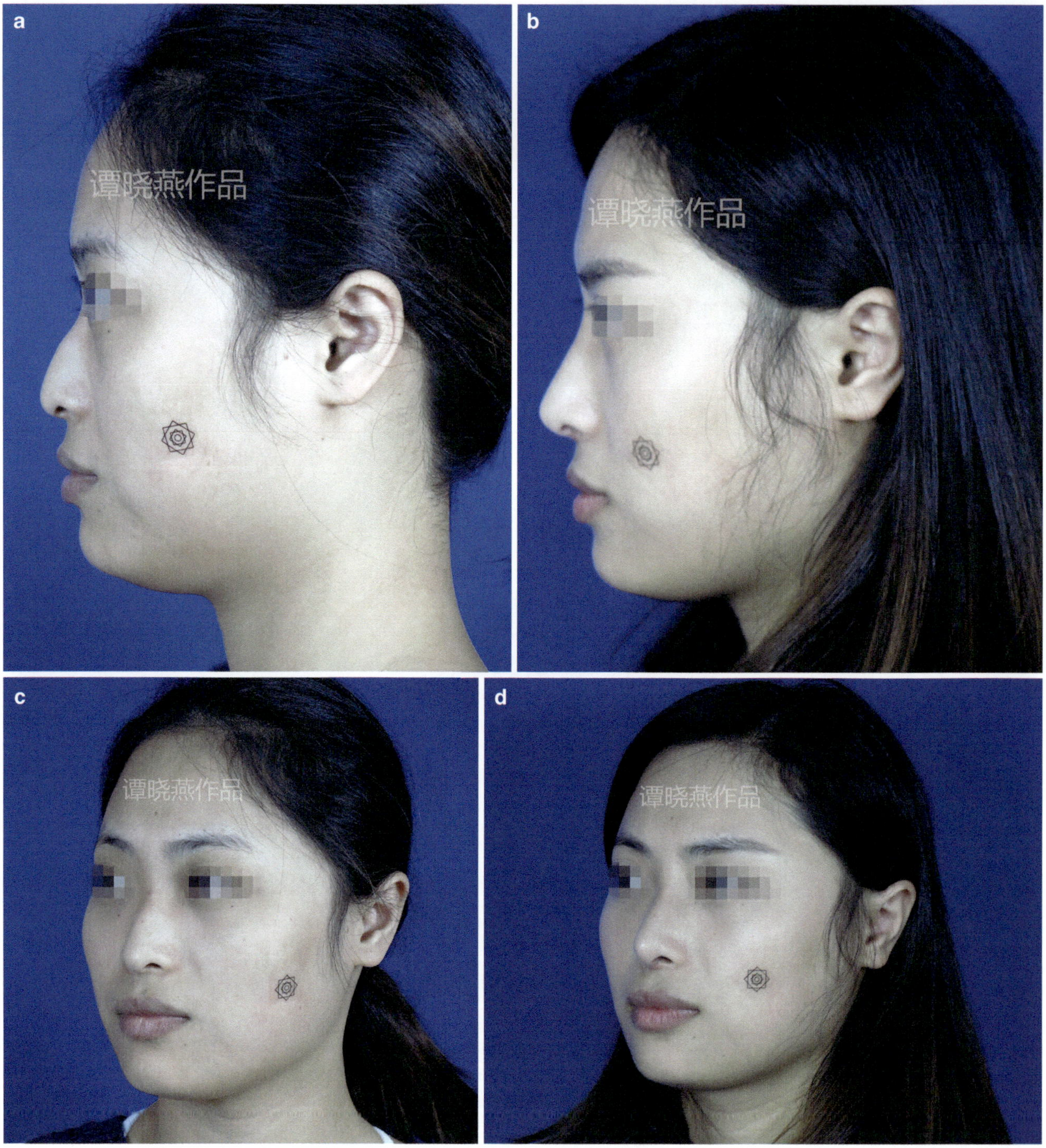

Fig. 5.30 (**a**–**f**) Pre- and post-operative comparison of comprehensive tip surgery. **a**, **c**, **e**: lateral; oblique lateral and Worm's eye view, pre-op; **b**, **d**, **f**: lateral; oblique lateral and Worm's eye view, post-op (dorsal hump correction and comprehensive tip reconstruction)

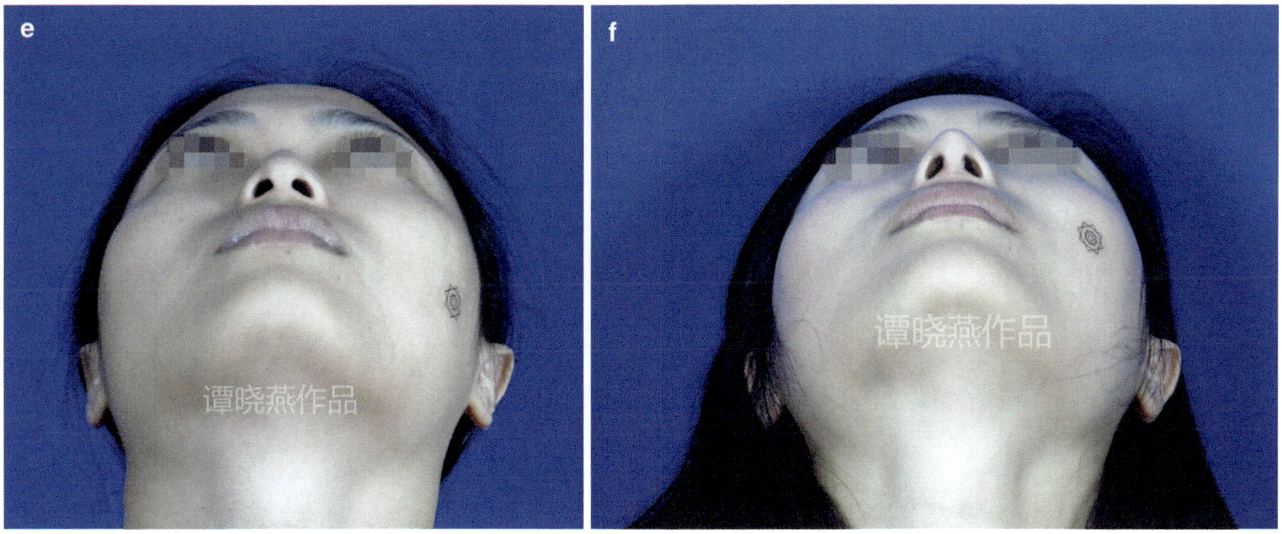

Fig. 5.30 (continued)

References

1. Yang Z-Y, Tan X-Y. Progress of plastic surgery on Asian people's nose and nose tip (in Chinese). Chin J Aesthet Plast Surg. 2012;23(4):240–3.
2. Yan-Yan S, Tan X-Y, Yang Z-Y. Autologous Cartilago Auricularis and Laminae Septi on nasal tip plastic surgery (in Chinese). Modern Pract Med. 2011;23(10):1152–3.
3. Wang W. Rhinoplasty and cosmetic surgery (in Chinese). Zhejiang Science and Technology Press; 2011.
4. Eren F, Öksüz S, Melikolu C, Karagöz H, Ülkür E. Saddle-nose deformity repair with microplate-adapted costal cartilage. Aesthet Plast Surg. 2014;38(4):733–41.
5. Hyun SM, Jang YJ. Treatment outcomes of saddle nose correction. JAMA Facial Plast Surg. 2013;15(4):280–6.
6. Li D, Zheng Y-S. Progress of treatment on crooked nose deformity (in Chinese). Chin J Plast Surg. 2011;27(2):155–7.
7. Xue Z-Q, Gao Z, Lu H. Composite reduction of crooked nose deformity (in Chinese). Chin J Plast Surg. 2011;27(2):129–30.
8. Cho GS, Jang YJ. Deviated nose correction: different outcomes according to the deviation type. Laryngoscope. 2013;123(5):1136–42.
9. Himy S, Zink S, Bodin F, Bruant-Rodier C, Wilk A, Meyer C. Calvarial bone grafting in augmentation rhinoplasties. Long-term results. Rev Stomatol Chir Maxillofac. 2009;110(5):256–62.
10. Heppt W. Techniques for correction of the nasal dorsum. Otorhinolaryngology. 2013;61(3):267–79.
11. Jin H-R, Won T-B. Nasal hump removal in Asians. Acta Otolaryngol. 2007;127(558):95–101.
12. Cakir B, Oreroglu AR, Daniel RK. Surface aesthetics in tip rhinoplasty: a step-by-step guide. Aesthet Surg J. 2014;34(6):941–55.

Part III

Plastic Surgery of Congenital Nasolabial Deformities

6 Unilateral Cleft Lip Repair

Bing Shi

6.1 Unilateral Micro-cleft Lip Repair

6.1.1 Invisible Incision Technique

1. Indications
   (i) The lip vermillion on the cleft side is not more than 1 mm higher than the non-cleft side.
   (ii) Deficient philtrum ridge and lip tubercle on the cleft side.
   (iii) Deviated nasal columella and widened base of the nose on the cleft side.
2. Surgical methods and procedures
   (i) Place the incisions in the lip vermillion, labial vestibule, or the nasal floor. This will allow the wound to appear concealed. Following the extensive dissection of the orbicularis oris muscle, the muscle from the cleft side is secured to the anterior nasal spine, while the muscle on the unaffected side is rotated downward. The philtrum ridge deficiency will be compensated by reconstruction of the orbicularis oris muscle.
   (ii) In cases where the alar base of the cleft side is wider than that on the unaffected side, a portion of skin from the alar base will be removed accordingly. The upper edge of the orbicularis muscle can be accessed through the same wound to be is dissected and reconstructed. In the case of the equal alar base widths, there will be no need to remove any skin. In such situations, the incisions can be placed either in the nasal or oral vestibules (Fig. 6.1).

The surgical approach begins with an incision made either within the deformed portion of the lip vermillion or on the nasal floor. Using the unaffected side as a guide, the orbicularis oris muscle of the cleft side is exposed and reconstructed.

An example of the surgical procedure (Fig. 6.2):

Administer local anesthesia and mark a C-shaped line on the nostril sill using Methylene Blue (Figs. 6.3 and 6.4).

Incise along the drawn lines toward the anterior nasal spine, and release the fibrous attachments. After which, deglove the orbicularis oris muscle and release the alar base on the cleft side. Using the same incision, free the malposed orbicularis oris muscle attachment on the unaffected side away from the piriform aperture and anterior nasal spine. This dissection should not exceed beyond the philtrum ridge of the unaffected side (Figs. 6.5 and 6.6).

Suture the end of the orbicularis oris muscles from the cleft side across the muscles on the unaffected side. The deviated columella is corrected by fixating the superior margin of the orbicularis oris muscles on the cleft side of the anterior nasal spine (Fig. 6.7).

Post-operative wound.

3. Points to note
   (i) Post-operative lip deviation: During the procedure, the orbicularis oris muscles on the cleft side must be fixated to the periosteum of the anterior nasal spine. This will ensure that the center of the lip will be aligned with the midline.
   (ii) Deficiency of the lip vermillion is not adequately corrected, causing a whistle deformity: The orbicularis oris muscle on the cleft side must be dissected and reconstructed, while the muscles from the unaffected side must be rotated inferiorly. This will create an appearance of a full lip tubercle avoids a post-operative whistle deformity [1].

B. Shi (✉)
Department of Cleft Lip and Palate Surgery, Vice Dean,
West China Stomatology College, Sichuan University, Chengdu, China

J. Liu, B. Shi (eds.), *Atlas of Lip and Nose Plastic and Cosmetic Surgery*, https://doi.org/10.1007/978-981-16-1911-3_6

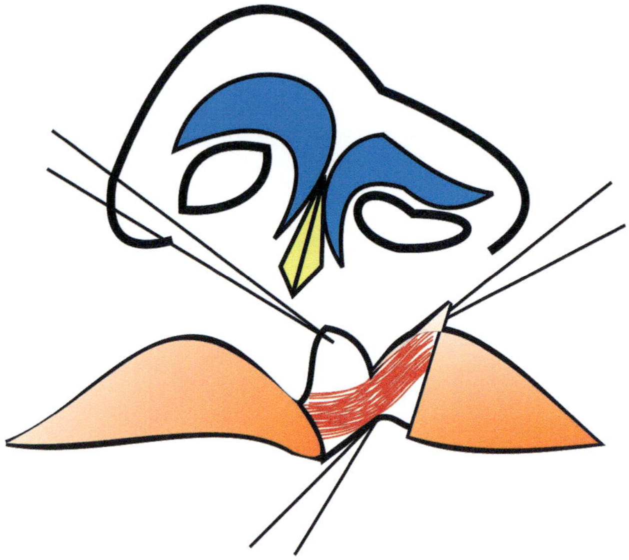

Fig. 6.1 Schematic diagram of the incisions

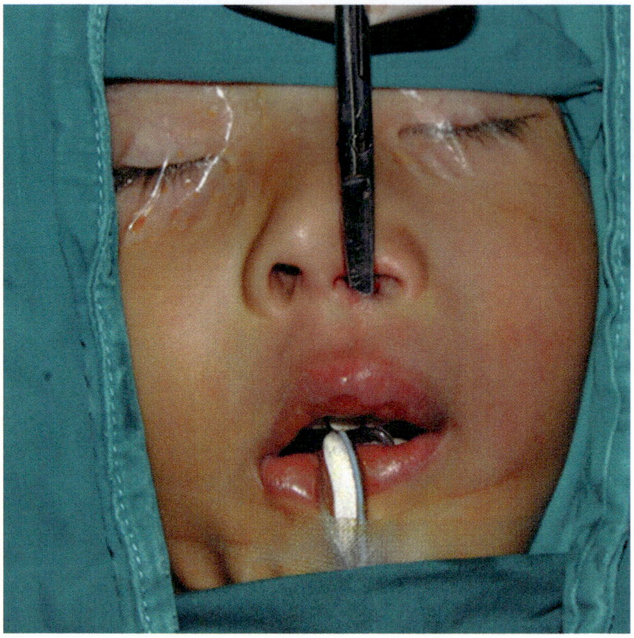

Fig. 6.3 Exposure

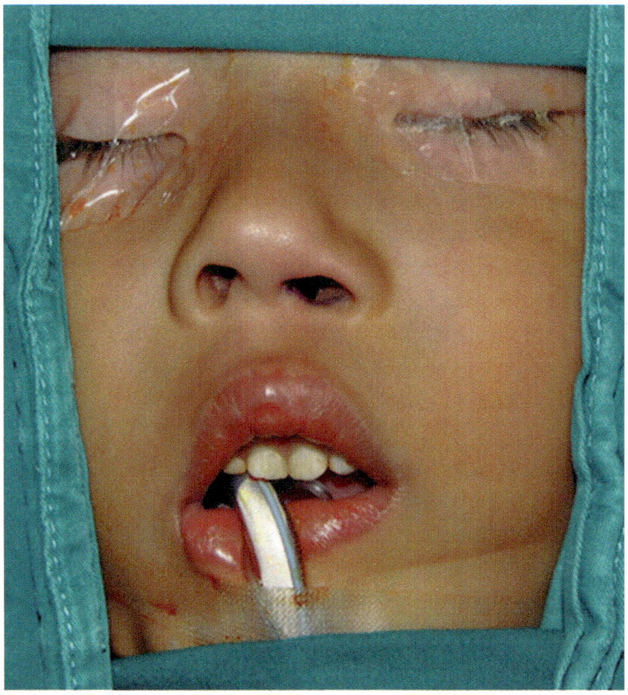

Fig. 6.2 Design of the surgical incision

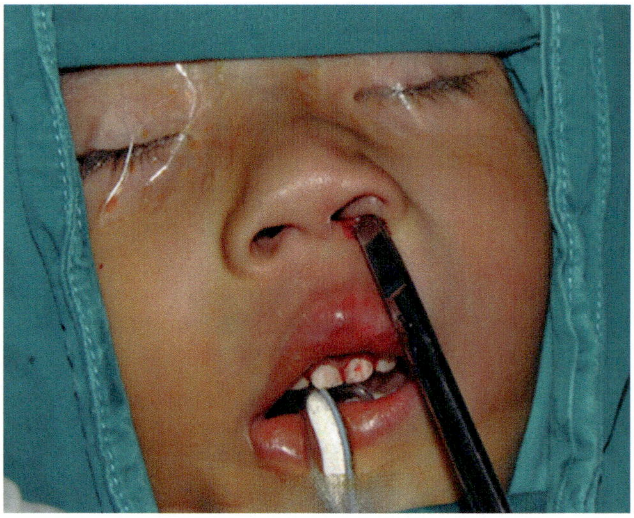

Fig. 6.4 Release of the alar base attachment

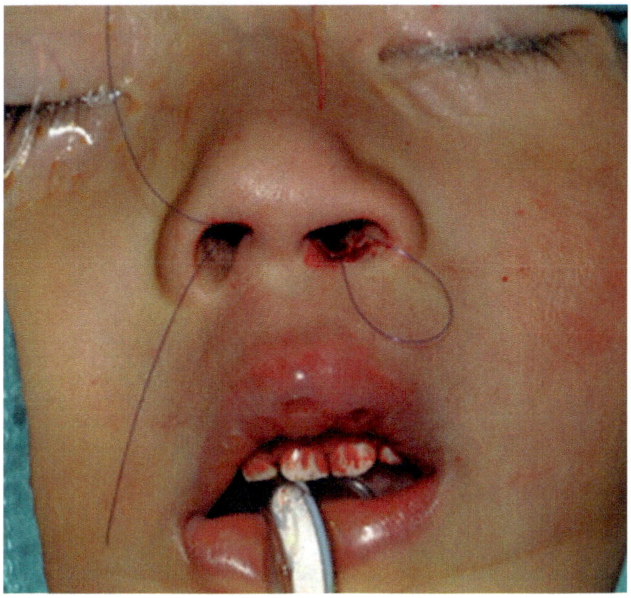

Fig. 6.5 Fixation of the orbicularis

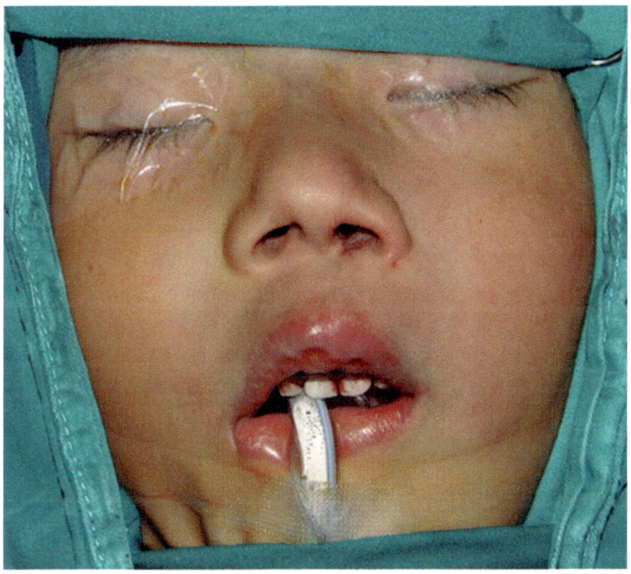

Fig. 6.6 Closure of the skin layer oris muscle

6.2 Z-Plasty Technique

1. Indications
   (i) The extension of the upper lip mucosa into the adjacent skin is almost the same length as the extension of the skin into the upper lip mucosa.
   (ii) Deficient philtrum ridge, indistinct lip tubercle, and micro-cleft on the inferior margin of the upper lip vermillion.
2. Surgical methods and procedures

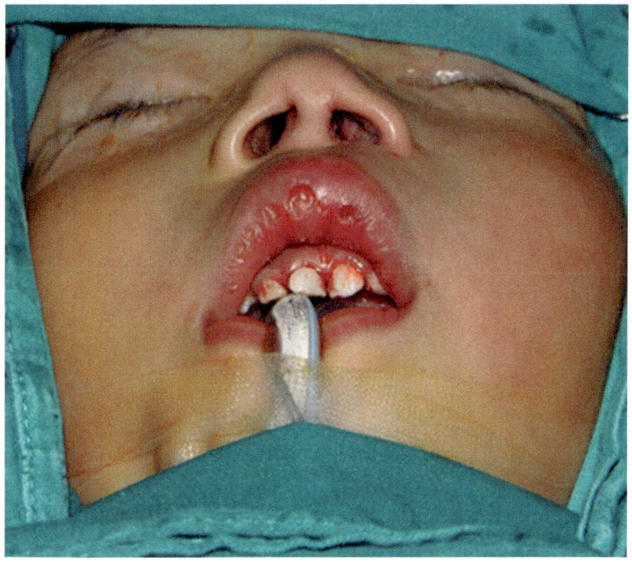

Fig. 6.7 Surgery completed

   (i) Make a Z-shaped incision along the mismatched vermillion border. Transpose the resultant two flaps to restore the normal appearance of the Cupid's bow.
   (ii) Place the incisions in the lip vermillion, labial vestibule, or the nasal floor. This will allow the wound to appear concealed. After the extensive dissection of the orbicularis oris muscle, the muscle on the cleft side is secured to the anterior nasal spine, while the muscle on the non-cleft side is rotated downward. The philtrum ridge deficiency will be compensated by the reconstruction of the orbicularis oris muscle.

An example of the surgical procedure:

The figure shows the peak of the Cupid's bow on the unaffected side (Point 2), the midpoint of the philtrum (Point 1), the highest point of the lip mucosa on the cleft side (Point 5), and the designated peak of the Cupid's bow on the cleft side (Point 3). Ensure that the distance from 1–2 = 1–3. Make a 2-mm incision from point 3 to point 1, following along the line of the lip. Point 4 is set along the vermillion border where the distance from this point to the alar base on the cleft side is equivalent to the distance from Point 2 to the alar base on the unaffected side. The most inferior point of the extension of the skin into the lip mucosa is marked as Point 6. The location of Point 3 is marked where the distance from 3–5 is equal to 4–6. The incisions are made between points 3–5, 4–6, and 5–6. The design of the lip vermillion incision appears similar to a unilateral cleft lip that has been stitched up. In this example, the bilateral alar base widths are equal and thus, the labial vestibular approach was chosen to dissect the orbicularis oris muscle (Fig. 6.8).

Incise according to the lines drawn, and expose the orbicularis oris muscle (Figs. 6.9 and 6.10).

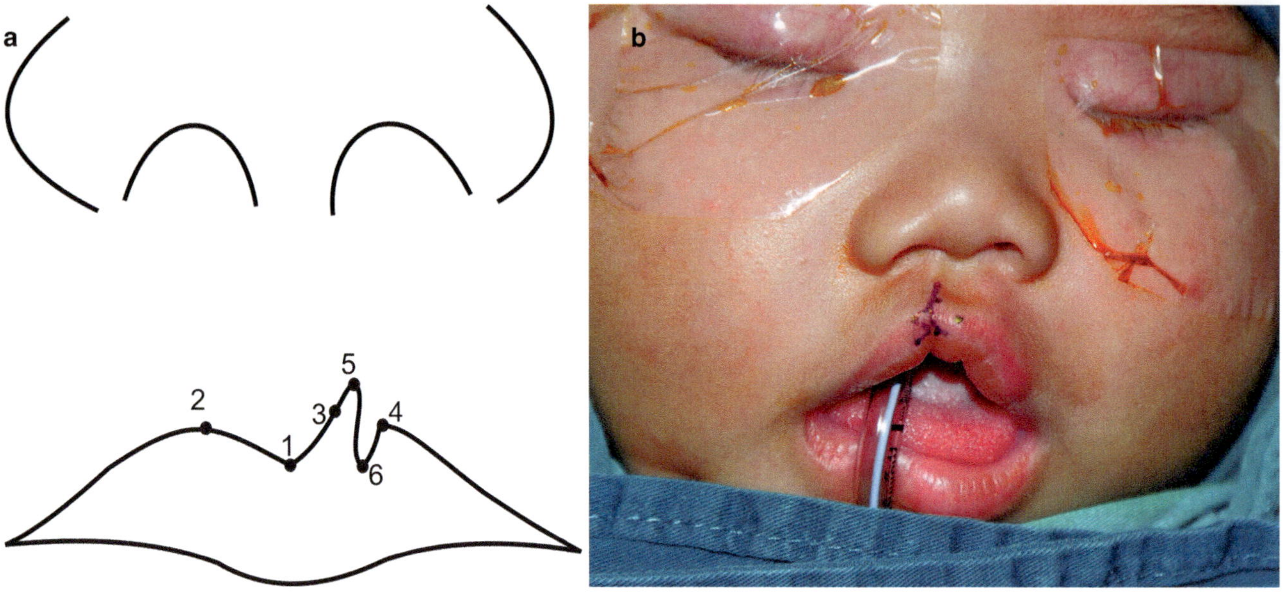

Fig. 6.8 (**a** and **b**) Schematic diagram of the surgical design

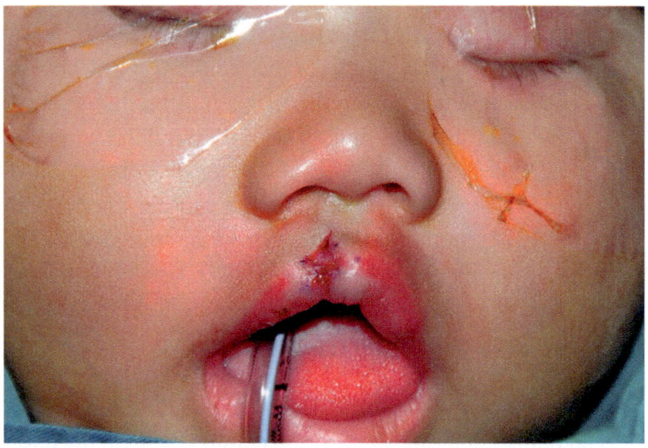

Fig. 6.9 Incision

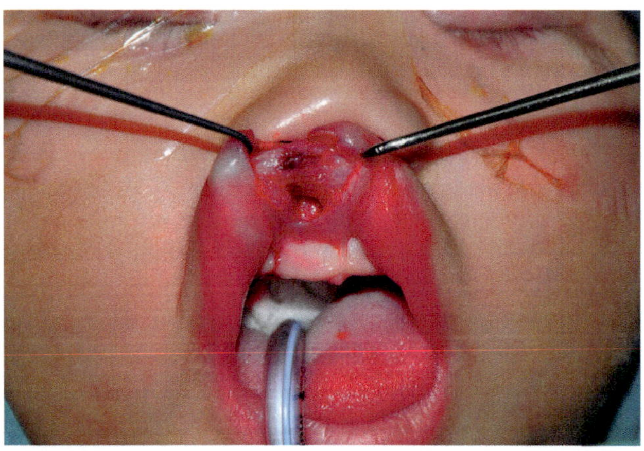

Fig. 6.10 Expose the orbicularis oris muscle

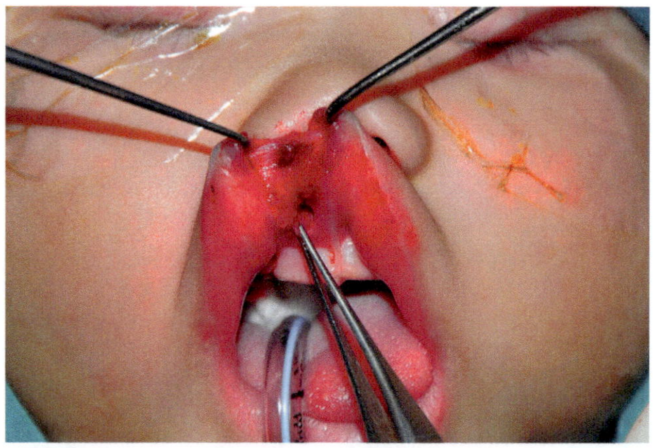

Fig. 6.11 Dissection of the muscle

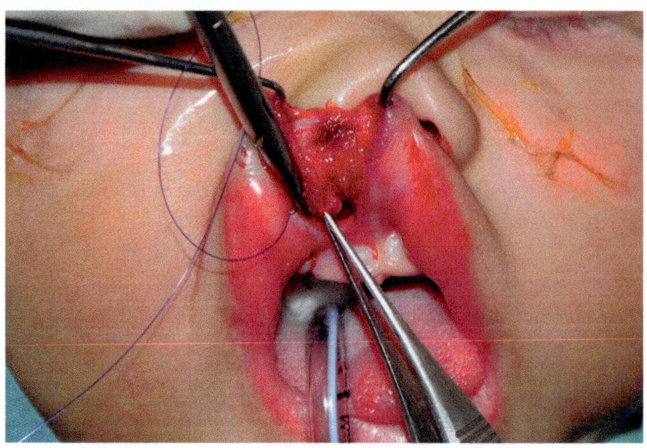

Fig. 6.12 Closure of the muscle layer

Cut the orbicularis oris muscle 2–3 mm lateral to the philtrum ridge of the cleft side. Following this, suture the muscle to its new position (Figs. 6.11 and 6.12).

The normal appearance of the peaks of the Cupid's bow is restored following transposition of the Z-Plasty flaps and closure of the subcutaneous layer (Figs. 6.13 and 6.14).

3. Points to note
    (i) Post-operative lip deviation: During the procedure, the orbicularis oris muscles on the cleft side must be fixated to the periosteum of the anterior nasal spine. This will ensure that the center of the lip will be aligned with the midline.
    (ii) Deficiency of the lip vermillion is not adequately corrected, resulting in a whistle deformity: The orbicularis oris muscle on the cleft side must be dissected and reconstructed, while the muscles on the unaffected side must be rotated inferiorly. This will create an appearance of a full lip tubercle and avoids a post-operative whistle deformity.

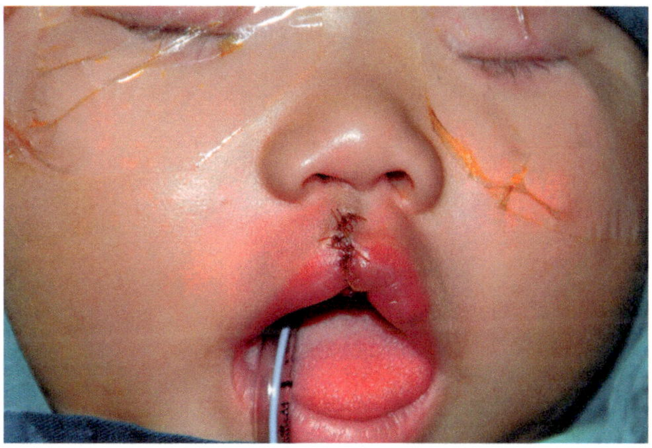

Fig. 6.13 Closure of the skin layer

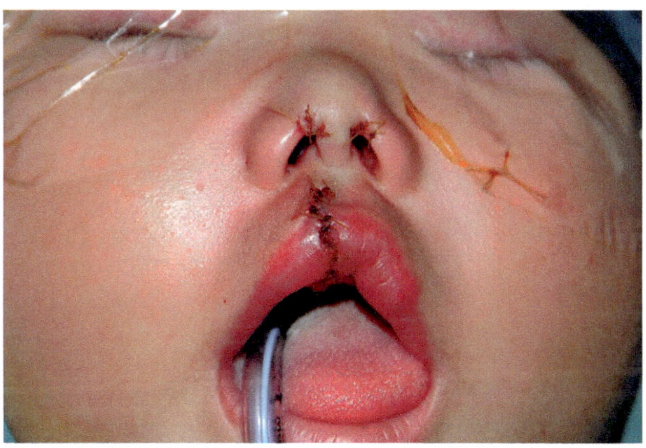

Fig. 6.14 Surgery Completed

6.3 Unilateral Incomplete Cleft Lip Repair

6.3.1 (Method A): Lower Triangular Flap Method

1. Indications
    (i) The height difference between the peak of the Cupid's bow on the cleft side and the non-cleft side must be within 2 mm.
    (ii) Deficient philtrum and lip tubercle on the affected side.
    (iii) Wide alar base on the cleft side and deviated nasal columella.
2. Surgical methods and procedures
    (i) The slope from the peak of the Cupid's bow is created by the transverse incision on the skin made from the planned peak of the cleft side toward the peak of the unaffected site. The gradient of the slope is dependent on the length of the transverse incision and the angle formed by the separation of the upper and lower parts of the transverse incision (α). In order not to disrupt the normal morphology of the philtrum ridge, the incision should not extend beyond the philtrum ridge of the unaffected side. If this condition can be met, the length of the incision should be equal to the height difference between the peaks of the Cupid's bow, and α = 60° should be achieved. However, when the end of the transverse incision is expected to exceed the philtrum ridge of the unaffected site, the length of the incision should be shortened, and α > 60° should be achieved.
    (ii) During the operation, the orbicularis oris muscle, skin, and mucosa on both sides of the incision should be separated. The dissection on the cleft side can be extended to the nasolabial fold. Whereas, the dissection on the unaffected side should not exceed beyond the philtrum ridge.

Determine the peak of the Cupid's bow on the unaffected side (point 2), the midpoint of the philtrum (point 1), and the peak of the Cupid's bow on the cleft side (point 3). Ensure that 1–2 = 1–3. Mark the end of the transverse incision as point 5. The distance between points 3–5 should be equal to the height difference between points 3–2, and point 5 should not exceed the philtrum ridge of the unaffected side. Determine the peak of the Cupid's Bow on the cleft side (point 4), the most lateral point of the columella along the cleft (point 6), the most medial point of the alar base along the cleft (point 6′), the point on the vermillion border medial to point 4 (point 5′) and the point on the skin superior and lateral to point 4 (point 3′). 3′–5′ = 4–5′ = 3–5, and 3′–6′ = 3–6 should be achieved (Fig. 6.15).

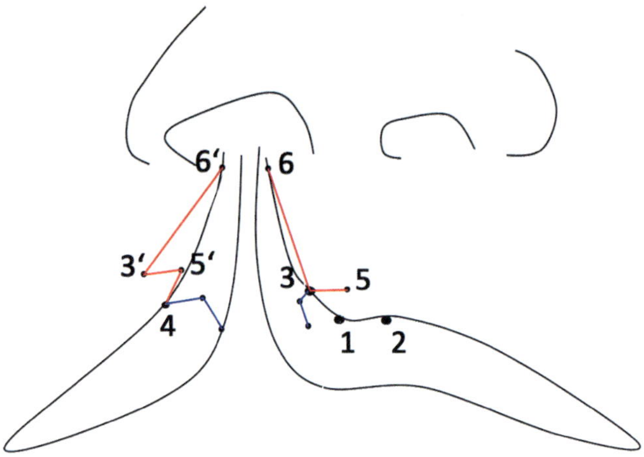

Fig. 6.15 Schematic diagram of the incisions

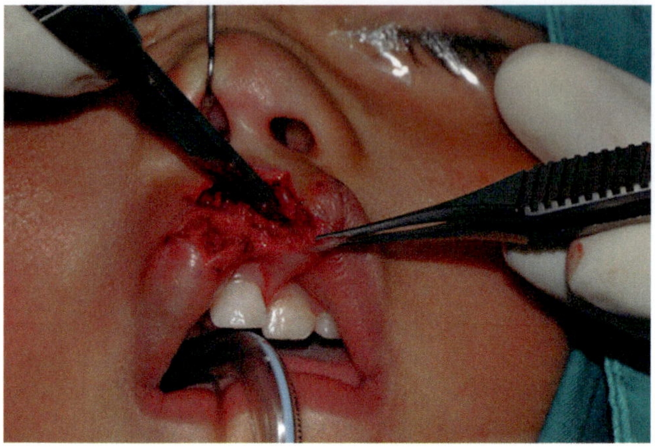

Fig. 6.17 Incision

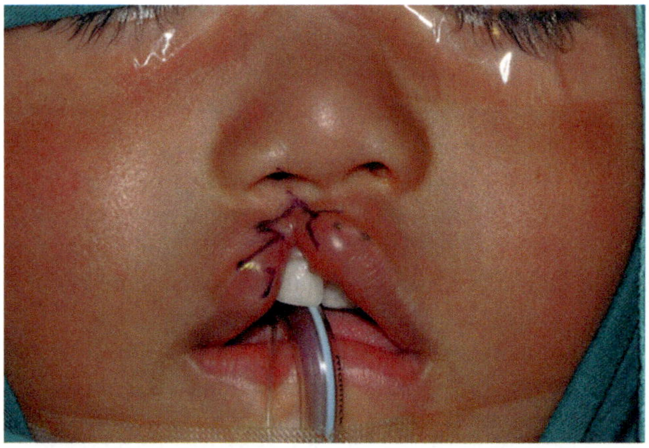

Fig. 6.16 Design of the surgical incisions

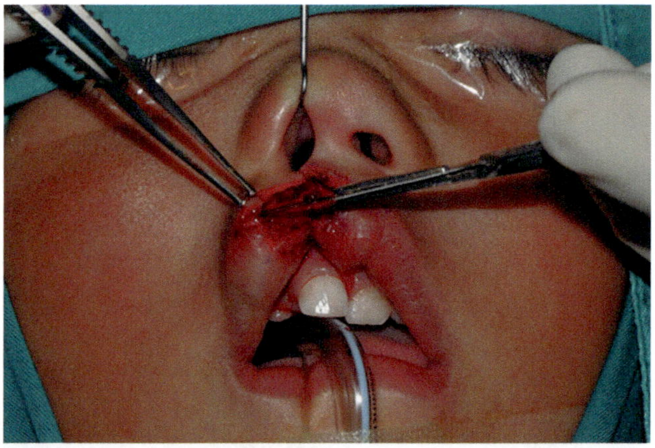

Fig. 6.18 Dissection of the muscle

An example of the surgical procedure (Figs. 6.16 and 6.17):

The incision is made according to the design drawn. The depth of the incision should only be limited to the mucosal and the submucosal layers (Figs. 6.18 and 6.19).

Sharply dissect the orbicularis oris muscle and deglove the mucosal and the skin layers. The dissection is sufficient when the superior margin of the orbicularis oris muscle on the cleft side can be easily pulled to the anterior nasal spine. Preserve the branch of the nasolabial artery as much as possible. Similarly, perform sharp dissection and deglove the orbicularis oris muscle on the unaffected side. After which free the malposed orbicularis oris muscle attachments away from the piriform aperture and anterior nasal spine. This dissection should not exceed the philtrum ridge of the unaffected side (Figs. 6.20 and 6.21).

Pull the orbicularis oris muscles on both sides of the lip horizontally toward the midline of the lip. Subsequently, close the muscles on both sides together avoiding significant tension (Figs. 6.22 and 6.23).

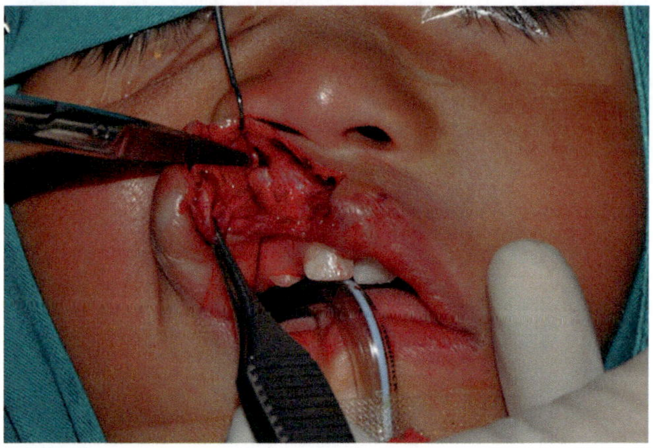

Fig. 6.19 Malposed muscle detached

3. Points to note
   (i) The peak of Cupid's bow on the cleft side is significantly lower: The transverse incision on the upper lip skin of the unaffected side should be the same length as the height difference between the peaks of Cupid's

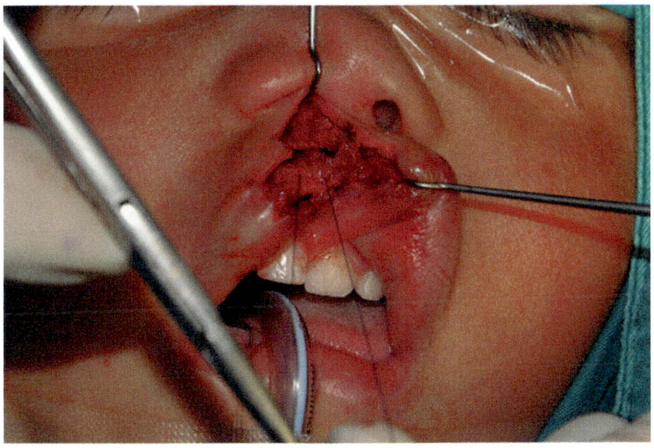

Fig. 6.20 Correction of the deviated

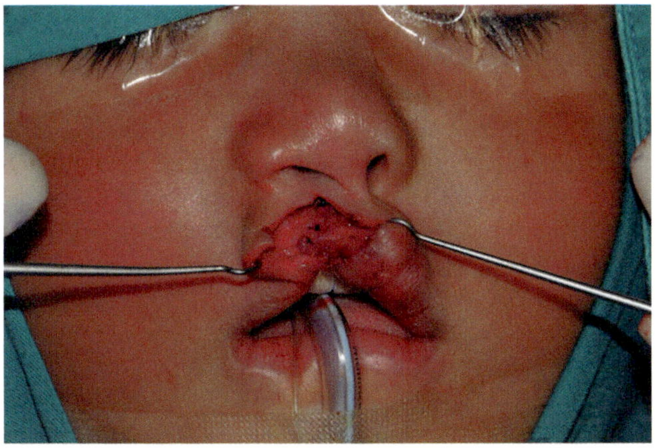

Fig. 6.21 Closure of the muscle layer columella

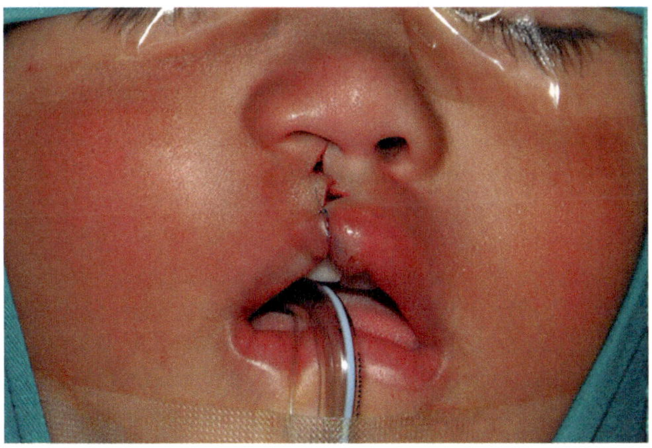

Fig. 6.22 Closure of the skin layer

bow. The triangular flap on the cleft side should also match the gap created on the contralateral side.

(ii) Whistle deformity and deviated upper lip after surgery: The dry mucosa of the lip on the cleft side should be aligned inferiorly to dry mucosa on the unaffected side. Make multiple, small, and continuous incisions instead of a single large incision during the repair of the inferior margin of the upper lip.

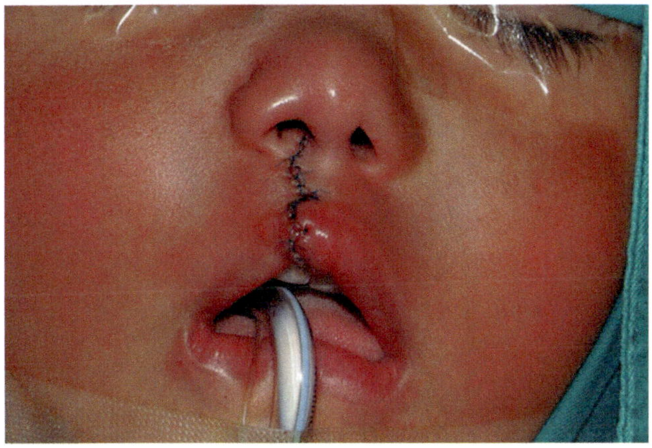

Fig. 6.23 Revision of the lip tubercle

6.3.2 (Method B): Huaxi's Principles

1. Indications
   (i) The difference in height of the peak of the Cupid's bow on the cleft side and the unaffected must be within 2 mm.
   (ii) Deficient philtrum ridge and lip tubercle on the cleft side.
   (iii) Wide alar base on the cleft side and deviated nasal columella.
2. Surgical methods and procedures
   (i) The critical points of this technique lie in the endpoint of the incision and achieving an equal incision length on both sides of the cleft.
   (ii) During the operation, the orbicularis oris muscle, skin, and mucosa on both sides of the incision should be separated. The dissection on the cleft side can extend to the nasolabial fold. Whereas, the dissection on the unaffected side should not exceed beyond the philtrum ridge.
   (iii) The post-operative wound should appear as one line extending from the columella to the peak of the Cupid's bow on the cleft side. Similar to the previous technique, there will be no scar on the nasal floor.

Huaxi Principles lie in determining point 5 accurately where points 5–2 = points 5–3 and, marking point x where points 3–x = points 4–7 while marking points 5–x = points 6–7. If points 6–7 are longer than points 5–x, a portion of skin can be excised starting from point x toward points 6–7 (Figs. 6.24 and 6.25).

An example of the surgical technique:

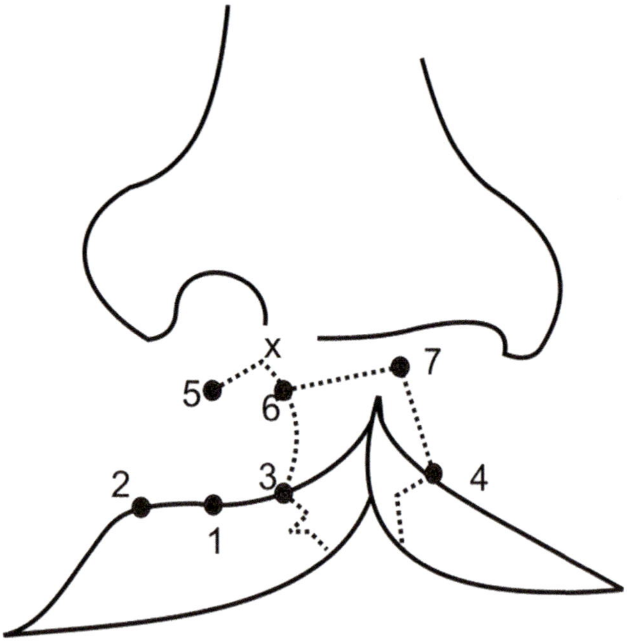

Fig. 6.24 Schematic diagram of the surgical design

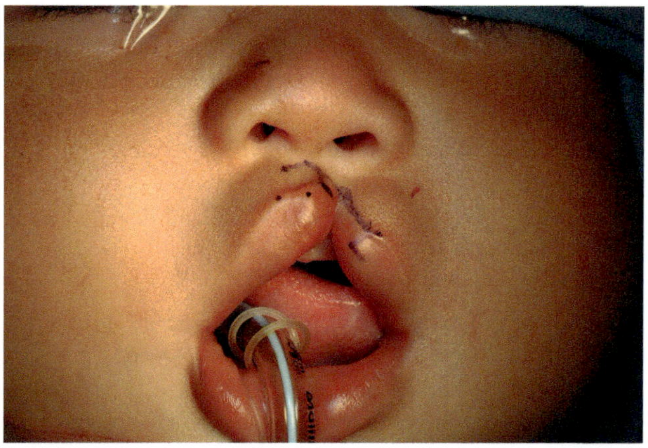

Fig. 6.25 Design of the surgical incision

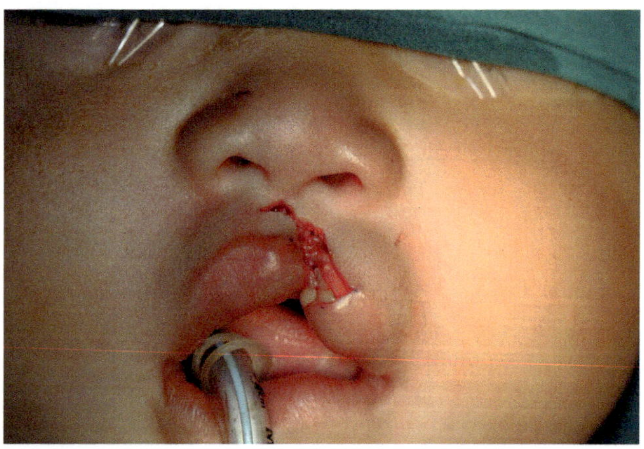

Fig. 6.26 Incision

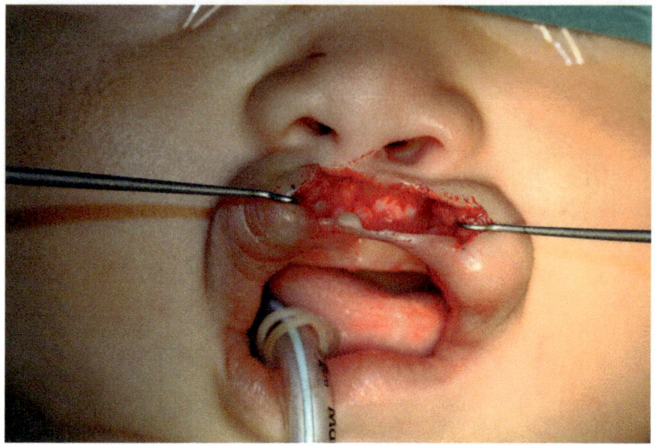

Fig. 6.27 Dissection of the orbicularis oris muscle

Make the incisions according to the diagram. The depth of the incision should only be limited to the mucosa and the submucosa (Fig. 6.26).

The orbicularis oris muscle was separated by sharp dissection of the adhesions, followed by degloving of the mucosal and the skin layers. The dissection is sufficient when the superior margin of the orbicularis oris muscle on the cleft side can be easily pulled to the anterior nasal spine. The branch of the nasolabial artery should be preserved as much as possible. Similarly, perform sharp dissection and deglove the orbicularis oris muscle away from the mucosal and the skin layers on the unaffected side. After which, free the malposed orbicularis oris muscle attachments away from the piriform aperture and anterior nasal spine. This dissection should not exceed the philtrum ridge of the unaffected side (Figs. 6.27, 6.28 and 6.29).

Pull the orbicularis oris muscles on both sides of the lip horizontally toward the midline of the lip. Subsequently, close the muscles on both sides together, avoiding significant tension (Figs. 6.30 and 6.31).

3. Points to note
   (i) The peak of Cupid's bow on the cleft side is significantly pulled lower: The transverse incision on the upper lip skin of the unaffected side should be the same length as the height difference between the peaks of Cupid's bow. The triangular flap on the cleft side should also match the gap created on the contralateral side.
   (ii) A lack of upper lip bulk on the cleft side, while both the philtrum ridge and fossa are not obvious: The upper margin of the orbicularis oris muscle on the cleft side should be fixated to the anterior nasal spine or the septal cartilage. The orbicularis oris muscle on the unaffected side should also be rotated downward. Suture the end of the orbicularis oris muscle on the

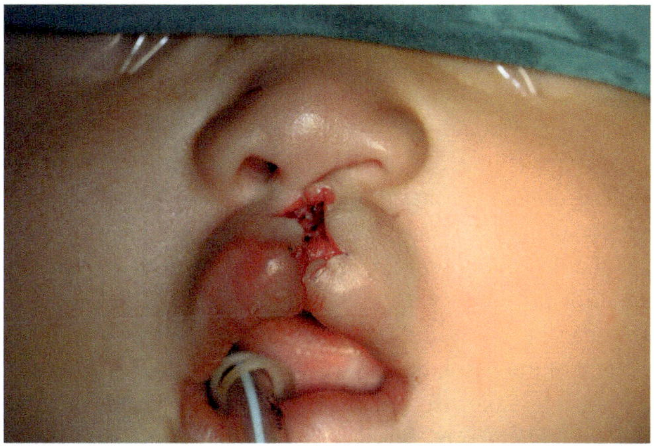

Fig. 6.28 Correction of the deviated

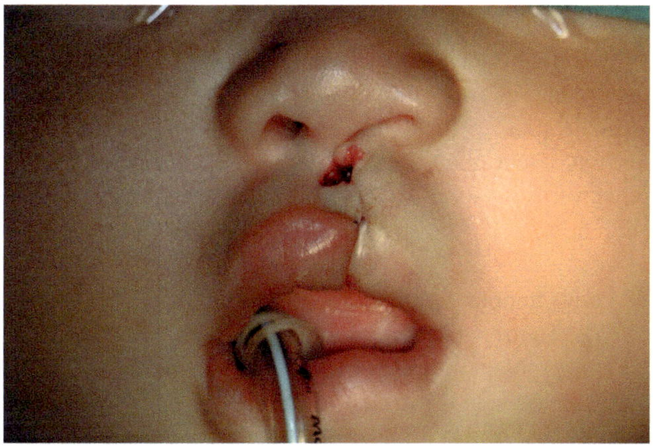

Fig. 6.29 Closure of the muscular layer columella

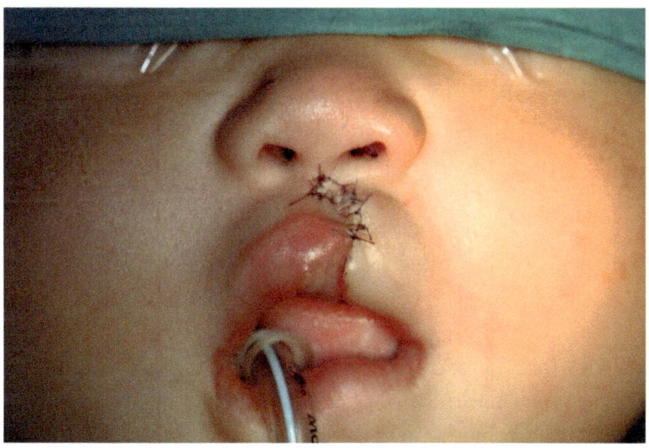

Fig. 6.30 Closure of the skin layer

unaffected side to the lower margin of the muscle on the cleft side.

(iii) Whistle deformity and deviated lip after surgery: The dry mucosa of the lip on the cleft side should be aligned inferiorly to the dry mucosa on the unaffected side. Make multiple, small, and continuous incisions instead of a single large incision during the repair of the inferior margin of the upper lip.

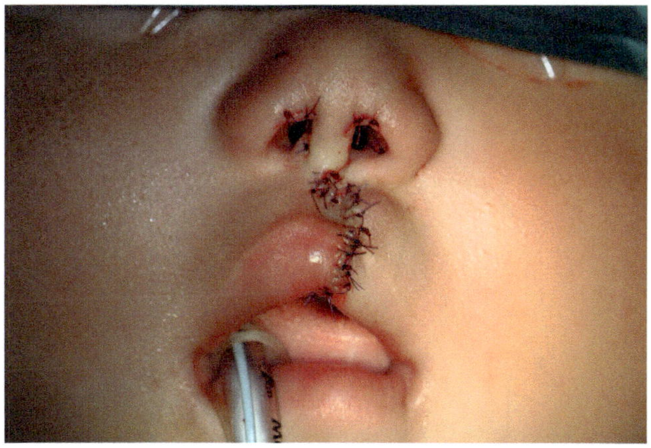

Fig. 6.31 Reconstruction of the lip mucosa

6.4 Unilateral Complete Cleft Lip Repair

6.4.1 Stepwise Downward Rotation Technique

1. Indications
   (i) Any degree of unilateral complete cleft lip.
2. Surgical methods and procedures
   (i) Rotation point of the peak of the Cupid's bow on the unaffected side: The endpoint of the incision affects the degree of downward rotation, and thus the slope of the Cupid's bow. It should not be altered by changing the shape of the incision or based on the angle bisector theory.
   (ii) Dissection of the orbicularis oris muscle: During the operation, the orbicularis oris muscle, skin, and mucosa on both sides of the incision should be separated. The dissection on the cleft side can be extended to the nasolabial fold. Whereas, the dissection on the unaffected side should extend to the bisecting angle.
   (iii) Stepwise downwards rotation: Pull the orbicularis oris muscle on the unaffected side downwards and rotate the skin, muscle, and mucosa layers respectively downward.

Determine the peak of the Cupid's bow on the unaffected side (point 2), the midpoint of the philtrum (point 1), and the peak of the Cupid's bow on the cleft side (point 3). Ensure that the points 1–2 = 1–3. Determine the base of the columella (point 6), Point 5 is sited within a plane bisecting the bilateral peaks of the Cupid's bow and where 2–5 = 3–5. Point 4 is on the vermillion border. Points 9 and 10 are on the alar base, and as such points 2–10 = points 4–9 (Fig. 6.32).

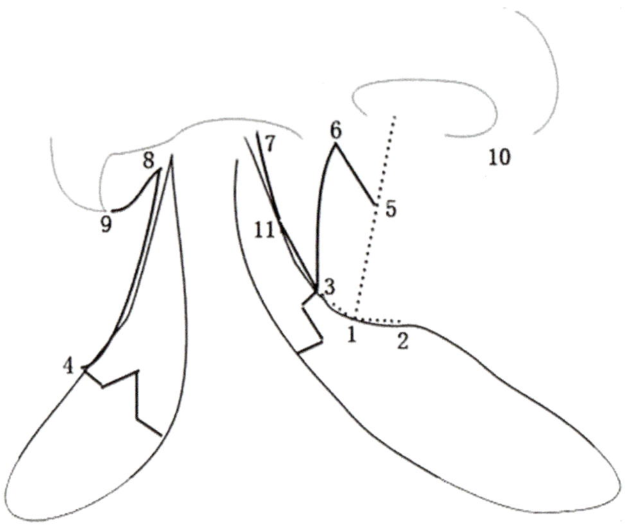

Fig. 6.32 Schematic diagram of the surgical design

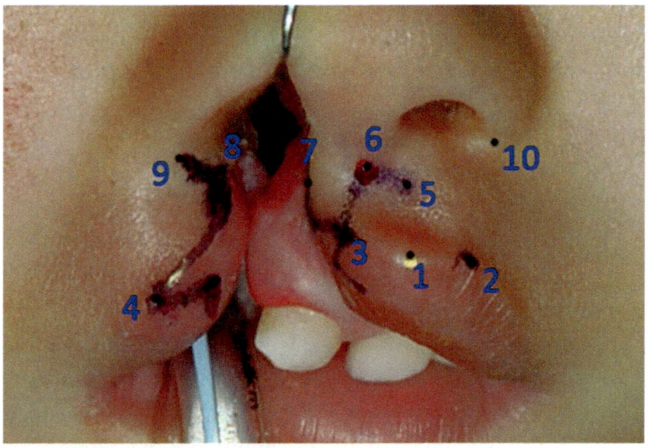

Fig. 6.33 Design of the surgical incisions

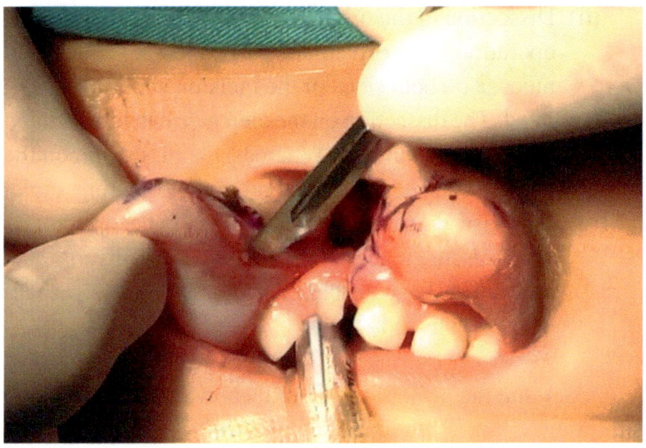

Fig. 6.34 Incision

An example of the surgical procedure (Figs. 6.33 and 6.34):

Make the incision according to the diagram. The depth of the incision should only reach the mucosa and the submucosa layers (Fig. 6.35).

The orbicularis oris muscle was separated by sharp dissection of the adhesions, followed by degloving of the mucosal and the skin layers. The dissection is sufficient when the superior margin of the orbicularis oris muscle on the cleft side can be easily pulled to the anterior nasal spine. The branch of the nasolabial artery should be preserved as much as possible. Likewise, perform sharp dissection and deglove the orbicularis oris muscle on the unaffected side. After which, free the malposed orbicularis oris muscle attachment away from the piriform aperture and anterior nasal spine. This dissection should not exceed the philtrum ridge of the unaffected side (Figs. 6.36 and 6.37).

Pull the orbicularis oris muscles on both sides of the lip horizontally toward the midline of the lip. Subsequently, close the muscles on both sides together, avoiding significant tension. Use a small hook to bring about a greater degree of downwards rotation of the muscle on the unaffected side (Fig. 6.38).

3. Points to note
   - (i) The repaired lip on the cleft side is too short: This problem may arise when the designated peak on the cleft side is too near to the base of the nose. It often occurs when the surgeon keeps the same distance from the peak of the Cupid's bow to the lip commissure. It can be avoided by maintaining equal distances from the alar base to the peak of the Cupid's bow on both sides.
   - (ii) Notching at the base of the columella: This can result from placing the endpoint of the incision within the columella. The rotation of the flap around this point will result in a notch at the base of the columella. Along the vertical axis, the point of rotation should be at the junction between the columella and the upper lip. Along the horizontal axis, the point should be 1/3 away from the cleft and 2/3 away from the unaffected side.
   - (iii) Insufficiency of the lip on the cleft side with indistinct philtrum ridge and fossa: The upper margin of the orbicularis oris muscle on the cleft side should be fixated to the anterior nasal spine or the septal cartilage. The orbicularis oris muscle on the unaffected side should also be rotated downward. Suture

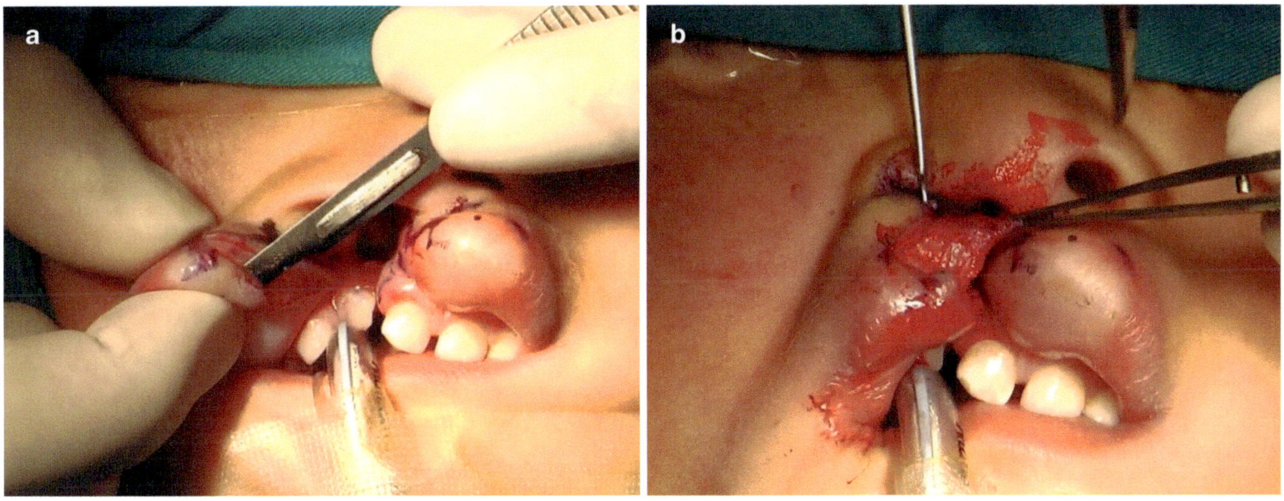

Fig. 6.35 (a and b) Degloving of the orbicularis oris muscle

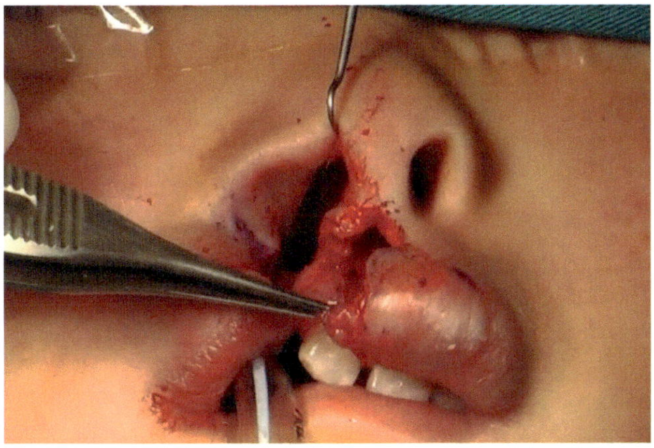

Fig. 6.36 Correction of the deviated

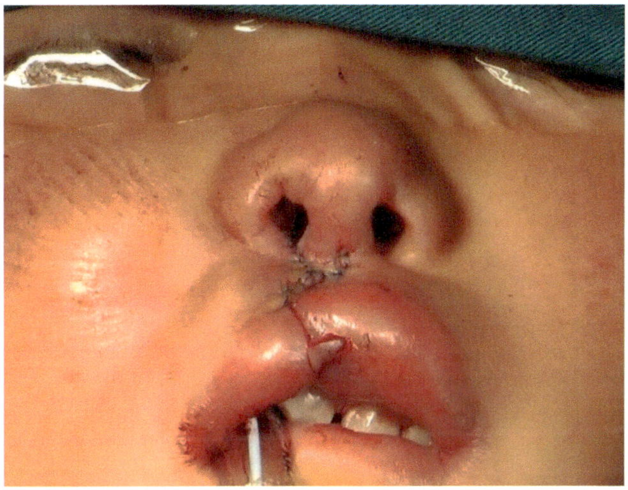

Fig. 6.38 Realignment and closure of the skin and mucosal layers

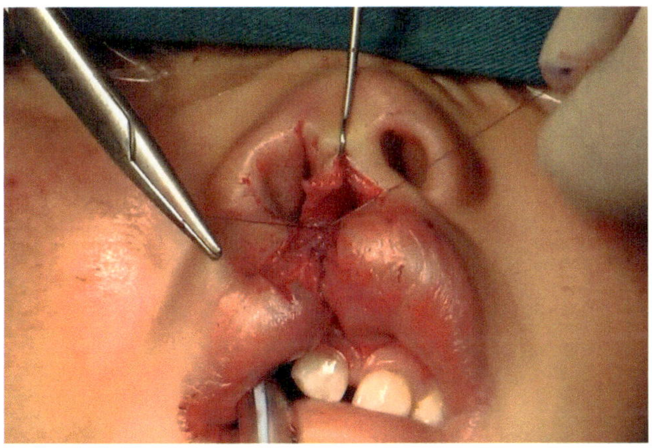

Fig. 6.37 Closure of the muscle layer Columella

the end of the orbicularis oris muscle from the cleft side across to the muscle on the other side.

(iv) Whistle deformity and deviated lip after surgery: The dry mucosa of the lip on the cleft side should be aligned inferiorly to the dry mucosa on the unaffected side. Also, make multiple, small, and continuous incisions instead of a single large incision during the repair of the inferior margin of the upper lip.

Reference

1. Bing S. Plastic surgery of cleft lip and palate (in Chinese). Chengdu: Sichuan University Press; 2004.

Bilateral Cleft Lip Repair

7

Chenghao Li and Bing Shi

7.1 Bilateral Micro-cleft Lip Repair

1. Indications
   (i) Symmetrical and asymmetrical bilateral micro-cleft lip repair.
   (ii) The clefts are limited to the lip mucosa with a linear groove on the skin of the lip due to the discontinuity of the orbicularis oris muscle.
   (iii) Distortions of either one or both of the peaks of the Cupid's bow, which is otherwise generally symmetrical. Additionally, the extension of the lip mucosa into the skin is minimal.
   (iv) Unilateral or bilateral widening of the base of the nose.
2. Surgical methods and procedures
   (i) Make a Z-shaped incision along the mismatched vermillion border. Transpose the resultant two flaps to restore the normal appearance of the Cupid's bow.
   (ii) Place the incisions in the lip vermillion, labial vestibule or the nasal floor. This will create an invisible wound. After extensive dissection of the orbicularis oris muscle, the muscle on the cleft side is secured to the anterior nasal spine, while the muscle on the unaffected side is rotated downward. The philtrum ridge deficiency will be compensated by reconstruction of the orbicularis oris muscle.

An example of the surgical procedure (Fig. 7.1):

Prior to the surgery, determine the landmark points and incision design. Using the linear groove of the vermilion of the lip as the mid axis, design Z-plasty flap incision. The design should consist of a triangular flap with angles between 45 and 75°, each on both sides of the axis. The incision on the skin should be limited to the lip mucosa extended into the skin. No other parts of the skin should be involved (Fig. 7.2).

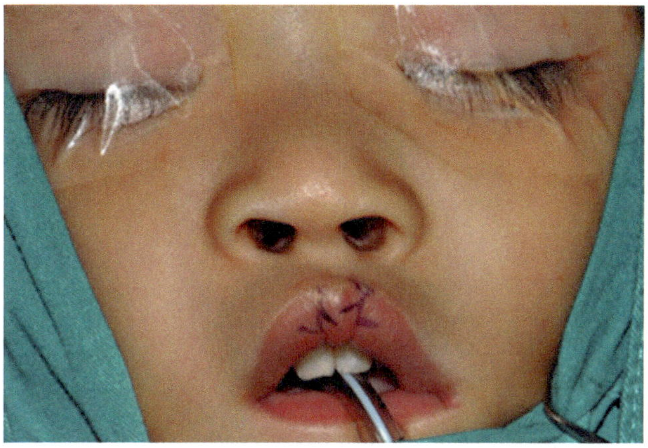

Fig. 7.1 Design of the surgical incisions

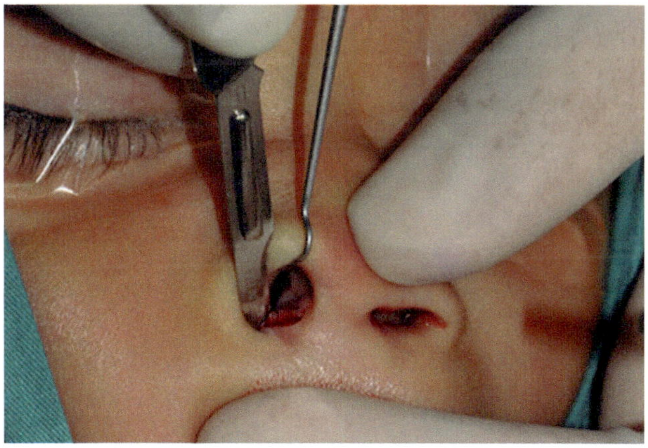

Fig. 7.2 Incision concealed within the nasal vestibule

Make an incision concealed within the nasal vestibule (Fig. 7.3).

Through approach in the nasal vestibule extend inferiorly to expose the orbicularis oris muscle underlying the skin of the lip. Dissect and deglove the muscle from the mucosal and

C. Li (✉)
Department of Cleft Lip and Palate Surgery, West China Stomatology Hospital, Sichuan University, Chengdu, China

B. Shi
Department of Cleft Lip and Palate Surgery, Vice Dean, West China Stomatology College, Sichuan University, Chengdu, China

J. Liu, B. Shi (eds.), *Atlas of Lip and Nose Plastic and Cosmetic Surgery*, https://doi.org/10.1007/978-981-16-1911-3_7

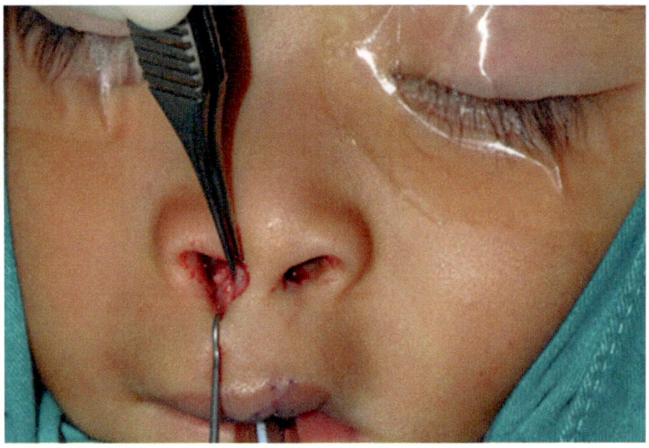

Fig. 7.3 Apposition and suturing

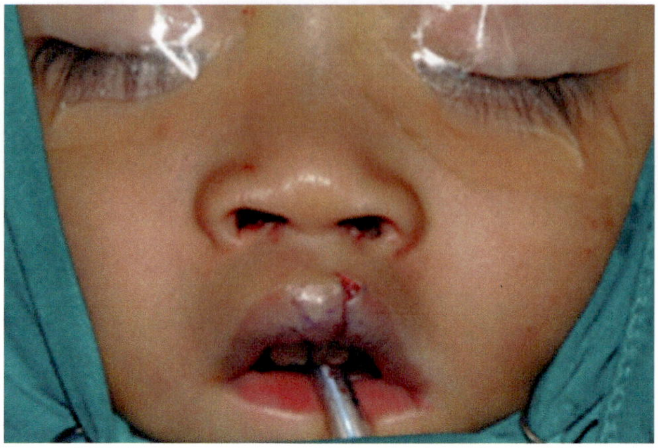

Fig. 7.5 Excision of the mucosa on the skin portion of the lip

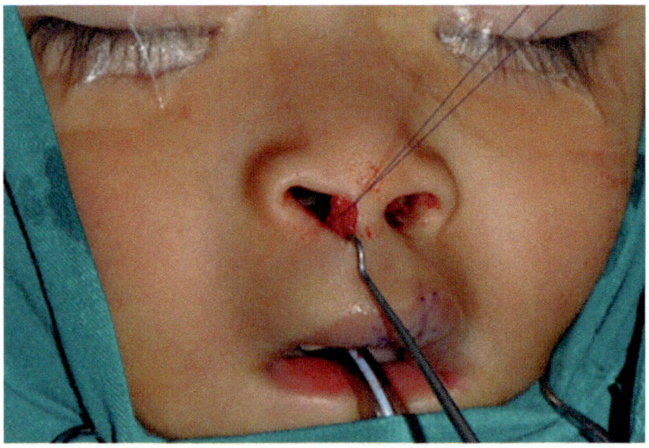

Fig. 7.4 Closure of the orbicularis oris muscle

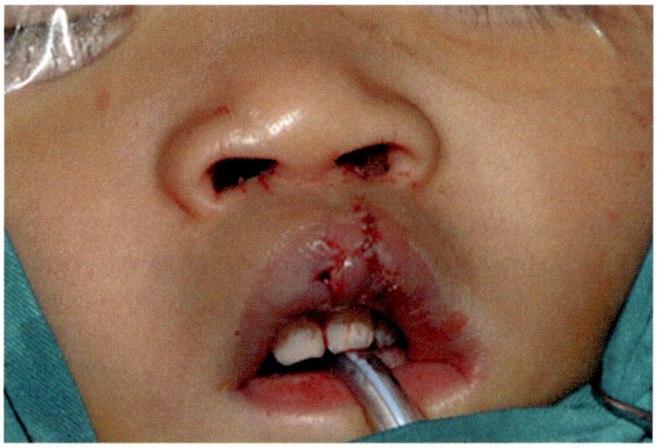

Fig. 7.6 Elimination of the notches on the lip mucosa

skin layers. The skin groove of the lip will disappear upon releasing the adhesion between the skin and the underlying layers (Fig. 7.4).

The continuity of the orbicularis oris muscle is reconstructed upon the closure of the muscle layer (Fig. 7.5).

Excise the mucosa that extends into the skin of the lip (Fig. 7.6).

The bilateral notches on the lip mucosa are repaired by transposing the Z-plasty flaps on each side (Fig. 7.7).

3. Points to note:
   (i) Approach inferiorly through the nasal vestibule will eliminate the scar due to incisions. Release the adhesions between the skin of the lip and the underlying layers. This will eliminate the linear groove on the skin.

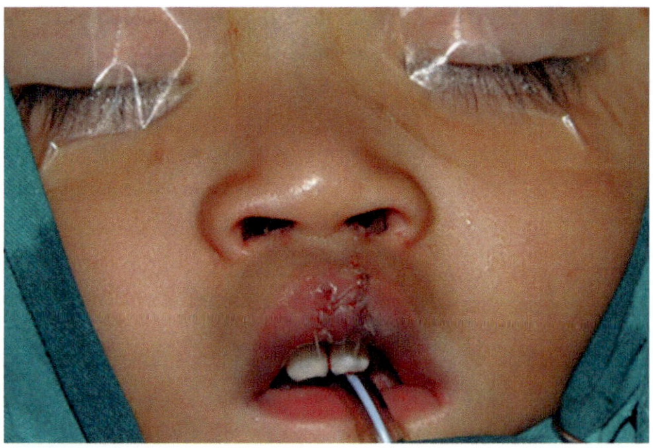

Fig. 7.7 Surgery completed

(ii) The continuity of the muscle layer will be restored by suturing and closure of orbicularis oris muscle. The width of the nasal base can also be adjusted with sutures.
(iii) Pay attention to the symmetry of the lips during the repair of the bilateral mucosal cleft.

7.2 Bilateral Incomplete Cleft Lip Repair

1. Indications
   (i) Congenital bilateral clefts of the upper lip.
   (ii) Asymmetrical bilateral clefts; whereby one side presents with a complete cleft while the other side presents with an incomplete or micro-cleft lip.
   (iii) Unilateral or bilateral widening of the base of the nose.
2. Surgical methods and procedures
   (i) Avoid damaging the peaks of the Cupid's bow on the cleft side as it is an important landmark and its absence may lead to poor results during the reconstruction process.
   (ii) Limit the dissection of the surgical site, and avoid unnecessary wide exposure.

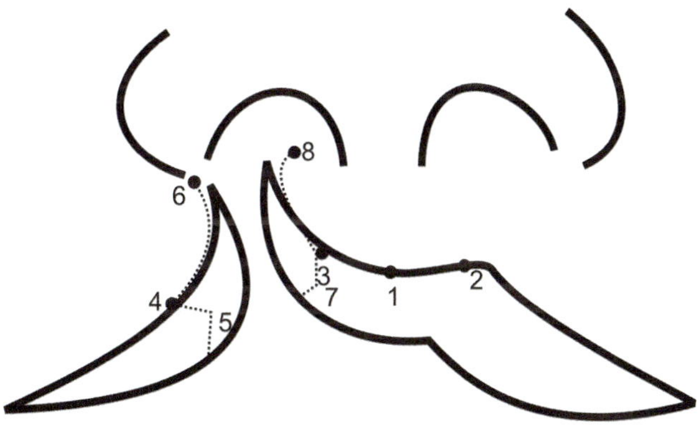

Fig. 7.8 Schematic designs of the incisions

Firstly, mark out the important landmarks of cleft lip repair: Peak of the Cupid's Bow on the micro-cleft side (point 2), the midpoint of the philtrum (point 1), planned peak of the Cupid's Bow on the medial side of the cleft (point 3), and on the lateral side of the cleft (point 4). Ensure that points 1–2 = 1–3. Mark point 5 and 7 on the lip mucosa below point 4 and 3, respectively. Point 6 is marked on the complete cleft side at the junction between the vermillion border and the base of the flattened alar. Point 8 is marked on the micro-cleft side at the junction of the vermillion border and base of the flattened columella. Ensure that points 3–7 = points 4–5 and points 3–8 = points 4–6 (Fig. 7.8).

An example of the surgical procedure (Fig. 7.9):

The incision is made according to the diagram. The depth of the incision should only reach the mucosal and submucosal layers (Fig. 7.10).

Incise according to the lines drawn, and expose the orbicularis oris muscle (Fig. 7.11).

Dissect and deglove the orbicularis oris muscle. Pull and advance the orbicularis oris muscles on both sides of the lip horizontally, avoiding significant tension (Fig. 7.12).

3. Points to note
   (i) Avoid damaging the landmarks that are crucial to the reconstruction process. The important landmark points and surgical design should be drawn clearly prior to the surgery. Make efforts to preserve the landmarks during the surgery.

7.3 Bilateral Complete Cleft Lip Repair

7.3.1 Technique to Reconstruct the Cupid's Bow

1. Indications
   (i) Congenital bilateral clefts of the upper lip extend to the base of the nose.

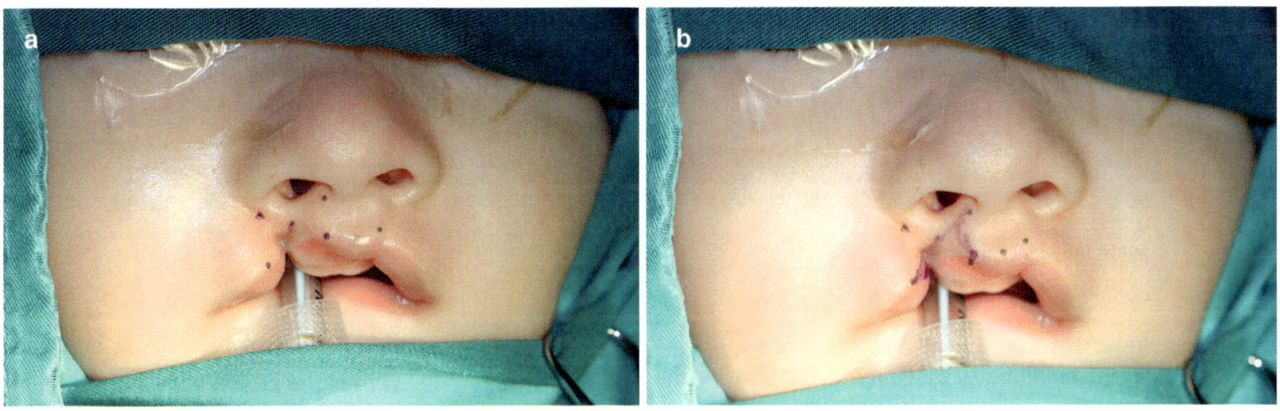

Fig. 7.9 (**a** and **b**) Design of the incisions

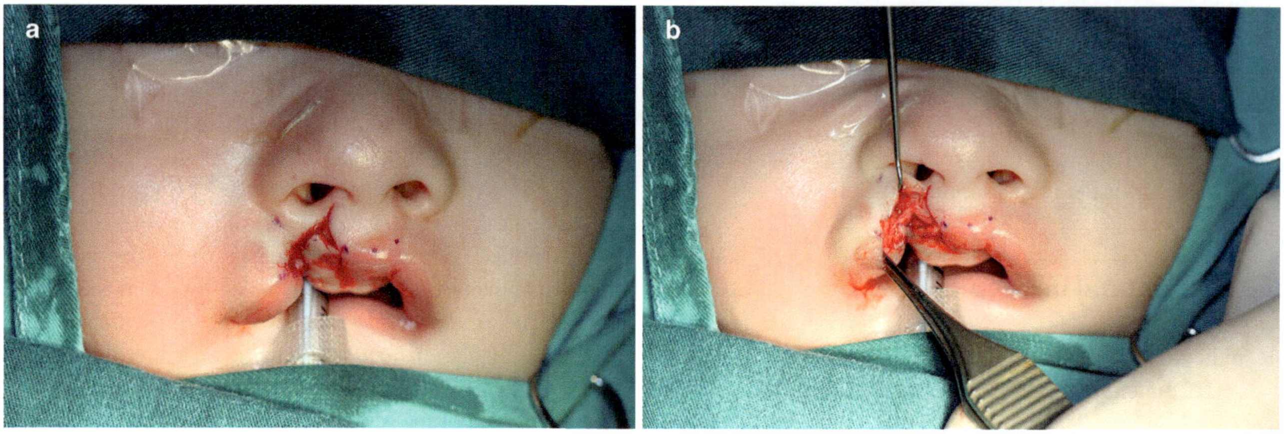

Fig. 7.10 (**a** and **b**) Incisions

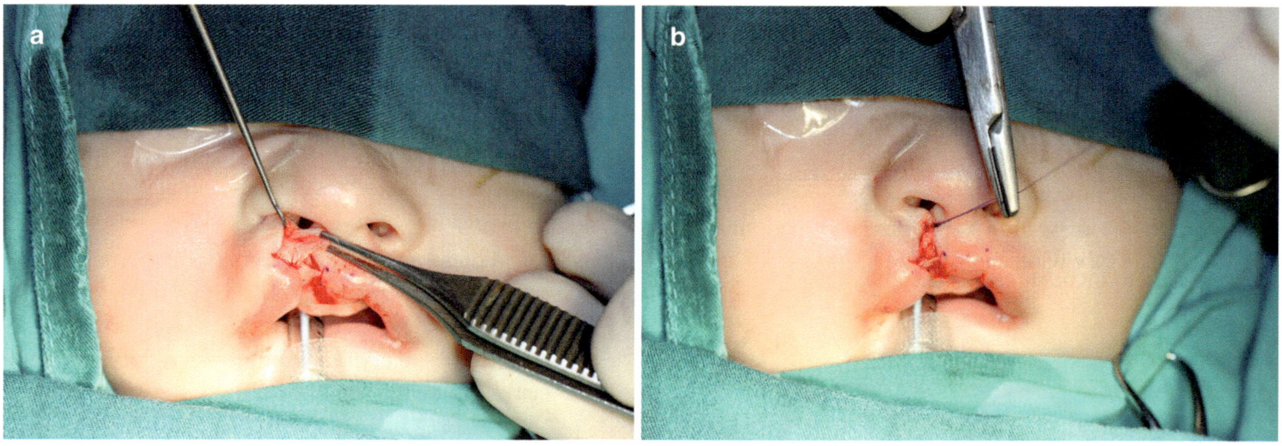

Fig. 7.11 (**a** and **b**) Degloving dissection and reconstruction of the orbicularis oris muscle

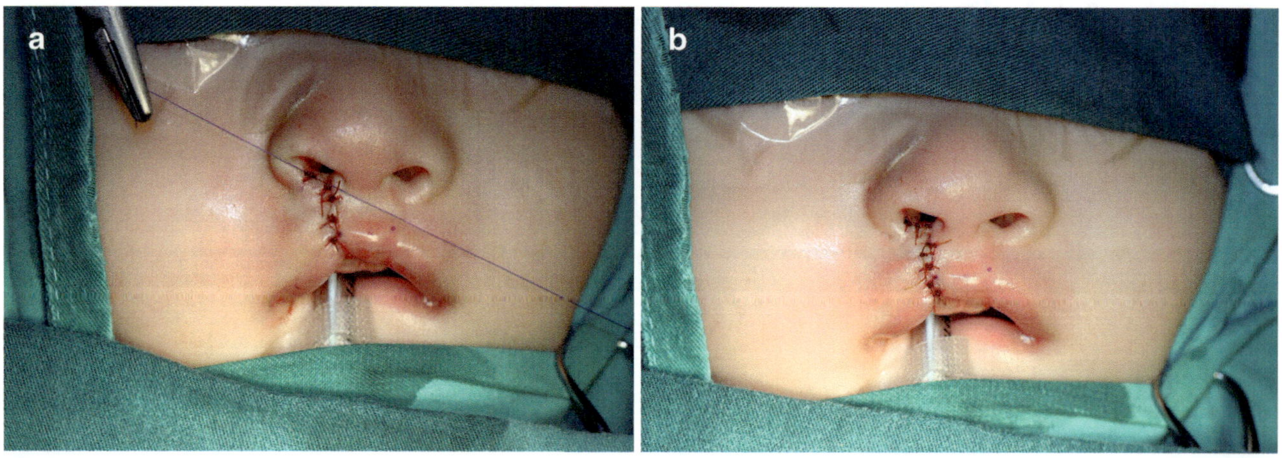

Fig. 7.12 (**a** and **b**) Surgery completed

(ii) Asymmetrical or symmetrical clefts.

(iii) Unilateral or bilateral widening of the base of the nose.

2. Surgical methods and procedures

(i) Use the length of the prolabium to estimate the length of the upper lip after the repair. The distance of bilateral peaks of the Cupid's bow should be 2–2.5 mm away from the midpoint of the philtrum.

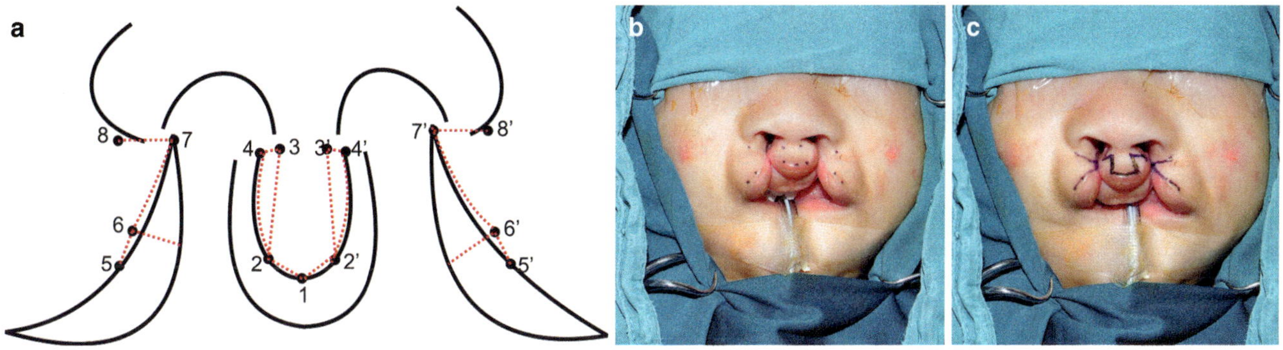

Fig. 7.13 Schematic designs of the incisions

(ii) Intentionally put the point for the peak of Cupid's bow and the point of the mid philtrum at a different distance from the Cupid's bow of the lateral lip. This will help to reconstruct the arch of Cupid's bow when the prolabium and lateral lips are sutured together.
(iii) The height of the lateral lips should be adjusted according to the height of prolabium during the operation.
(iv) The lip tubercles are reconstructed by suturing the lower 1/3 of the orbicularis oris muscle together on both sides.
(v) Include closure of the subcutaneous layer on both sides of the prolabium to allow healing by primary intention. This will facilitate the reconstruction of the philtrum ridge.

An example of the surgical procedure (Fig. 7.13):

Design of the front lip incisions: Generally, the width of the prolabium is designed to be about 4–5 mm. The most inferior point of the vermillion border on the prolabium is defined as point 1. As such, points 1–2 = 1–2′ and points 1–2 + 1–2′ = 4–5 mm. Points 3 and 3′ are then marked, whereby points 2–3 = 2′–3′ and the width of point 3–3′ is slightly less than the distance of point 2–2′. At the vermillion border lateral to points 3 and 3′, mark the points 4 and 4′. The incision can be executed with a slight curvature along 2–1–2′, 3–2, 3′–2′, 3–4, and 3′–4′, respectively.

Surgical design of the lateral lips: The planned peak of the Cupid's bow should be selected at the thicker portion of the lateral lips, while the midpoint of the planned philtrum should be at 2–3 mm above this point, i.e., points 5 with 5′ and points 6 with 6′. However, the distance between points 5 and 5′ to their respective oral commissure and alar base should be equal. Note that points 5–6 = 5′–6′ = 2–3 mm. Point 6 can be located at 1–2 mm above the vermillion border if the length of the prolabium is shorter. The incision will be made along 7–8, 7–6–5, 7′–8′, and 7′–6′–5′.

Following the lines drawn, incise the skin and mucosal layers. Proceed with sharp dissection of the orbicularis oris muscle and deglove it from the skin and mucosal layers. Preserve the branch of the nasolabial artery as much as possible. Through the medial side of the alar base, cut open the attachment of the alar to the maxilla, and the attachment of the malposed orbicularis oris muscle to the alar. The orbicularis must be completely degloved from the skin and oral mucosa. Ensure that the muscles from the lateral lip can be pulled freely to the midline (Figs. 7.14 and 7.15).

Incise the skin and mucosa of the prolabium following the premarked design. Remove only epidermis on both sides of prolabium (within lines 2–3–4 and 2′–3′–4′). Using a small hook elevate prolabial skin and subcutaneous tissue. Start the dissection from the submucosa of the prolabium and continue upward to the base of the nasal columella. This forms a prolabial skin flap pedicled to the columella (Fig. 7.16).

Pull the bilateral orbicularis oris muscles horizontally toward the midpoint of the prolabium, avoiding significant tension. This will restore the continuity of the orbicularis oris muscle (Fig. 7.17).

Suture the skin and mucosa.

3. Points to note.

- The length of the prolabium and lateral lip components are not equal: The length of the reconstructed upper lip should always be based on the length of the prolabial portion. Thus, the length of the lateral lip components should be adjusted accordingly prior to closure. A crescent-shaped incision can be used to remove some skin tissue of the lateral lip at the base of the nose. This will help to keep the length of the lateral lips consistent with that of the prolabial portion.
- Delayed healing of the surgical site as a result of excessive wound tension: When raising the prolabial flap, only the epidermis on both sides of the prolabium should be removed. Retain as much subcutaneous tissue as possible. The subcutaneous layer supports the wound and facilitates primary wound healing of the reconstructed lips [1, 2].
- Post-operative whistle deformity: The reconstruction of the orbicularis oris muscle does not just involve suturing the muscle from both sides together in the midline. A

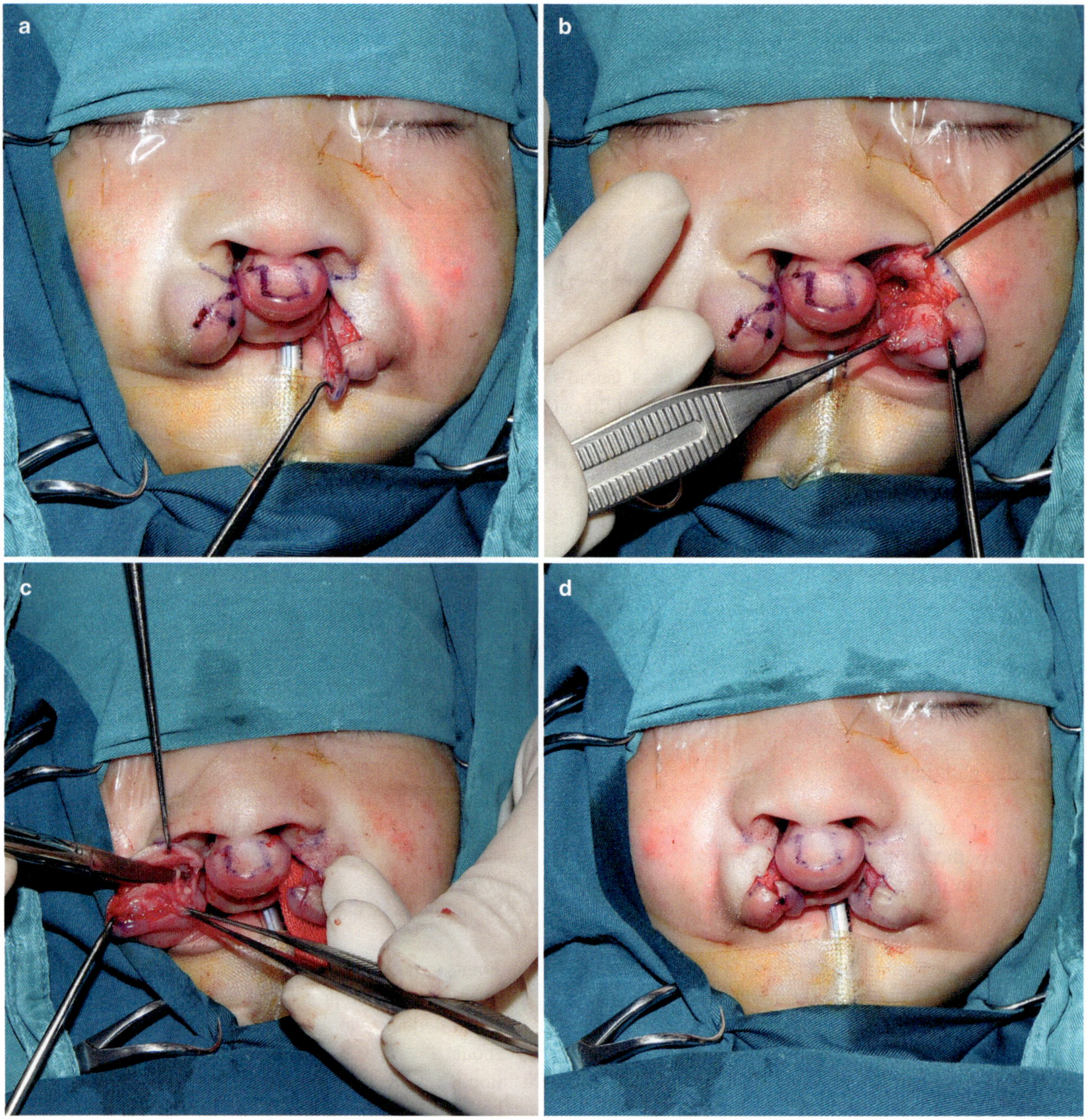

Fig. 7.14 Formation of the lateral lip flaps and dissection of the orbicularis oris muscle

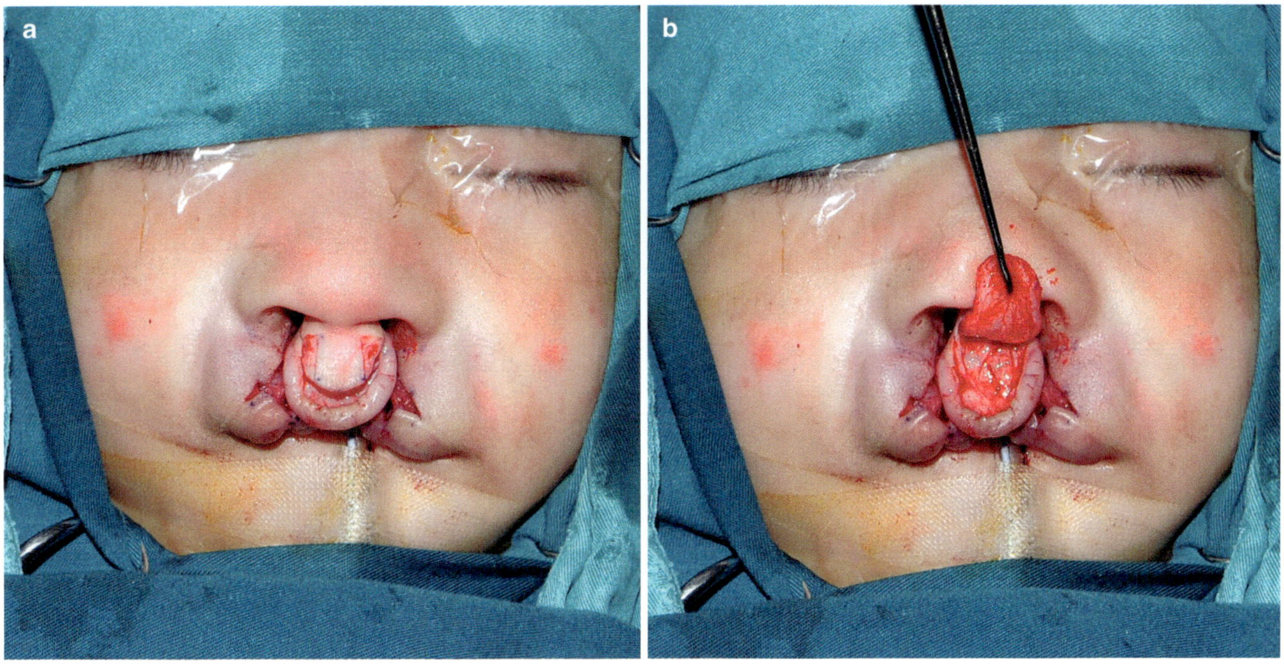

Fig. 7.15 Formation of the prolabium flap

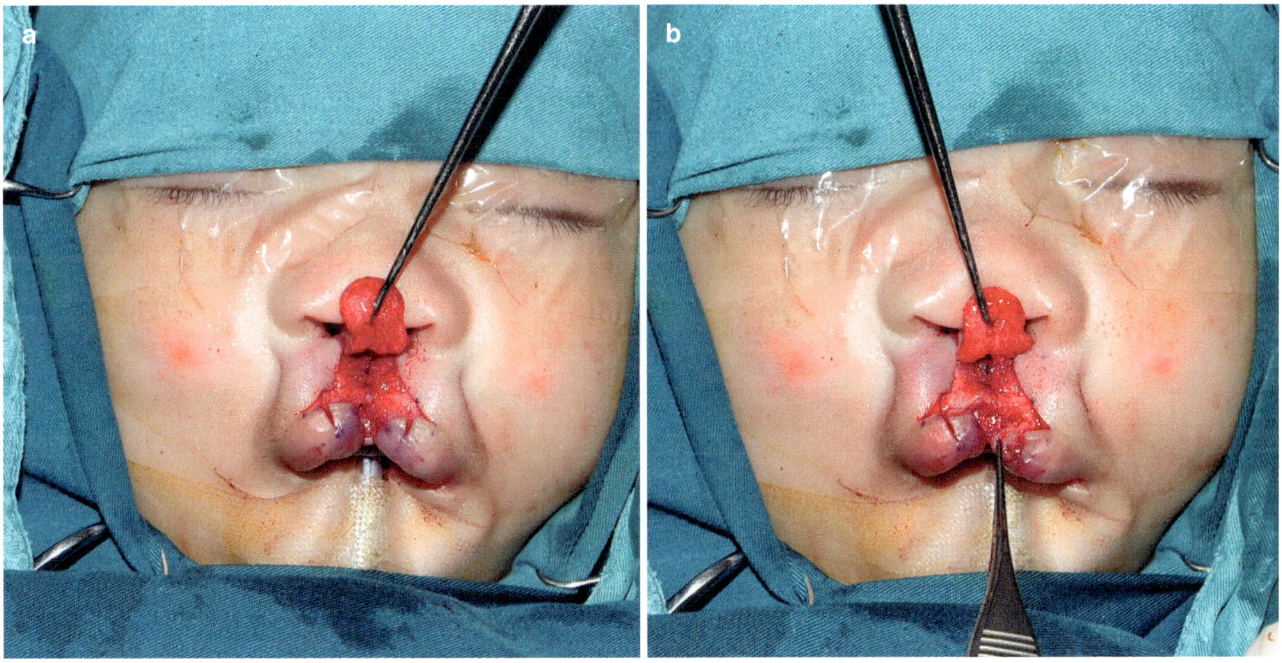

Fig. 7.16 Connecting the orbicularis oris muscle from both sides

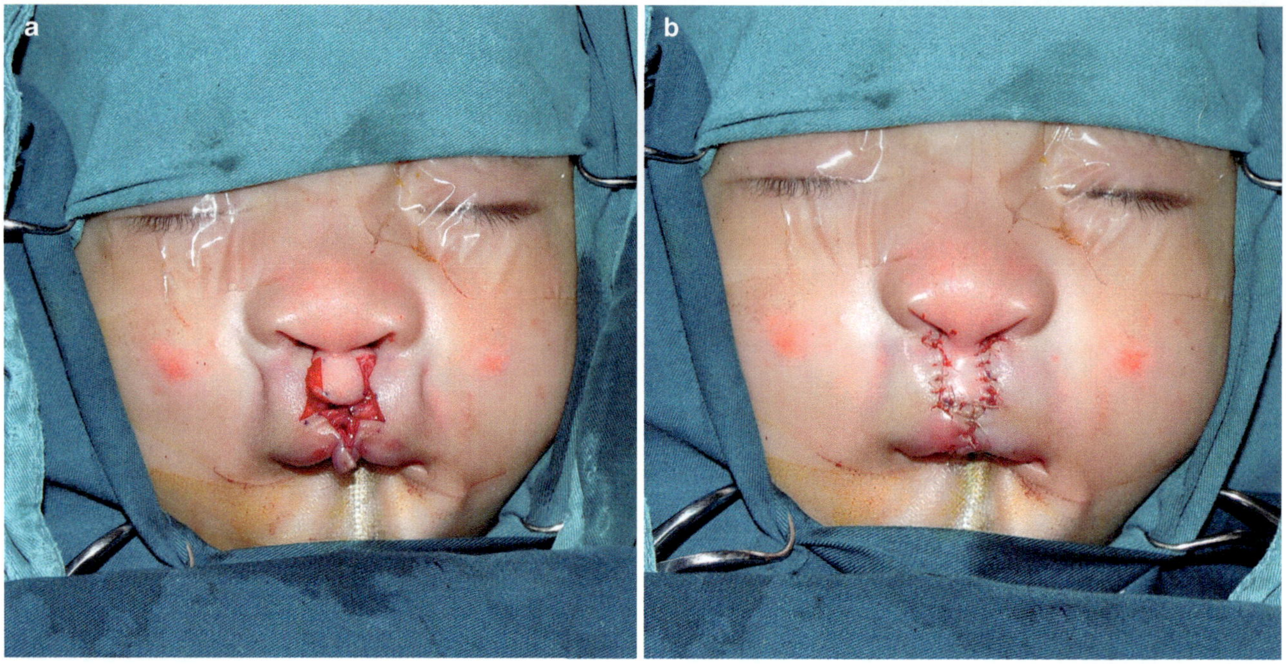

Fig. 7.17 Surgical Completed

horizontal incision should also be executed on the lower third of the muscle to create a separate muscle flap on each side. The lip tubercle is formed by the closure of the separate muscle flaps at the midline. Additionally, the lower lip margin should be repaired with small bilateral labial mucosal flaps.

References

1. Bing S. Plastic surgery of cleft lip and palate (in Chinese). Chengdu: Sichuan University Press; 2004.
2. Molendijk J, Pendleton C, Rachwalski M, et al. Harvey Cushing's contributions to plastic surgery: bilateral cleft lip repair. Cleft Palate Craniofac J. 2014;51(1):105–9.

Repair of Secondary Deformities of Unilateral Cleft Lip Surgery

8

Qian Zheng

8.1 Reconstruction of the Lip Tubercle

1. Indications
   (i) There is no distinct lip tubercle and the lip mucosa is hypertrophic on one side.
   (ii) There is a depression on the lip and the lip mucosa is hypertrophic on one side.
   (iii) Deviation of the lip tubercle.
2. Surgical methods and procedure
   (i) Depending on the hypertrophic degree of the lip mucosa, determine the width and length of the mucosal rotation flap.
   (ii) The flap should be pedicled to the center of the lip and rotated toward the lip tubercle. This makes the lip tubercle appear fuller and eliminates depressions on the lip.

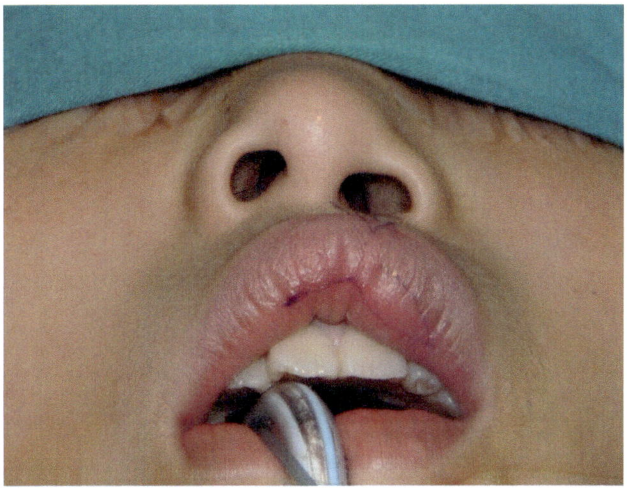

Fig. 8.1 Design of the surgical incisions

An example of the surgical procedure (Fig. 8.1):

Design a fusiform lip mucosal flap based on the hypertrophic degree of the lip mucosa on the affected side. The tip of the fusiform flap should be located at the junction of the dry and wet lip mucosa. The dimensions of the flap also take reference from the shape of the contralateral side to ensure the symmetrical thickness of the upper lip after the flap rotation. After the incision passes through the most protruded point of the hypertrophic mucosa, gradually direct the inner incision toward the dry-wet lip mucosa junction. Then extend the incision slightly shorter than the flap length, toward the opposite side and along the junction. This allows the flap to have adequate tissue and gives the lip tubercle a more prominent appearance (Fig. 8.2).

Incise the mucosal layer according to the pre-marked design. Make sure the flap has at least 2 mm of submucosal tissues to prevent damage to the labial artery (Fig. 8.3).

Rotate the lip mucosal flap to the contralateral side. Make sure that both sides of the upper lip are symmetrical and the lip tubercle is at the midline (Fig. 8.4).

Finally, suture and close the mucosal layer.

Classic Example (Figs. 8.5, 8.6, 8.7):

3. Points to note
   (i) Decide the required width and length of the lip mucosal rotation flap according to the degree of lip mucosa hypertrophy on the affected side. The ratio of length to width should be less than 4:1.
   (ii) The inner incision of the lip mucosal rotation flap should extend to the intended site of the new lip tubercle. This will allow the flap pedicle to be located toward the external portion of the mouth. By doing so, the creases of the rotation can be concealed.

Q. Zheng (✉)
Department of Cleft Lip and Palate Surgery, West China Stomatology Hospital, Sichuan University, Chengdu, China

J. Liu, B. Shi (eds.), *Atlas of Lip and Nose Plastic and Cosmetic Surgery*, https://doi.org/10.1007/978-981-16-1911-3_8

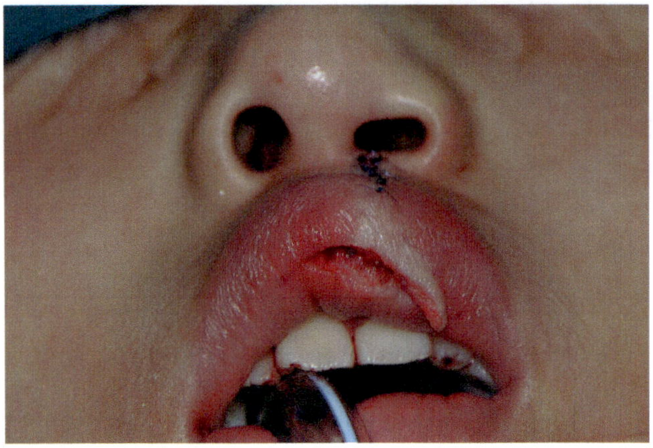

Fig. 8.2 Raise the mucosal and submucosal layers to complete the rotation flap

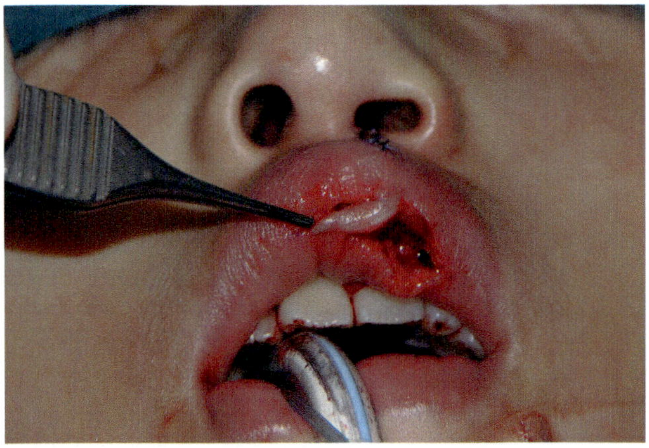

Fig. 8.3 Rotate the flap to the contralateral side to form a new lip tubercle

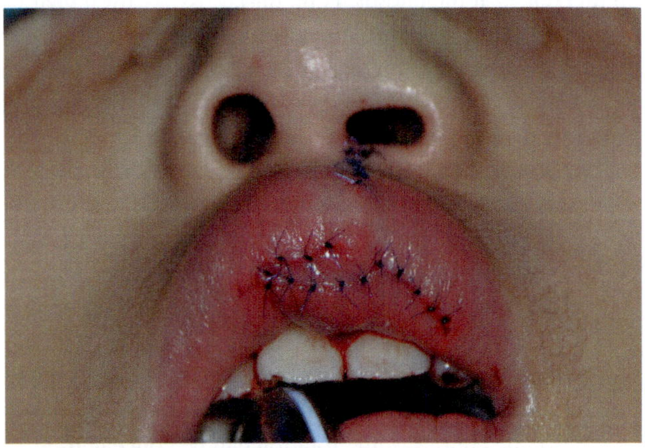

Fig. 8.4 Closure of the mucosal layer

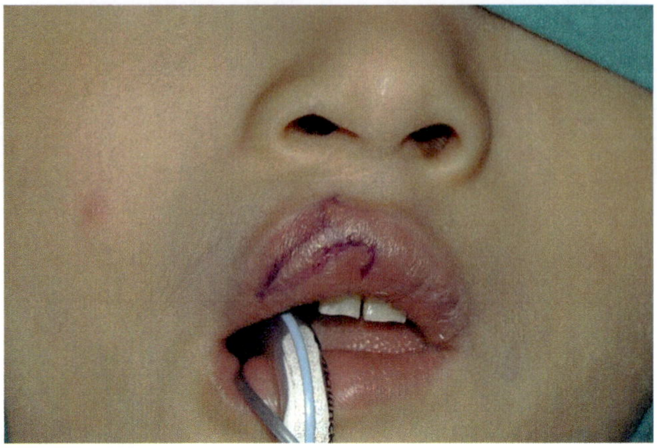

Fig. 8.5 The lip tubercle is not distinct pre-operatively

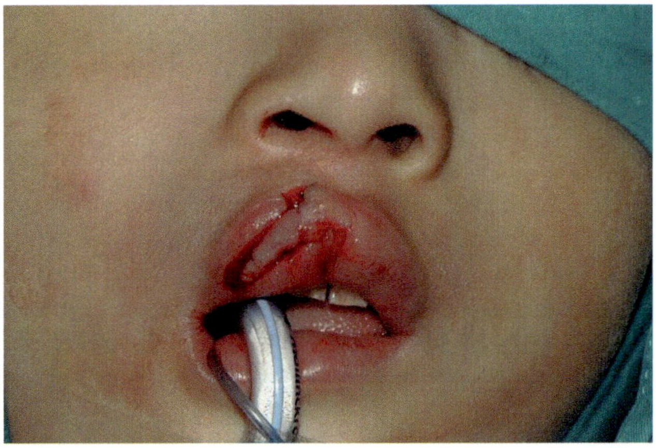

Fig. 8.6 Design of the incisions

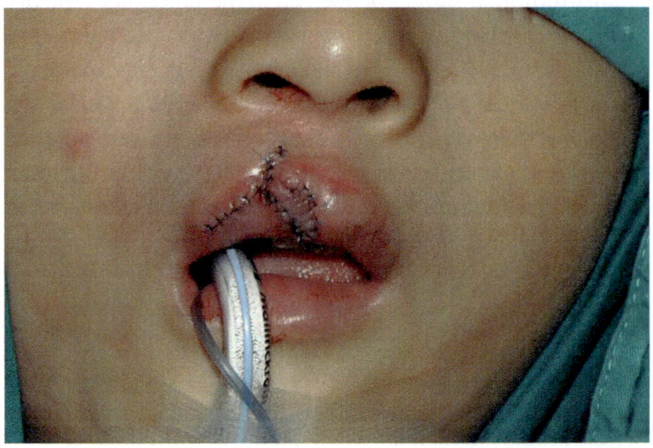

Fig. 8.7 Postoperative outcome

8.2 Correction of a Deviated Philtrum Ridge (Fossa)

1. Indications
   (i) The midline of the upper lip does not coincide with the facial midline and is inclined toward the cleft side.
   (ii) The philtrum ridge on the unaffected side is deviated toward the cleft side.
2. Surgical methods and procedure
   (i) After dissecting the orbicularis oris muscle, tie the upper part of the muscle from the cleft side to the periosteum of the anterior nasal spine to form a stable anchorage. Next, pull and suture the upper part of the orbicularis oris muscle from the unaffected side to the repositioned muscle on the cleft site. This will correct both the philtrum ridge and midline of the upper lip. The main focus of this surgical approach is the dissection of the orbicularis oris muscle. The incision of the skin of the upper lip should be kept as small as possible. In specific cases, this surgical approach can be combined with incisions through the nasal floor, nasal vestibule, or lip mucosa.

An example of the surgical procedure (Fig. 8.8):

In this patient, the philtrum is inclined toward the cleft side, the margin of the lip mucosa has a notch defect, and the alar on the cleft side is collapsed. The surgical approach consists of an incision on the lip mucosa from the inferior margin of the lip to the notch defect. In addition, a C-shaped incision is made along the alar, columella, and the nasal base on the cleft side (Fig. 8.9).

Access the orbicularis oris muscle through the incisions made on the base of the nose and on the lip mucosa. Next, dissect and deglove the muscle away from the skin and mucosal layers. Subsequently, release the malposed orbicularis oris muscle attachments from the anterior nasal spine and the piriform aperture of the cleft side (Figs. 8.10 and 8.11).

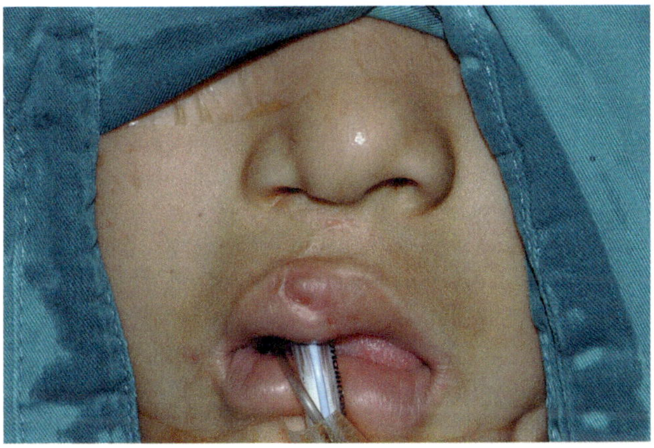

Fig. 8.8 The pre-operative philtrum ridges are deviated toward the cleft side

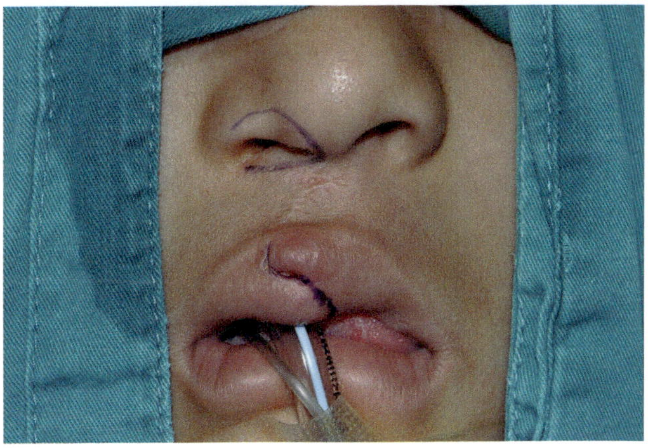

Fig. 8.9 Design of the surgical incisions

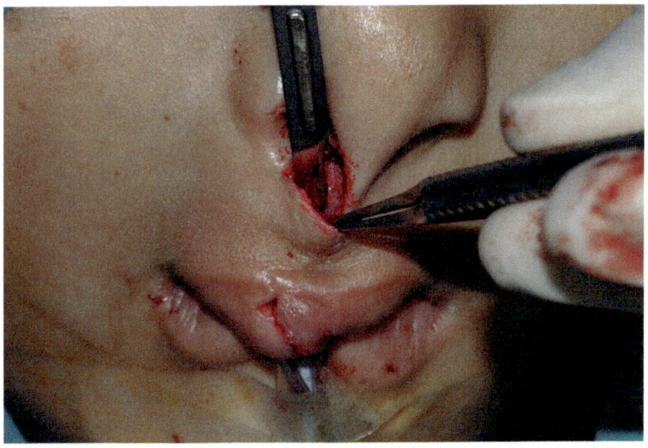

Fig. 8.10 Dissection of the orbicularis oris muscle via the incision made on the nasal base

Cut the orbicularis oris muscle 2 mm lateral to the philtrum ridge on the affected side (Fig. 8.12).

Pull the muscle bundle from the cleft side to the anterior nasal spine and use a 3–0 suture to secure it to the periosteum. Ensure equal height on both sides of the upper lip, and avoid obvious upward movement of the alar base on the cleft side. Shift the upper part of the muscle bundle from the unaffected side toward the muscle bundle on the cleft side and suture them together. This aligns the middle and bottom parts of the philtrum to the midline. Adjust the remaining muscle bundles on the unaffected side inward and downward. Use the muscle bundles from the cleft side to fill up the space created from the aforementioned maneuver. Complete the reconstruction of the orbicularis oris muscle by tying both ends of the muscle bundles together (Figs. 8.13 and 8.14).

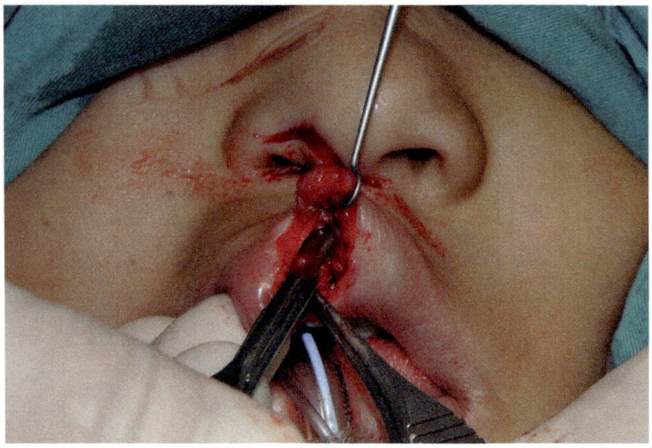

Fig. 8.11 Dissection of the orbicularis oris muscle via the incision made on the lip mucosa

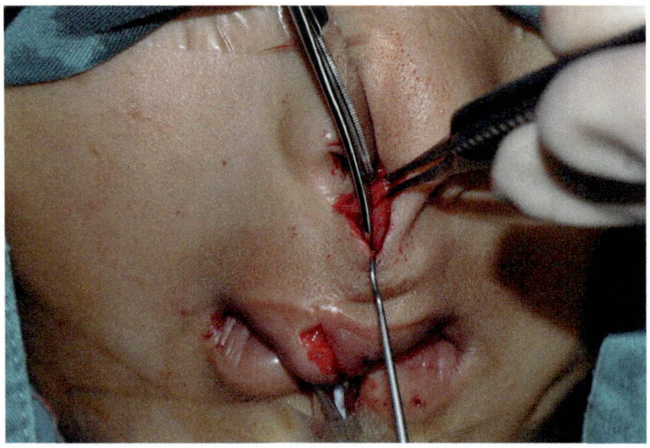

Fig. 8.12 Cutting of the orbicularis oris muscle

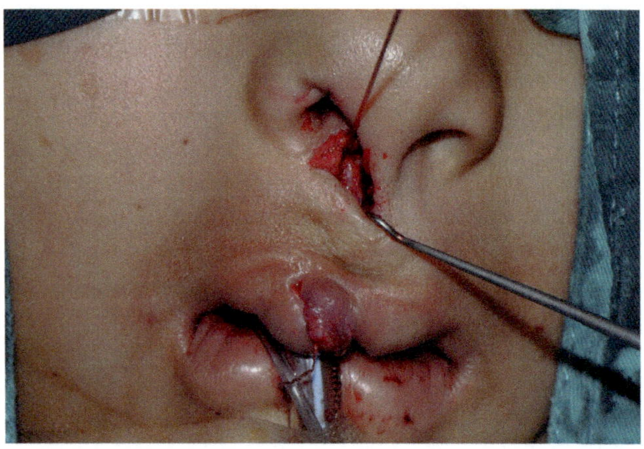

Fig. 8.13 Suture the orbicularis oris muscle from the cleft side to the periosteum of the anterior nasal spine

3. Points to note
   (i) This approach of using the orbicularis oris muscle to realign the philtrum ridge may not suitable for cases in which the philtrum ridge is severely deviated. In such situations, an Abbe flap may be required to reconstruct the central portion of the philtrum.

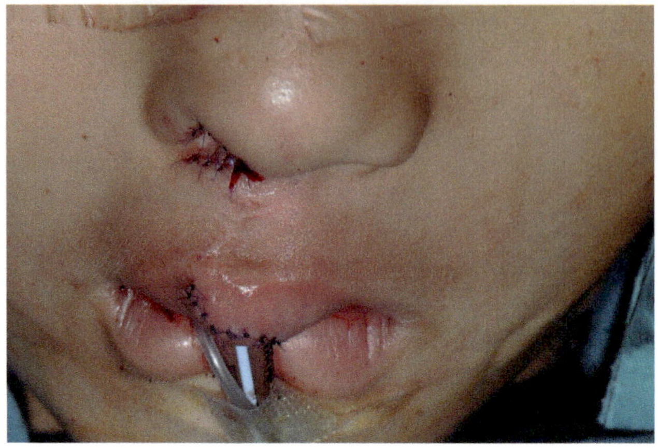

Fig. 8.14 The deviation of the philtrum ridge is corrected to a certain extent

8.3 Correction of an Excessive Peak of the Cupid's Bow

8.3.1 Oblique Flap Technique

1. Indication
   (i) The peak of the Cupid's bow on the cleft side is higher and flatter as compared to the unaffected side.
2. Surgical methods and procedures
   (i) Make an oblique inter-positional flap from the skin portion of the lip at the peak of the Cupid's bow on the affected side. The interposition of the flap will push the lip mucosa inferiorly and as a result will correct the excessive peak of the Cupid's bow.

An example of the surgical procedure (Fig. 8.15):

Draw the inferior section of the incision along the vermillion border (White roll) from the peak of the Cupid's bow on the cleft side to the center of the philtrum. Next, draw the superior section of the incision from the peak of the Cupid's bow on the cleft side toward the direction of the nasal columella with an angle of approximately 60°. Make sure that both sections are of equal length. Complete the oblique flap design by connecting the two sections with another line. The dimensions of the flap should be according to the size of the tissues required to adequately push the peak of the Cupid's bow on the cleft side inferiorly (Fig. 8.16).

Perform subsurface dissection between the skin, mucosa, and orbicularis oris muscle to loosen the lip mucosa on the cleft side and allow it to rest downward. Interpose the skin

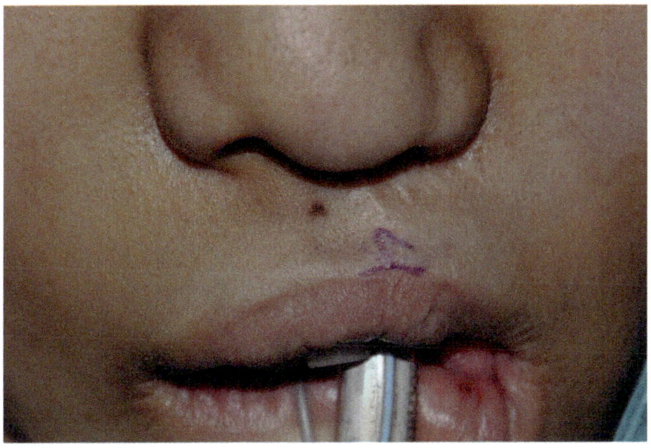

Fig. 8.15 Design of the surgical incisions

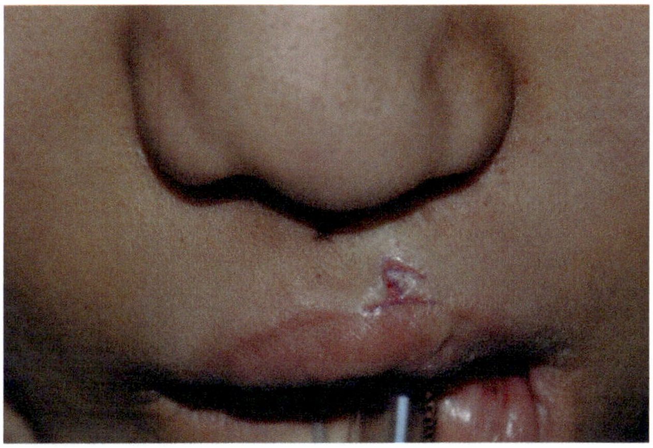

Fig. 8.16 Incise the white roll and skin of the upper lip

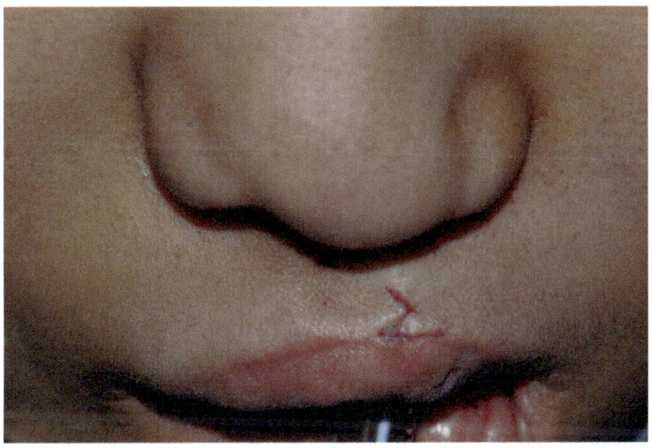

Fig. 8.17 The oblique flap is used to fill the space created after descending the peak of the Cupid's bow

flap to fill the space created on the cleft side after the inferior shift of the peak of the Cupid's bow (Fig. 8.17).

Suture the subcutaneous layer and adjust the oblique skin flap. Finally, close the skin layers (Fig. 8.18).

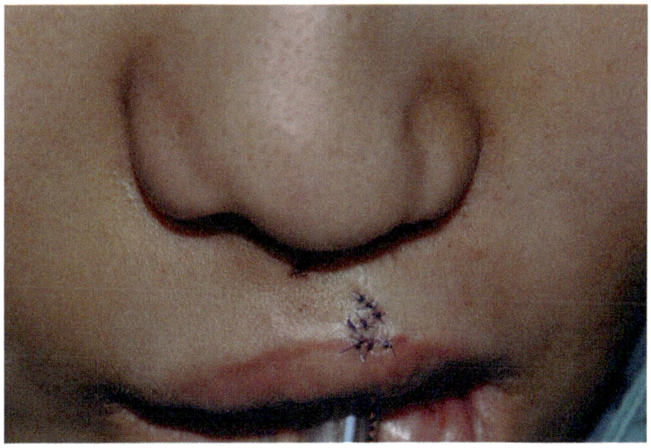

Fig. 8.18 Surgery completed

Classic Example (Figs. 8.19, 8.20, 8.21):

3. Points to note:
   (i) This method is suitable for patients with a higher peak of the Cupid's bow on the cleft side as compared to the unaffected side.

8.3.2 Downward Rotation Technique

1. Indications
   (i) The peak of the Cupid's bow on the cleft side was not sufficiently adjusted to the inferior position and extends into the portion of the skin on the upper lip.
2. Surgical methods and procedures
   (i) Following the principles of primary cleft lip repair: Reconstruct the orbicularis oris muscle and rotate the excessive peak of Cupid's bow downward.

An example of the surgical procedure (Fig. 8.22):

Following the principles of primary cleft lip repair: Determine the peak of the Cupid's bow on the unaffected side (point 2), the center of the philtrum (point 1), and the peak of the Cupid's bow on the cleft margin (point 3). Ensure that points 1–2 = 1–3. Mark the base of the nasal columella (point 6). Point 5 can be pinpointed by determining it accurately where points 5–2 = points 5–3. The distance from points 2 and 4 to the alar base on each side must be equal. Point 7 is the junction between the scar of the upper lip and the nasal base. Point 8 is at the alar base of the cleft side. Connect 3–6–5, 3–7, 4–7, and 7–8 with curvilinear lines.

Incise the skin layer according to the lines drawn and excise the scar on the skin portion of the lip (Fig. 8.23).

Dissect the orbicularis oris muscle from the skin and mucosal layers. Release the malposed orbicularis oris muscle attachments from the piriform aperture and anterior nasal spine on the cleft side (Fig. 8.24).

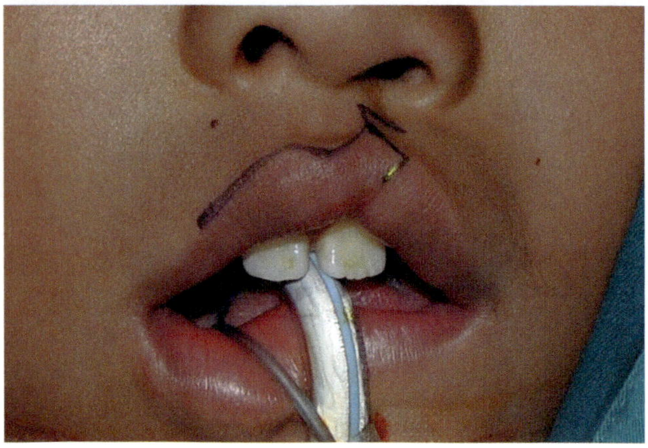

Fig. 8.19 Design of the surgical incisions

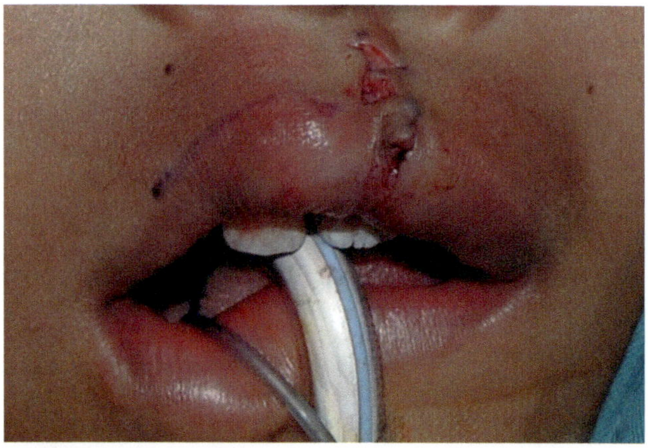

Fig. 8.20 The oblique skin flap is used to push the peak of the Cupid's bow inferiorly

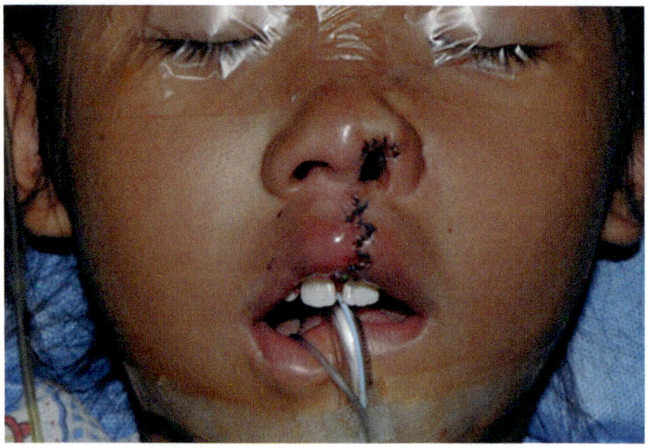

Fig. 8.21 Postoperative outcome

Pull the muscle bundle from the cleft side to the anterior nasal spine and use a 3–0 suture to secure it to the periosteum. Ensure equal height on both sides of the upper lip and no obvious upward movement of the alar base on the cleft side (Fig. 8.25).

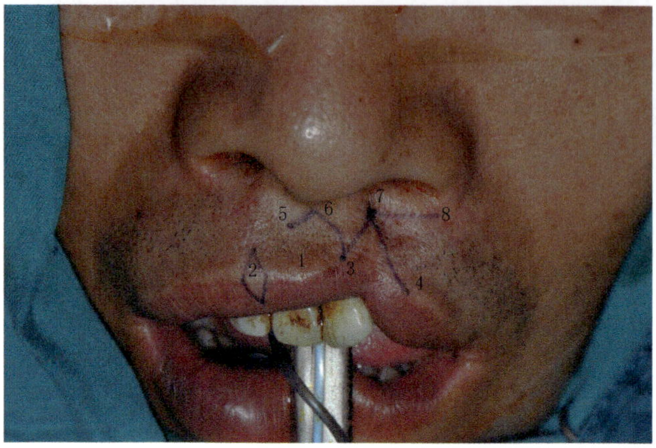

Fig. 8.22 Design of the surgical incisions

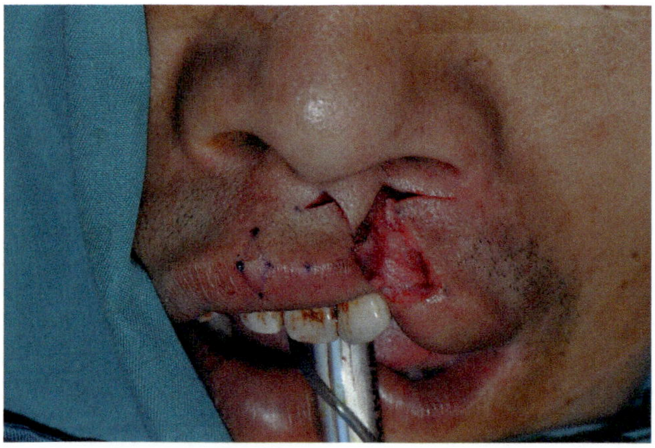

Fig. 8.23 Incise the skin layer

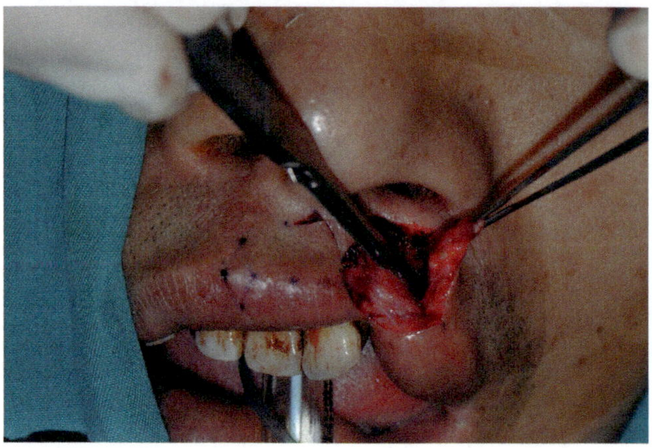

Fig. 8.24 Dissection of the orbicularis oris muscle

Pull the muscle bundles from the unaffected side inward and downward. Use the muscle bundles from the cleft side to fill up the space created as the result of the pulling maneuver. Complete the reconstruction of the orbicularis oris muscle by closing both ends of the muscle

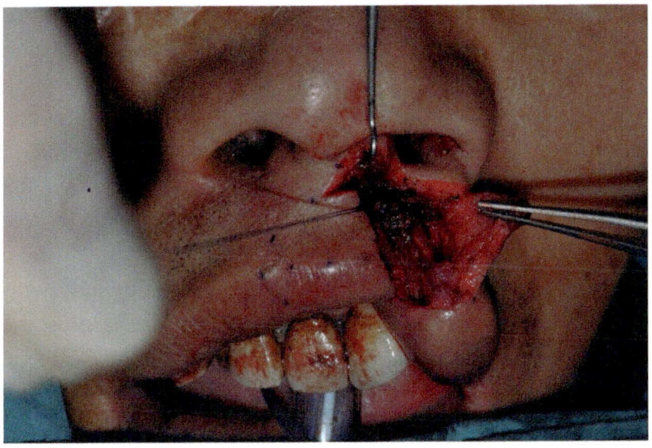

Fig. 8.25 Secure the upper part of the orbicularis oris muscle from the cleft side to the periosteum of the anterior nasal spine

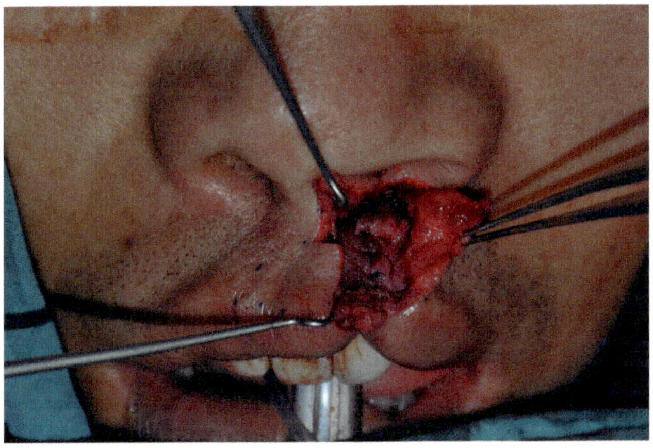

Fig. 8.26 Appose and close the ends of the orbicularis oris muscle bundles together

bundles together with 5–0 PDS interrupted suture ties (Fig. 8.26).

Use 6–0 resorbable sutures to close the subcutaneous layer at points 3 and 4. Start the closure from the bottom to the top. Remove excess subcutaneous tissue and close the skin with 6–0 cosmetic sutures.

Similarly, for the flap region close the subcutaneous layer first, alter the flap as required, and close the skin layer with cosmetic sutures (Fig. 8.27).

At the junction of dry and wet lip mucosa, insert a triangular flap from the cleft side into the opposite side to reconstruct the shape of the lip (Fig. 8.28).

3. Points to note:
   (i) As the nature of the surgery involves changing the position of the peak of the Cupid's bow on the cleft side, it is easy to result in a midline deviation of the upper lip. During the reconstruction process, secure the orbicularis oris muscle from the cleft side to the anterior nasal spine to ensure that the central portion of the lip is in the midline [1, 2].

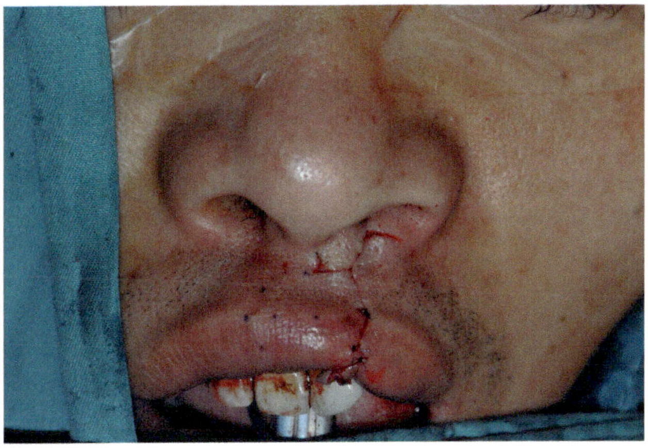

Fig. 8.27 Close the subcutaneous layer starting from the bottom to the top

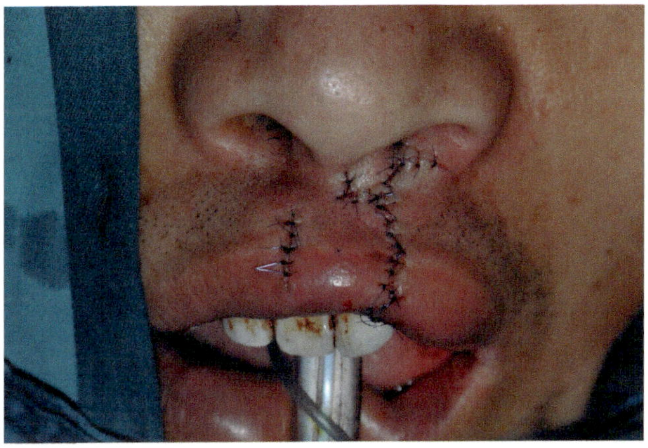

Fig. 8.28 Repair the lip mucosa

8.4 Correction of Excessive Upper Lip Length

1. Indications
   (i) The lip is longer on the cleft side than on the unaffected side.
2. Surgical methods and procedures
   (i) Dissect the orbicularis oris muscle extensively, and secure the muscle bundle from the cleft side to the anterior nasal spine. On the cleft side, cut away some portions of orbicularis oris muscle near the base of the nose as required. This will help to lift up the lip on the cleft side. Maintain the incisions in concealed areas as much as possible, and avoid unnecessary cutting of the skin on the cleft side. Specific to each case, the incision can be made through the base of the nose, the margin of the lip mucosa, oral mucosa, etc.

An example of the surgical procedure:

In this case, the alar on the cleft side was collapsed. A proposed approach would be a C-shaped incision on the cleft side involving the margin of the alar base, columella, and base of the nose. This will help in correcting the shape of the nose. The lip of this patient was also hypertrophic on the cleft side, and the lip tubercle was deviated. A lip mucosal flap was proposed to transfer excess tissues and reconstruct the lip shape. Approach and complete the reconstruction of the orbicularis oris muscle through the incisions on the nasal floor and the lower margin of the lip on the cleft side (Fig. 8.29).

Through the incisions made on the base of the nose and the lower margin of the lip, dissect the orbicularis oris muscle extensively. The superior border of the dissection is the base of the nose and anterior nasal spine, the mesial border may extend till the philtrum fossa, the lateral border is till the rim of the piriform aperture and the alar base, and the inferior border extends up to the most inferior rim of the orbicularis oris muscle (Fig. 8.30).

Dissect between the orbicularis oris muscle and the skin and between the muscle and the lip mucosa. Release the attachment of the malposed orbicularis oris muscle from the anterior nasal spine and the piriform aperture on the cleft side (Fig. 8.31).

Identify the orbicularis oris muscle underlying the philtrum ridge on the cleft side. Cut the muscle at about 3 mm from the philtrum ridge on the cleft side. This permits a greater amount of muscle of the unaffected side to be rotated toward the lip tubercle and allows the latter to appear fuller. In addition, the shorter length of the muscle bundle allows the lip to be lifted up on the cleft side. Pull and secure the muscle bundle from the cleft side to the anterior nasal spine. Make sure that both sides of the upper lip are of equal length without any obvious upward movement of the alar base on the cleft side. If the upper portion of the muscle on the cleft side is excessively thick, it can obstruct the lifting of the upper lip. In such situations, the muscle can be trimmed as appropriate. Using either 3–0 silk or nylon sutures, anchor the muscle bundle from the cleft side to the periosteum of the anterior nasal spine and nasal base. Pull the muscle bundle from the unaffected side downward and inward. After this, take the muscles from the cleft side and insert it into the space formed. Complete the reconstruction of the orbicularis oris muscle with 5–0 PDS interrupted sutures (Figs. 8.32 and 8.33).

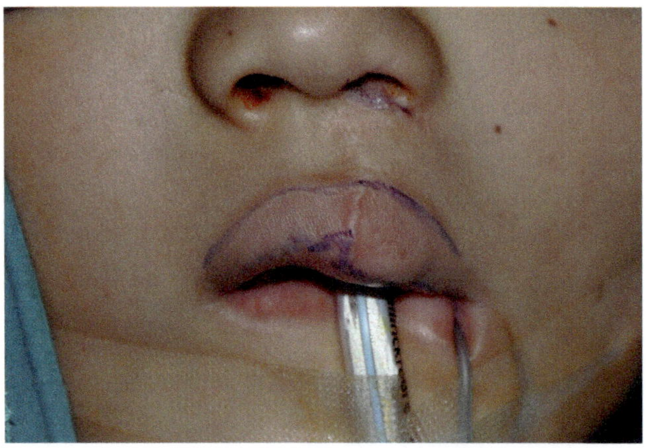

Fig. 8.29 Design of the surgical incisions

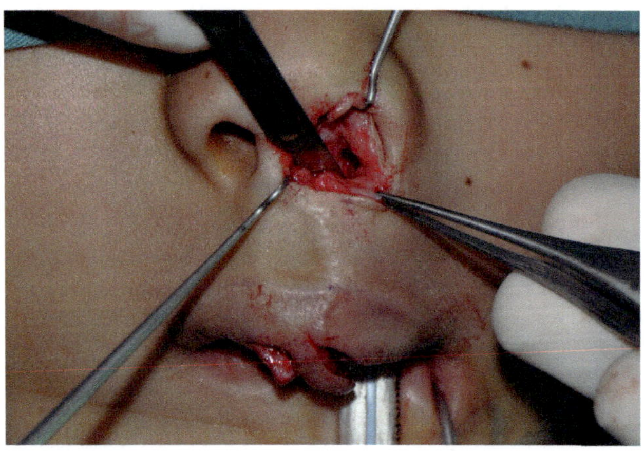

Fig. 8.30 Dissection of the orbicularis oris muscle

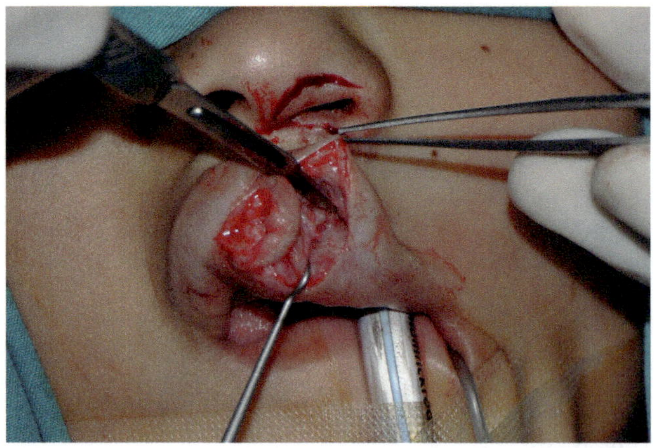

Fig. 8.31 Dissection of the orbicularis oris muscle

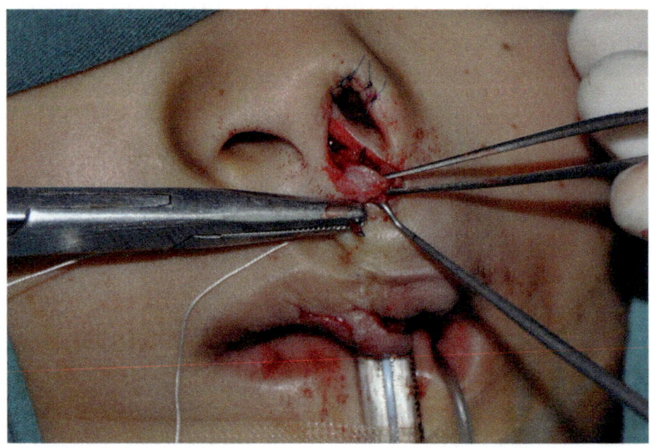

Fig. 8.32 Secure the upper part of the orbicularis oris muscle from the cleft side

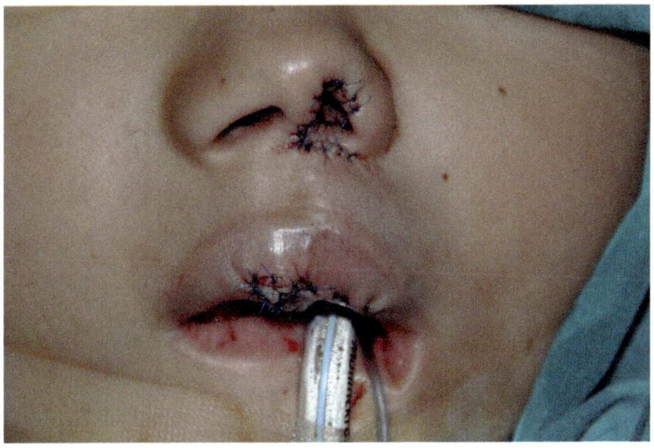

Fig. 8.33 Surgery Completed

3. Points to note:
   (i) It is necessary to extensively dissect the alar base of the cleft side in order to prevent its upward movement when the upper lip is lifted. This will allow the muscle and the skin of the alar base to move separately and thus, prevents the upward shift of the alar base.
   (ii) Postoperative relapse can be reduced by the use of 1 to 2 non-absorbable sutures to anchor the orbicularis oris muscle to the periosteum of the anterior nasal spine and the nasal base.
   (iii) If it is too thick, the upper portion of the muscles on the cleft side may be trimmed as required.

References

1. Bing S, Zheng Q. Composite treatment of cleft lip and palate (in Chinese). Military Science Publishing House; 2011.
2. Bing S, Sheng L. Salyer's Atlas of cleft lip and palate surgery (in Chinese). Military Science Publishing House; 2007.

9 Repair of Secondary Deformities of Bilateral Cleft Lip Surgery

Qian Zheng

9.1 Correction of Whistle Deformity of the Lip

1. Indications
   (i) The central portion of the lip mucosa is deficient, and the lip tubercle may even be absent.
   (ii) The lateral portion of the lips is hypertrophic.
   (iii) The philtrum is too wide and rounded.
   (iv) Large and thick scars on one or both sides of the philtrum ridge.
2. Surgical Methods and Procedures
   (i) Excise the scars on the sides of the philtrum ridge, and trim the excess width of the philtrum. Rotate the deep layers of the orbicularis oris muscle 90° inwards and downwards, bulking up the lip tubercle in the process. Finally, raise bilateral local flaps from the lip mucosa and advance them towards the midline. This will create the appearance of a fuller lip tubercle.

An Example of the Surgical Procedure:

The width of the philtrum is based on the width of the columella. Mark the planned peak of the Cupid's bow on the vermillion border as points 1 and 2. Do the same for the contra-lateral side and mark them as points 3 and 4. Lastly, mark the wet-dry lip mucosa junction of the prolabium as points 5 and 6 (Fig. 9.1).

Excise the scars on the philtrum ridges and the extended portion of skin into the lip mucosa (Fig. 9.2).

Incise the mucosa along the dry-wet lip junction of the prolabium. Expose the deep layers of the orbicularis oris muscle underneath the skin portion of the lip. Rotate the muscle 90° inwards and downwards to fill up the lip tubercle (Fig. 9.3).

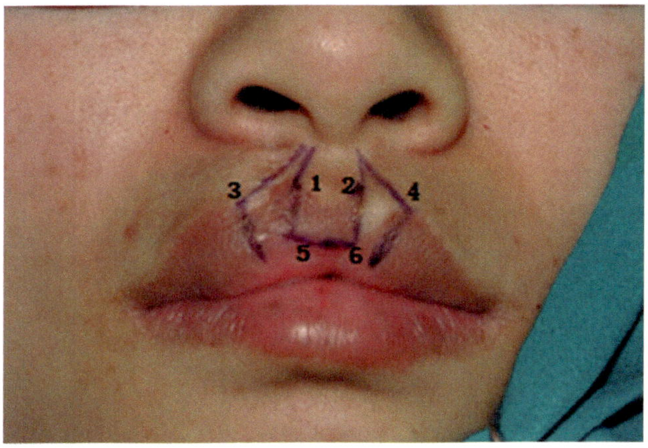

Fig. 9.1 Design of the surgical incisions

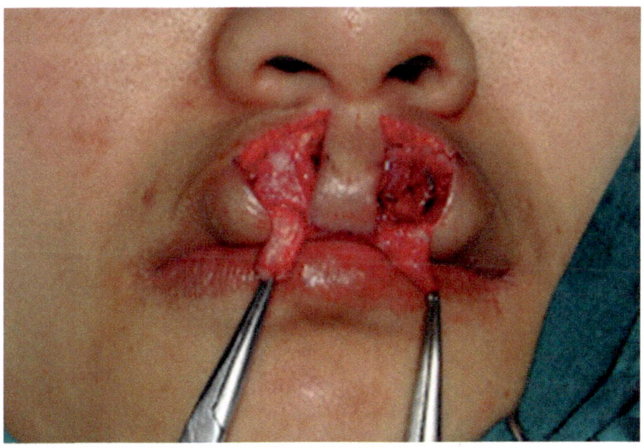

Fig. 9.2 Excise the scars on the bilateral philtrum ridges

On each side, appose and suture the planned peaks of Cupid's bow from the prolabium and lateral lip together. This will reconstruct the arch of the Cupid's bow (Fig. 9.4).

Advance the bilateral myomucosal flaps towards the midline. Next, close the mucosal flaps together in a zig-zag manner to create a plump lip tubercle (Fig. 9.5).

Classic Example:

Q. Zheng (✉)
Department of Cleft Lip and Palate Surgery, West China Stomatology Hospital, Sichuan University, Chengdu, China

J. Liu, B. Shi (eds.), *Atlas of Lip and Nose Plastic and Cosmetic Surgery*, https://doi.org/10.1007/978-981-16-1911-3_9

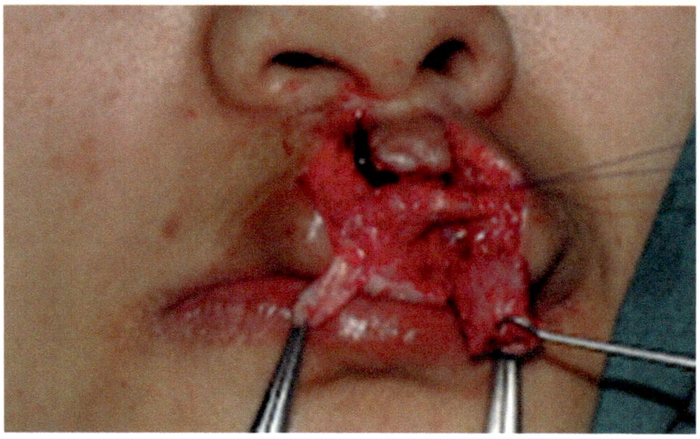

Fig. 9.3 Rotation of the orbicularis oris muscle flaps

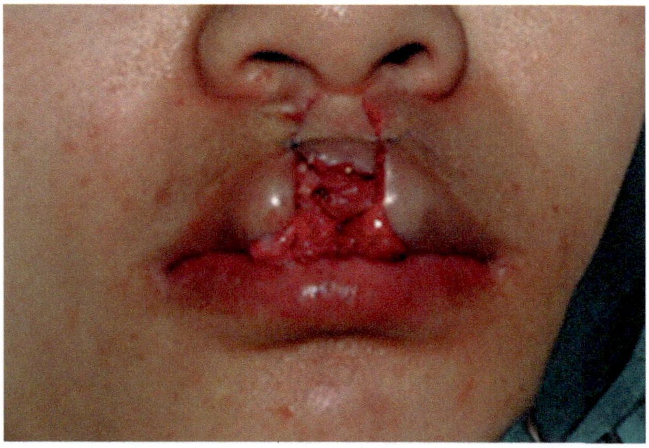

Fig. 9.4 Apposition and closure

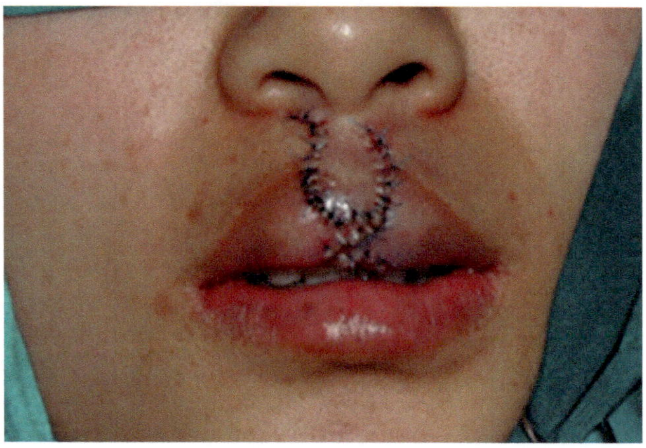

Fig. 9.5 Surgery Completed

Excise the scars on the sides of the philtrum ridge, and trim the excess width of the philtrum. After which, rotate the lip mucosa and the underlying layers 90°, bulking up the lip tubercle in the process (Figs. 9.6 and 9.7).

3. Points to Note
   (i) The incision length of the lateral lip and the front lip is often different. First, match the peaks of Cupid's bow and then suture upwards from this point. Lastly, cut away excess skin of the lateral lip components at the region near the base of the columella.
   (ii) The dry mucosa of the prolabium can be removed, provided that there is enough mucosa on both sides of the lip to cover the wound after lip tubercle reconstruction.
   (iii) Make full use of the myomucosal flaps from both sides of the lip to reconstruct the surface of the lip tubercle. The apposition of the myomucosal flaps in the midline will allow the lip tubercle to appear more natural.

9.2 Reconstruction of the Philtrum Ridges (Fossa)

1. Indications
   (i) The philtrum fossa is too wide and round.
   (ii) There is a bulge at the central portion of the philtrum fossa.
   (iii) The scars at the sides of the philtrum ridges are pronounced.
   (iv) The upper lip does not appear to be overly tight.
2. Surgical Methods and Procedures
   (i) Excise the scars on the sides of the philtrum ridge, and trim the excess width of the philtrum. Make an incision on both sides of the lip, and from the lateral and medial side of the incision dissect and deglove the orbicularis oris muscle. Fold the ends of the muscle from each side and suture them together. This will bulk up the tissues at the interface between the prolabium and lateral lips (the philtrum ridges).
   (ii) Reconstruct the philtrum fossa and ridges by closing the subcutaneous layers of the prolabium and lateral lips together.
   (iii) Cutaway a portion of submucosal and muscular tissues at the center of the deep surface of the orbicularis oris muscle. Next, suture the superficial muscle tissues to the periosteum of the anterior maxilla to form the philtrum fossa.

An Example of the Surgical Procedure:

On each side, draw the lateral section of the incision along the scar. Make the medial incision by modeling it after the normal appearance of a philtrum, where the upper part is narrower and the lower part is wider. The width of the upper part

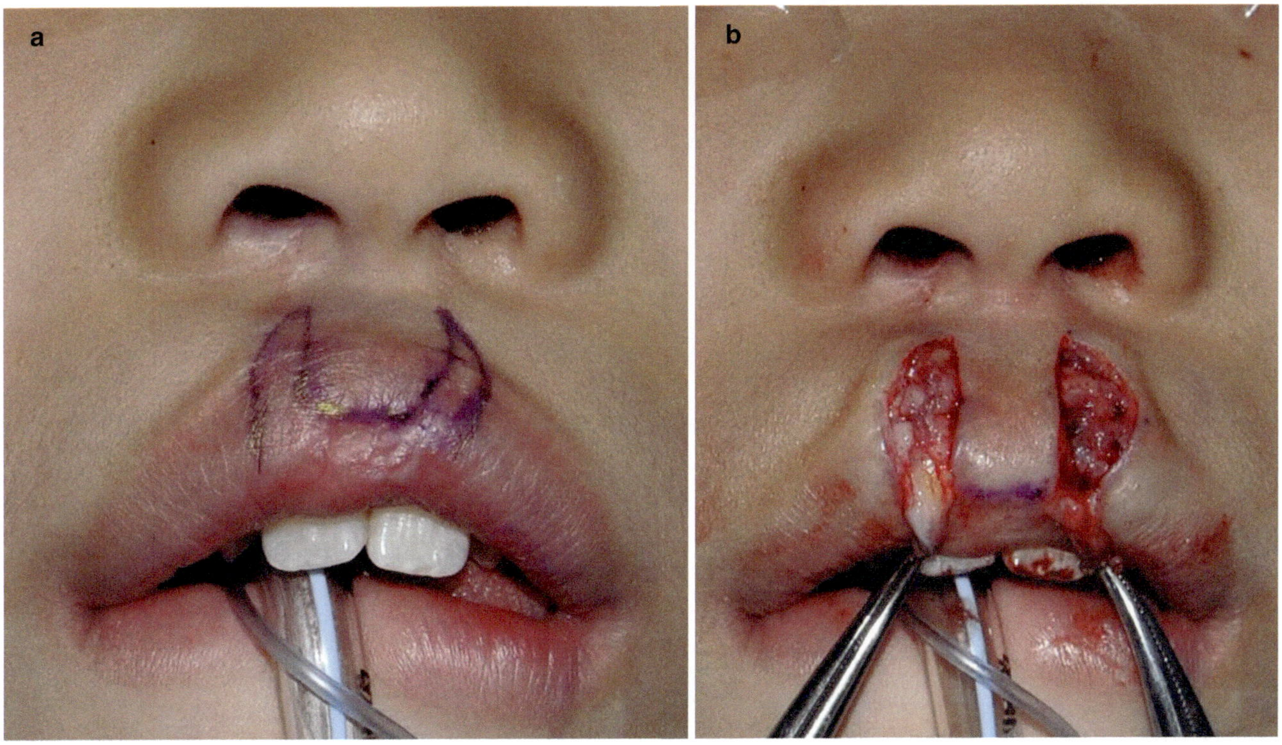

Fig. 9.6 (**a** and **b**) Excise the scars and trim the excess width of the philtrum

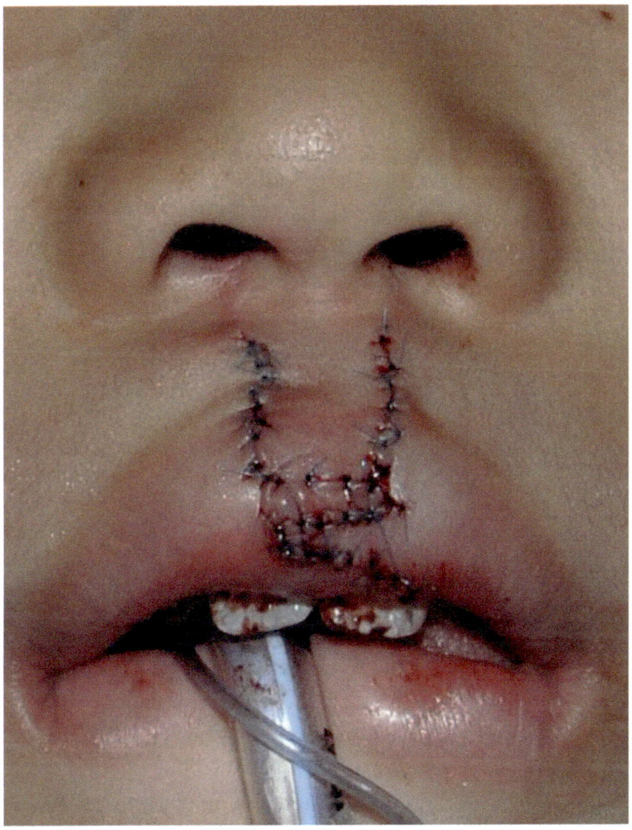

Fig. 9.7 The lip mucosa rotated 90° to cover over the lip tubercle

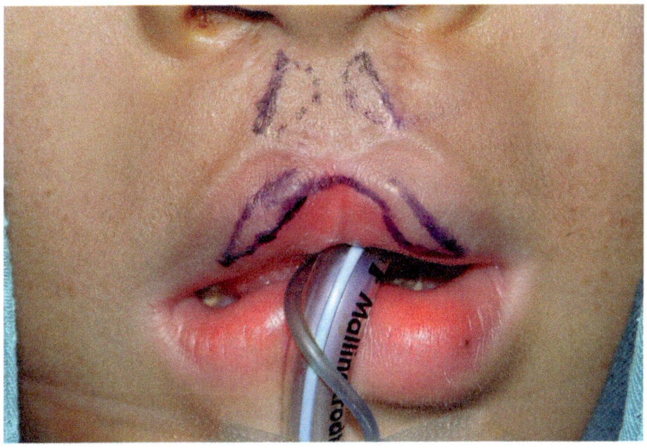

Fig. 9.8 Design of the surgical incisions

of the philtrum is based on the width of the columella (Fig. 9.8).

Excise the scars on both sides of the philtrum. Resect only the skin layer and preserve the deeper tissue layers (Fig. 9.9).

On each side, fold the deeper tissue layers of the lateral lips and suture it (Fig. 9.10).

Create the bulge of the philtrum ridge by tying the orbicularis oris muscle of the lateral lips to the muscle of the prolabium using horizontal mattress sutures (Figs. 9.11 and 9.12).

Classic Example (Figs. 9.13, 9.14, 9.15):

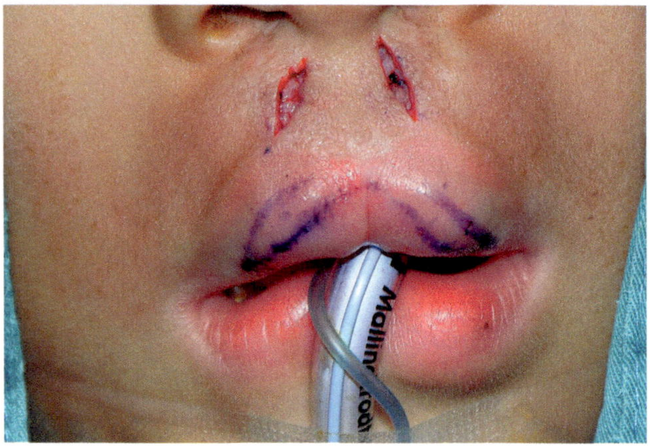

Fig. 9.9 Resection of the bilateral scars on the philtrum

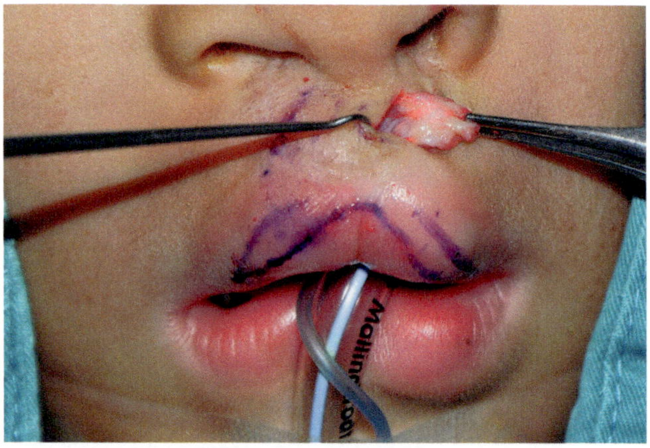

Fig. 9.10 Fold the tissues of the lateral lips

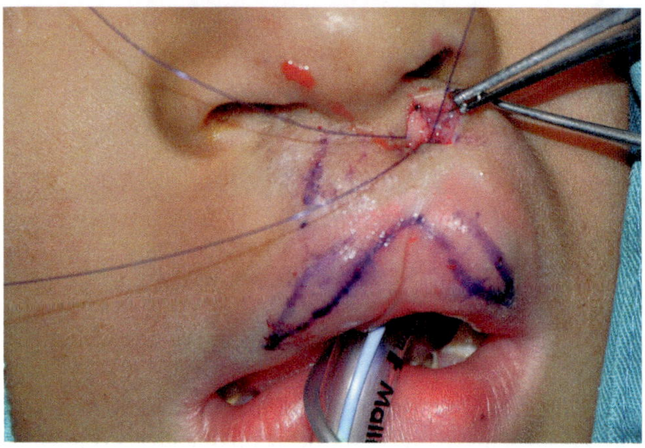

Fig. 9.11 Horizontal mattress suture

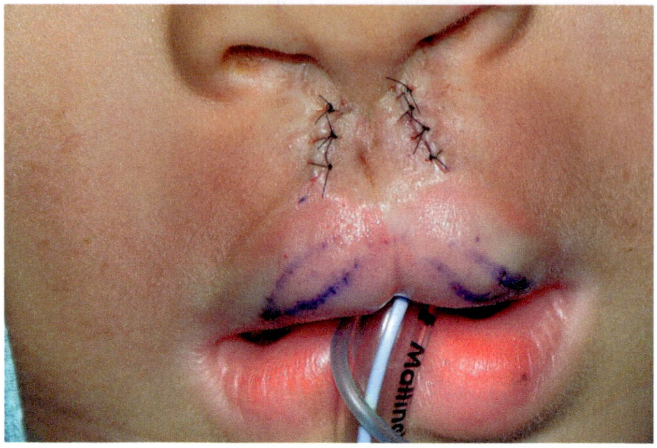

Fig. 9.12 Reconstructed philtrum fossa

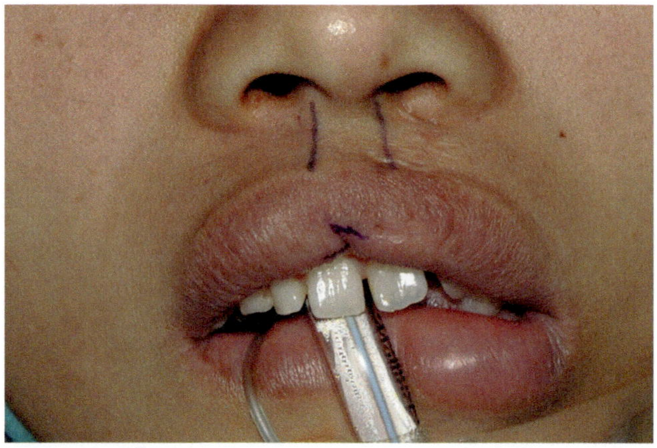

Fig. 9.13 In this case, the philtrum is too wide. Excise the scar tissues to regain a normal philtrum width

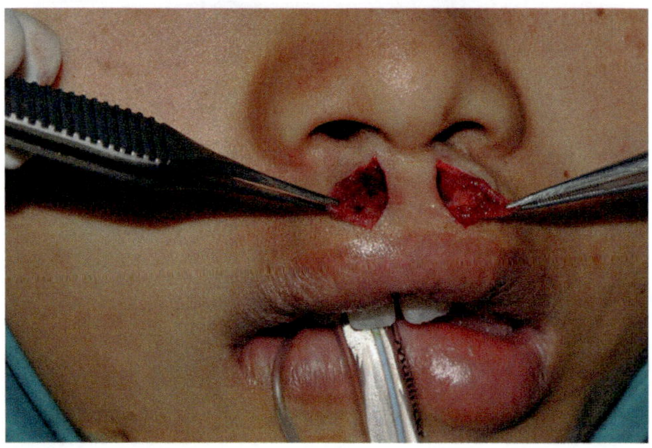

Fig. 9.14 Fold and suture the deep layers of the lateral lips

3. Points to Note
   (i) When closing the deep layers of the prolabium and the lateral lips using horizontal mattress sutures, ensure that the needle entry point is at an equal distance on each side of the incision. Upon completion of the closure, check that the skin margins are everted to produce a natural-looking philtrum ridge.

(ii) Suture the superficial tissues of the philtrum to the periosteum of the anterior maxilla at the midline. This is to prevent deviation of the philtrum.

9.3 Correction of a Tight Upper Lip

1. Indications
   (i) The repaired upper lip is too tight, and the lower lip has an obvious protrusion.
   (ii) The scar on the prolabium is so thick that excision and closure will result in an overly tight lip.
   (iii) Severe whistle deformity of the prolabium that will require lower lip tissue transfer to compensate for the deficiency.
   (iv) Adolescents (over the age 15 years old) with good compliance and tolerance.
2. Surgical Methods and Procedures
   (i) Depending on the case, choose between excising the scars on the prolabium, or making a full thickness incision at the midline of the lip. Next, release the upper lip from the underlying attachments and examine the resultant defect. Based on the average philtrum width and shape, design a full thickness lower lip flap (Abbe flap) to replace the defect and reconstruct the upper lip.

An Example of the Surgical Procedure:

Upper lip Incision Design: Mark the intended peaks of the Cupid's bow at the white roll of the lip. Draw the incision line from this point to the most upper end of the pre-existing scar, at the point closest to the base of the columella. This should be done for both sides of the lips (Figs. 9.16 and 9.17).

Lower Lip Abbe Flap: Mark two points side by side at the center of the lower lip. The distance between the two points should be according to the average width of the upper philtrum (for adults, that is approximately 11 mm). The shape of the Abbe flap is based on the normal appearance of the philtrum.

Dissect and separate the bilateral vessels supplying the lower lip. Cut the vessel on one side while preserving the other (Fig. 9.18).

Excise the irregular philtrum tissues (Fig. 9.19).

Rotate the Abbe flap 180° to replace the missing upper lip tissues (Figs. 9.20, 9.21, 9.22).

Classic Example (Figs. 9.23 and 9.24):

3. Points to note
   (i) The inferior lip artery is generally parallel to the vermillion of the lower lip. At the junction between the lip mucosa and the orbicularis oris muscle, the artery is close to the white roll and the oral mucosa, about 2–3 mm away from the lip mucosa. When raising the Abbe flap, it is safe for vertical incisions of the skin below the white roll to be cut to full thickness

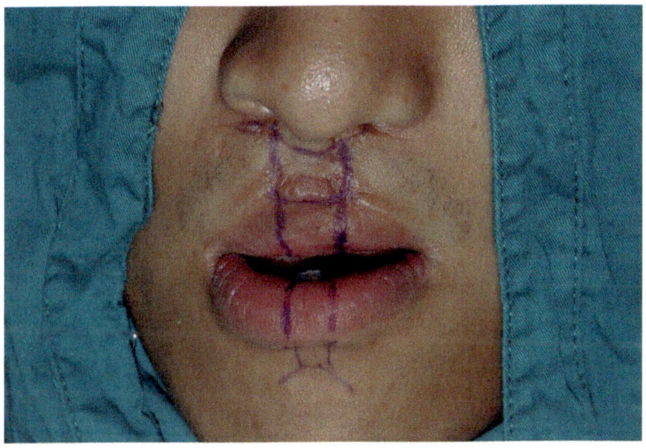

Fig. 9.16 Design of the surgical incisions

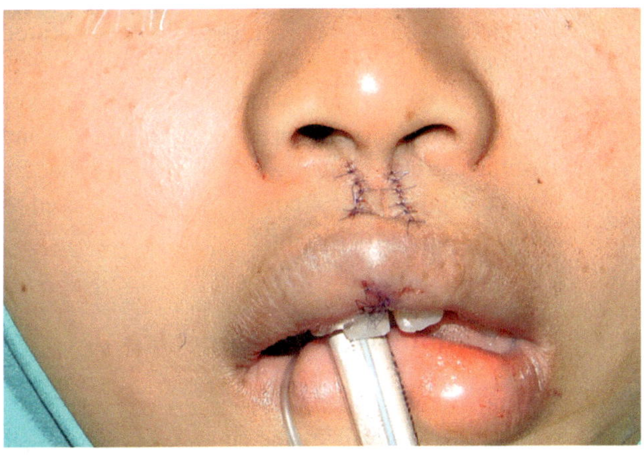

Fig. 9.15 Use Z-plasty flaps to get rid of the groove on the lower margin of the lip

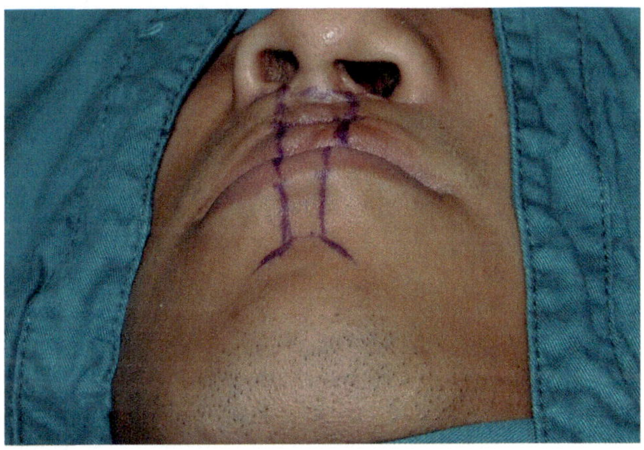

Fig. 9.17 Design of the surgical incisions

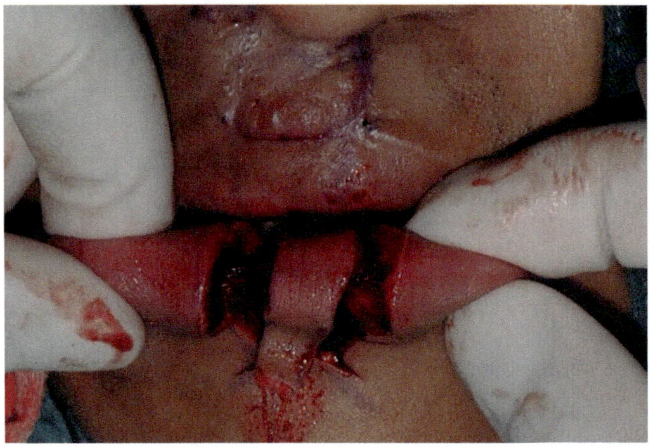

Fig. 9.18 Preparation of the vascularized pedicle

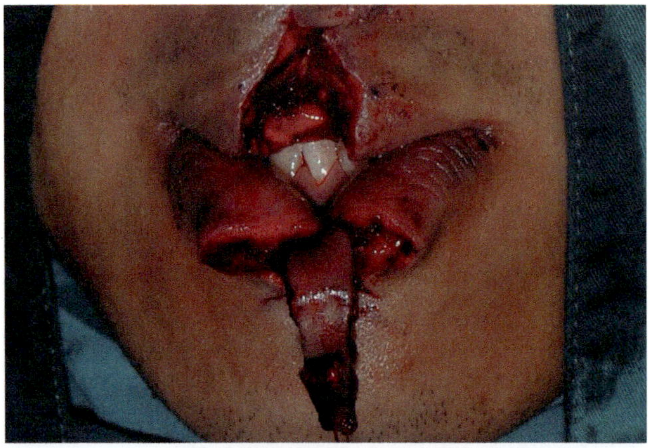

Fig. 9.19 After excising the scars on the upper lip

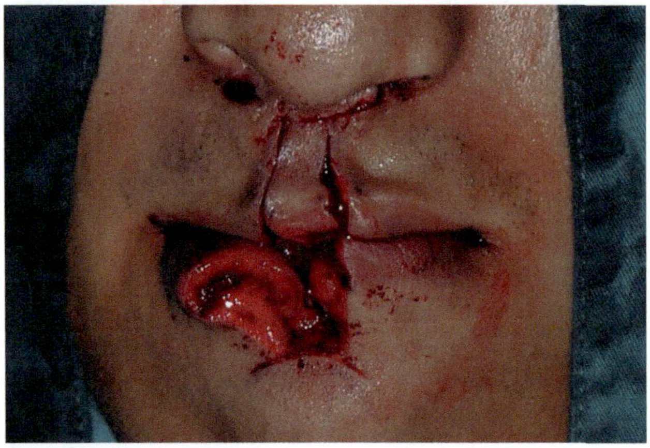

Fig. 9.20 Abbe flap rotation

through to the oral mucosa. However, care must be taken during dissection of the lip mucosa area, especially note that the depth of the incision should not exceed 2 mm. During the preparation of the vascularized pedicle, it is advised to first expose the vessels on both sides before severing the artery. Traction of the artery on one side can help to locate the pedicle on the other side. The muscle bundles surrounding the artery should be retained on the side of the Abbe flap. The diameter of the pedicle should be about 2 mm, as excessive thickness will hinder the rotation and placing of the flap. Conversely, if it is too thin, the blood vessel may become deformed and obstructed. Vascular pedicles that are too thin are also not conducive for retrograde venous blood flow [1, 2].

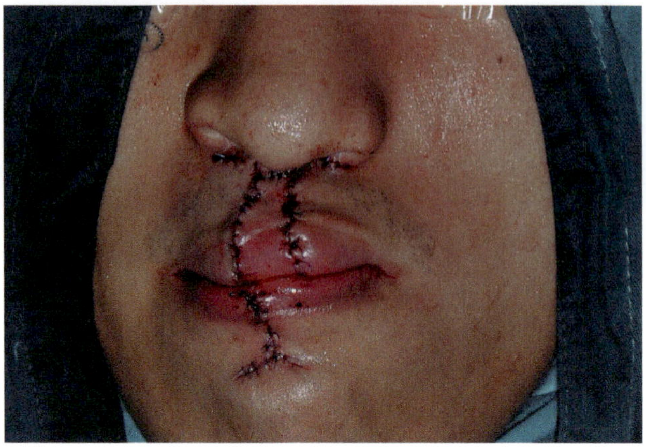

Fig. 9.21 Apposition and suturing

(ii) Upon rotation, use sutures to fix the Abbe flap to its approximate location. The suturing should be done on the inner side first before the outer, and on the bottom before the upper. First, fixate the oral mucosa on the most distal part of the flap, as well as the muscle flap with 2–3 sutures. Then match the height of the peaks of the Cupid's bow to their appropriate position. The flap may then be sutured to the lateral lips from the bottom to the top. The closure of the muscle layer with 2–3 sutures is to avoid the formation of dead space and hematoma. However, it should not be sutured too tightly.

(iii) Avoid excessive pulling when closing the margins of the flap as it can result in arterial compression and insufficient blood supply. Some remaining mucosa can be exposed. Local compression can be used to stop post-operative bleeding.

9.4 Correction of a Short Upper Lip

1. Indications
   (i) The anterior part of the repaired lip is too short compared to the lateral part of the lips.
2. Surgical Methods and Procedures

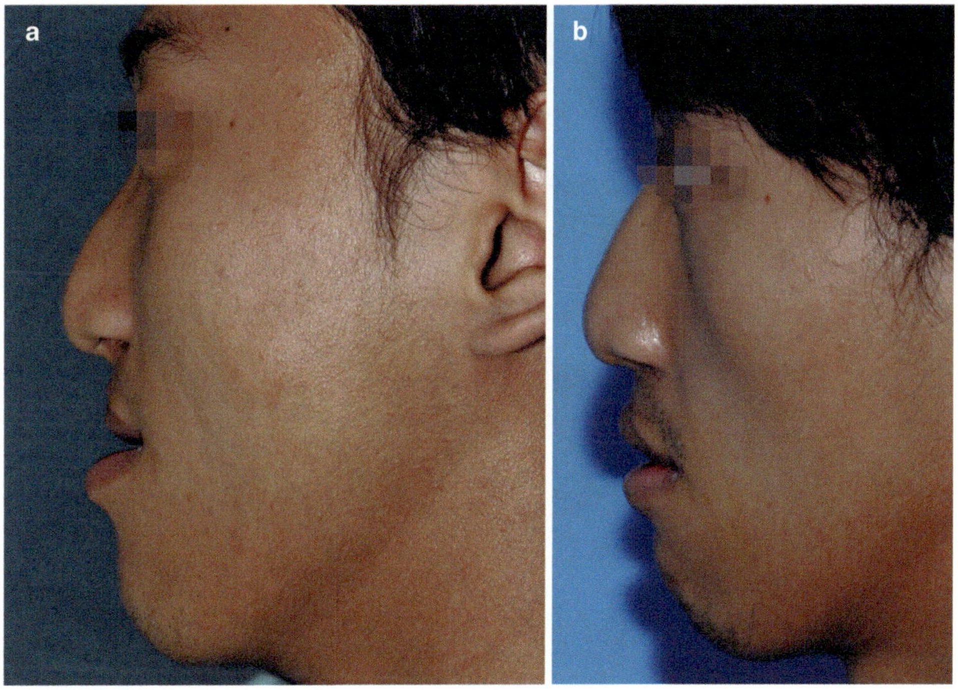

Fig. 9.22 (**a** and **b**) Comparison between the pre-operative and post-operative profile

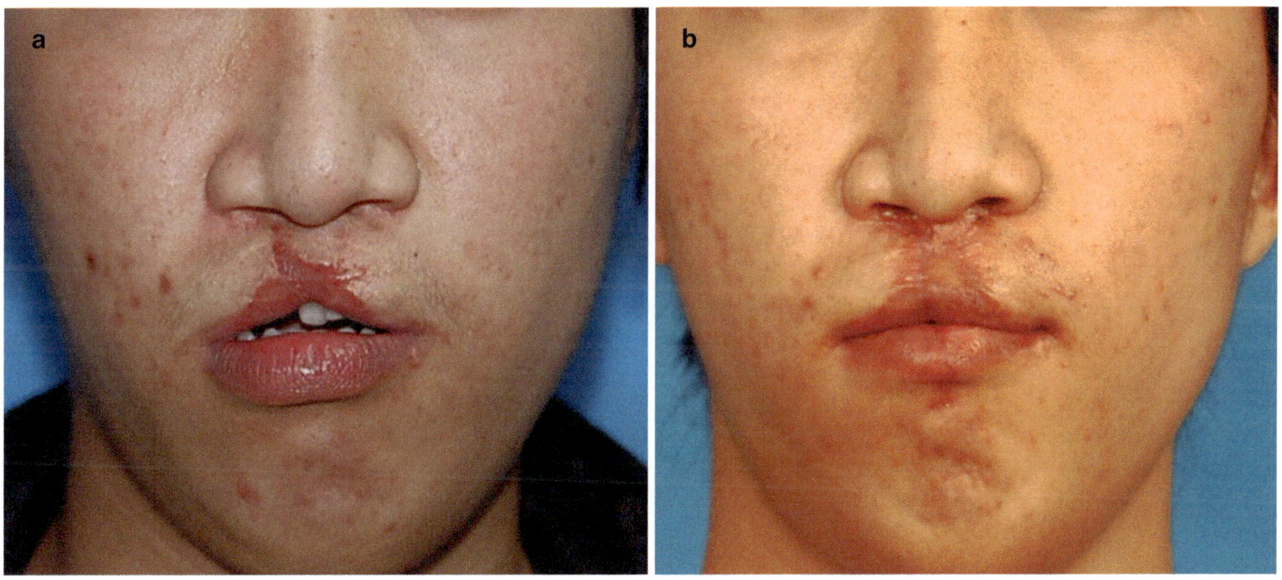

Fig. 9.23 (**a** and **b**) Comparison of the pre-operative and post-operative frontal view

(i) Incise the skin of the philtrum below the base of the columella. Pull the cut portion inferiorly and align it with the lateral lips to reconstruct the Cupid's bow. Fill the defect at the superior part of the philtrum with the tissues from the lateral lip.

An example of the Surgical Procedure:

The transverse incision is made inferior to the base of the columella, across to the nasolabial junction, and a small distance away from the alar base. The vertical incisions are made along the edge of the scars at the philtrum ridge. Upon reaching the peaks of the Cupid's bow, turn the incisions inwards until the incisions meet at the center of the lower lip margin (Fig. 9.25).

Cut the skin of the philtrum below the base of the columella and reposition the patch inferiorly (Fig. 9.26).

Release the orbicularis oris muscle away from the periosteum of the anterior nasal spine (below the base of the columella) (Fig. 9.27).

Reconstruct the Cupid's bow by shifting the patch of skin inferiorly and matching it with the lateral lip (Fig. 9.28).

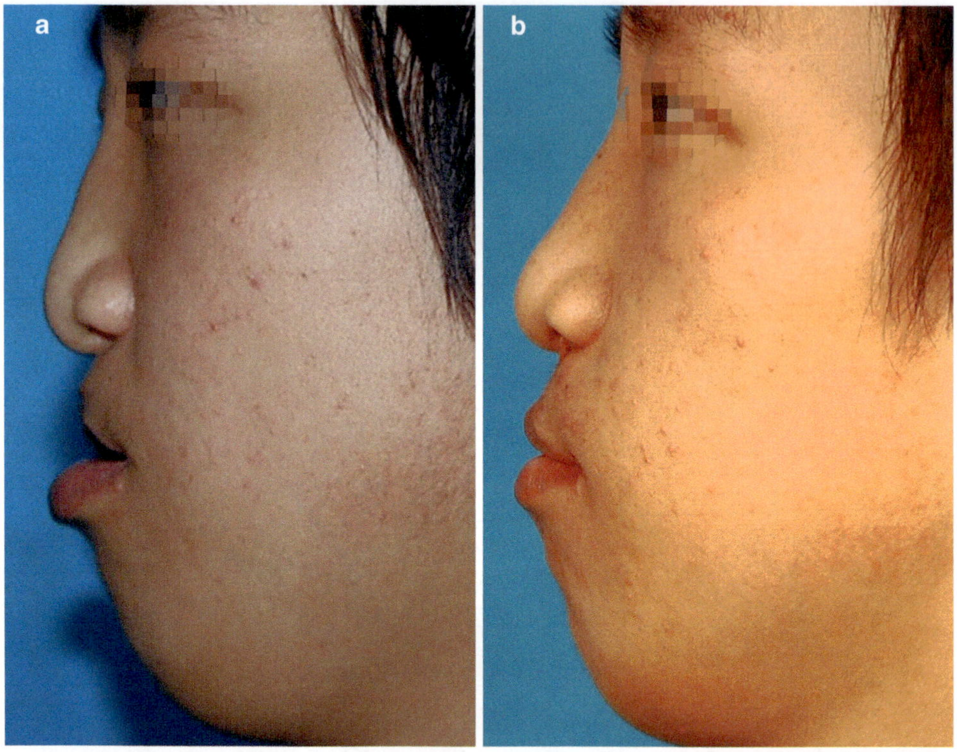

Fig. 9.24 (**a** and **b**) Comparison of the pre-operative and post-operative profile

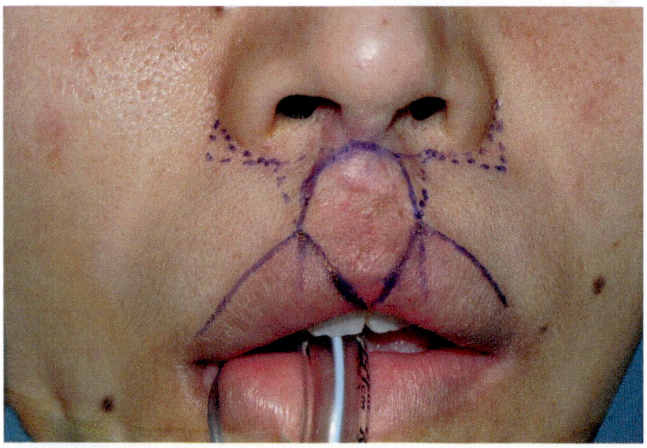

Fig. 9.25 Design of the surgical incisions

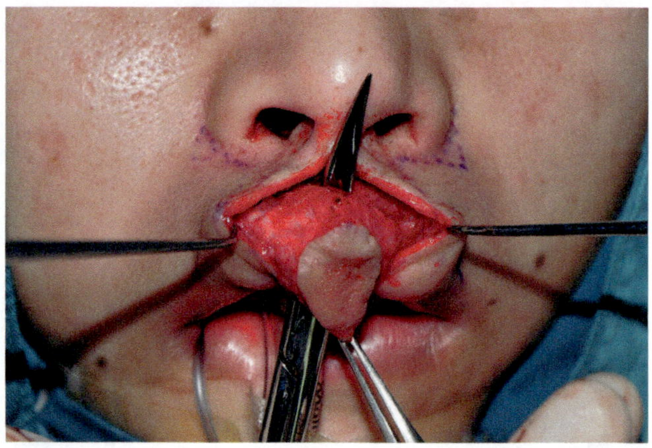

Fig. 9.27 Release the orbicularis oris muscle

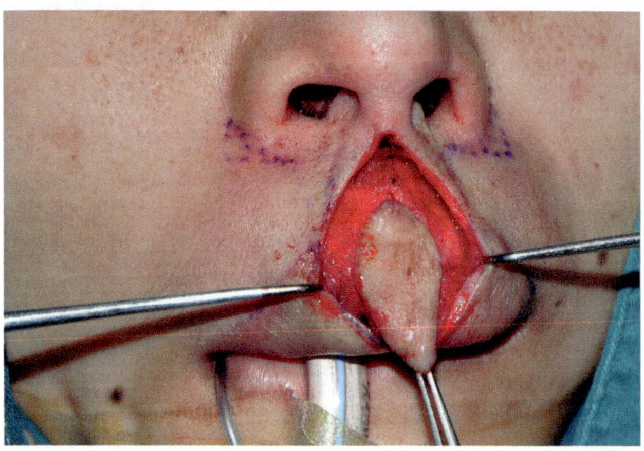

Fig. 9.26 Reposition the philtrum skin patch inferiorly

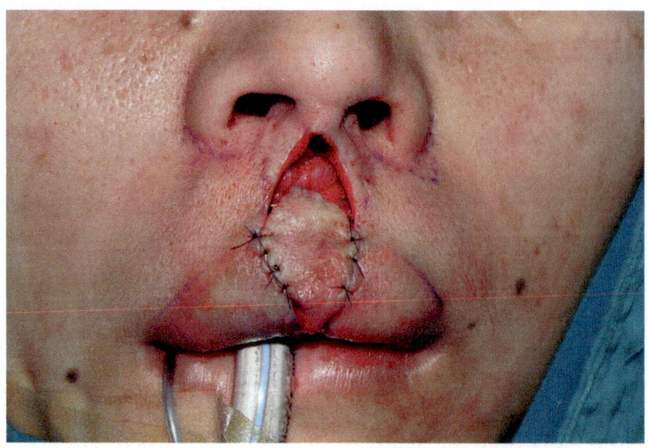

Fig. 9.28 Reconstruction of the Cupid's Bow

Pull the tissues from the lateral lips towards the midline and close the defect on the superior part of the philtrum (Fig. 9.29).

Classic Example (Figs. 9.30, 9.31, 9.32, 9.33):

3. Points to Mote
   (i) Keep the vertical incisions within the subcutaneous tissues and the superficial layer of the orbicularis oris muscle. Maintain the connection of the orbicularis oris muscle from the lateral lip to the philtrum area to ensure adequate blood supply to the philtrum skin flap.
   (ii) The anterior maxilla is the main vascular supply to the philtrum skin flap. Therefore, do not strip the orbicularis oris muscle from the surface of the bone when severing it from the anterior nasal spine.
   (iii) The purpose of the incisions around the philtrum is to allow it to be shifted inferiorly without hindrance. It is necessary to be vigilant about the blood supply to the flap, and to avoid extensive incisions, as poor wound healing, large scars, and even necrosis of the skin flaps may result.

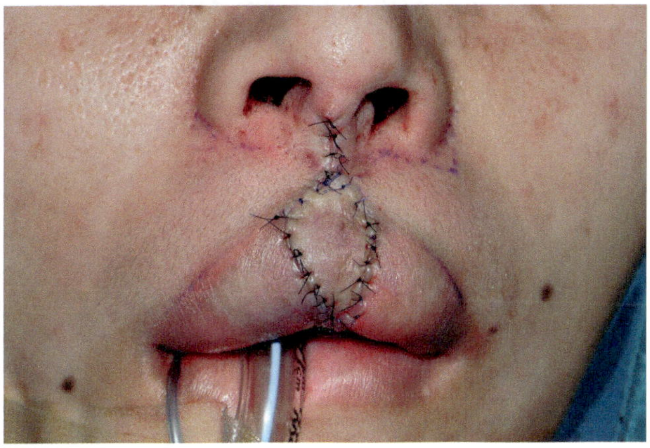

Fig. 9.29 Advancement of the lateral lip towards the midline

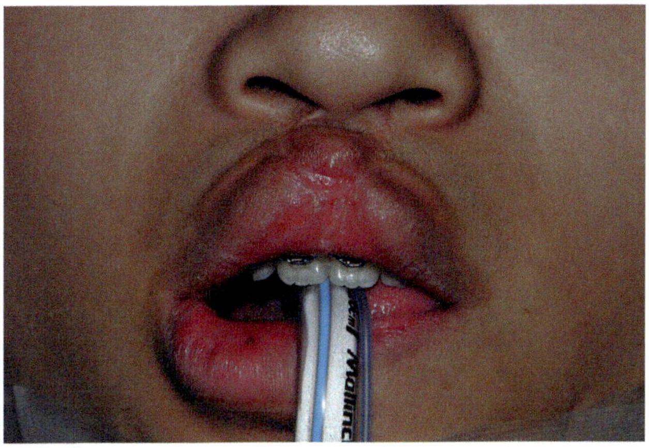

Fig. 9.30 The median lip tubercle is divided into three, the Cupid's bow is disrupted and skin of the philtrum is short

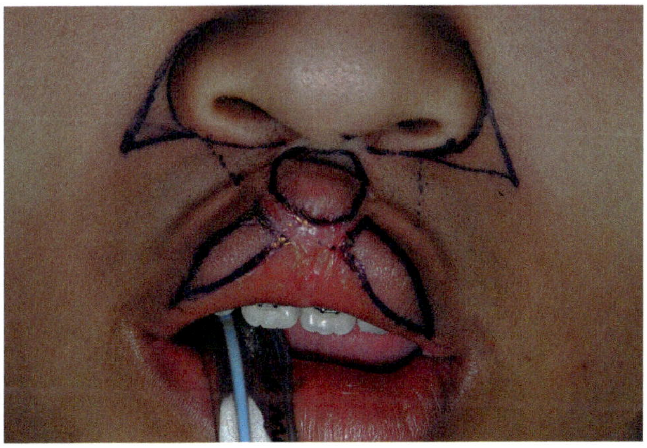

Fig. 9.31 Rotate the tissues of the nasolabial groove inwards and downwards to prolong the upper part of the philtrum

9.5 Correction of a Long Upper Lip

1. Indications
   (i) The lateral portion of the repaired lip is too long on either one or both sides.
2. Surgical Methods and Procedures
   (i) Lift the orbicularis oris muscle up by removing part of the muscle and the overlying tissue layers under the nasal base.

An Example of the Surgical Procedure:

The vertical incisions are made along where the normal philtrum ridges would be but slightly slanted to allow the top of the philtrum to be narrower than the bottom. The horizontal incisions are hidden at the nasolabial junction, stopping at the medial ends of the alar (Fig. 9.34).

Make full-thickness incisions along the philtrum ridges and at the nasolabial junction. Expose and deglove the orbicularis oris muscle (Fig. 9.35).

Lift the bilateral orbicularis oris muscle upwards and secure them to the periosteum of the anterior nasal spine (Fig. 9.36).

Make transverse incisions on each side of the lateral lip to remove the upper part of the orbicularis oris muscle and the overlying tissue (Fig. 9.37).

Through bilateral alar Tajima "Reverse U" incisions, suture the bilateral alar cartilages together to correct the flattened alars (Fig. 9.38).

Classic Example (Figs. 9.39, 9.40, 9.41, 9.42, 9.43):

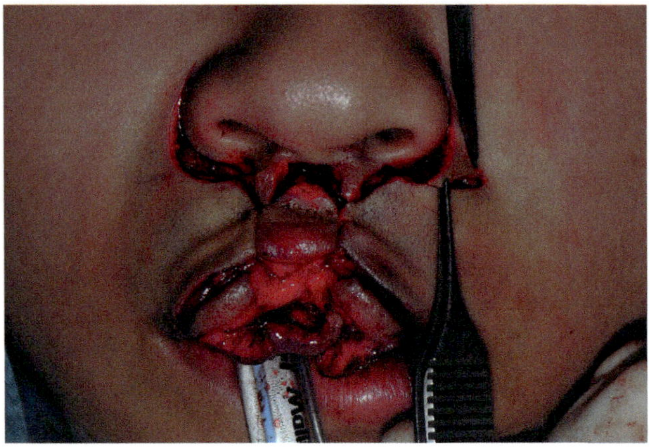

Fig. 9.32 Cut away the peri-alar skins to allow the skin flap to have greater mobility

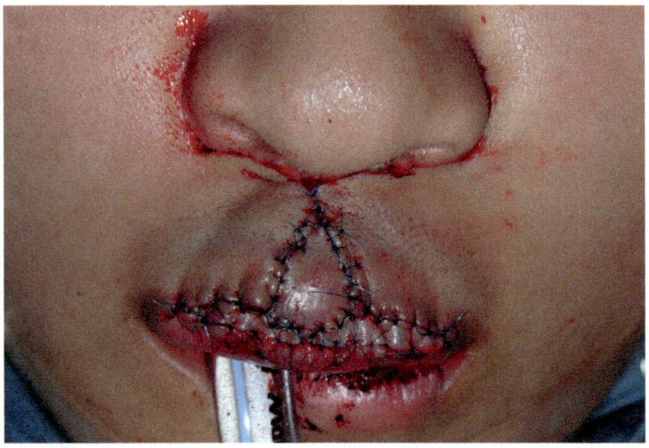

Fig. 9.33 Surgery completed

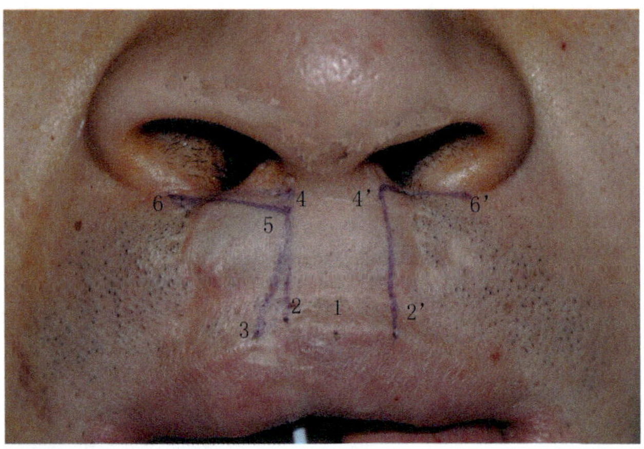

Fig. 9.34 Design of the surgical incisions

3. Points to Note:
   (i) The lifting of the orbicularis oris muscle must be equal on both sides. Otherwise, it will lead to an asymmetrical Cupid's bow.
   (ii) After lifting the orbicularis oris muscle, it should be secured to the periosteum of the anterior maxilla.

9.6 Repair of Alveolar Cleft with Bone Graft

In some cases, a tight upper lip may be the result of a palatal and alveolar bone cleft. The lip becomes severely retruded due to poor development of the maxilla. The usual approach for managing tight upper lips is not advisable in these cases and will lead to a poor outcome. Very often it is necessary to proceed with an alveolar bone graft, followed by orthodontic therapy or orthognathic surgery.

1. Indications
   (i) Cleft type: Linear cleft (width < 5 mm).
   (ii) The incisor foramen does not have a large fistula.
   (iii) The mucosa lining of the cleft is intact: There is no ectopic tooth within the cleft.
2. Surgical Methods and Procedures
   (i) Palatal Incision: First, make vertical incisions along the sides of the alveolar cleft. At the alveolar crest region, turn the incisions horizontally and apical to the gingival papilla. This will form 2 P-shaped palatal flaps on each side of the cleft (Fig. 9.44a). The vertical incisions may be placed further within the cleft, and towards the buccal side if the cleft is too wide.
   (ii) Buccal Incision: Similarly, first make the incisions along the two sides of the cleft and then continue horizontally along the gingiva of two more teeth. The labium frenulum should not be excessed in the incisions, and dental papilla should be reserved. Join the buccal incision with the palatal incision at the alveolar crest (Fig. 9.44a).
   (iii) Incision Within the Cleft: Make triangular incisions on the inner walls of the cleft (on the alveolar process). The apex of the triangle is towards the alveolar crest. This forms N-shaped nasal flaps on each side to close the nasal cavity defect. The remaining tissues are turned outwards to the buccal side to form L-shaped flaps (Fig. 9.44b).
   (iv) Closure of the Wound: Rotate the distal N-flap 90° to the nasal cavity and suture it vertically with the palatal tissues. Then close the distal and medial N-flaps together. Finally, close the palatal and buccal flaps to close the cleft (Fig. 9.44c).

An example of the Surgical Procedure (Figs. 9.45, 9.46, 9.47):

When inserting the bone graft, do not apply force along the long axis of the teeth (Figs. 9.48, 9.49, 9.50, 9.51, 9.52, 9.53).

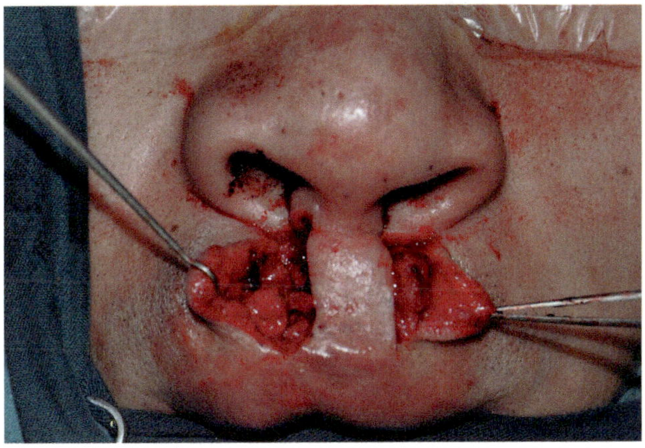

Fig. 9.35 Degloving dissection of the orbicularis oris muscle

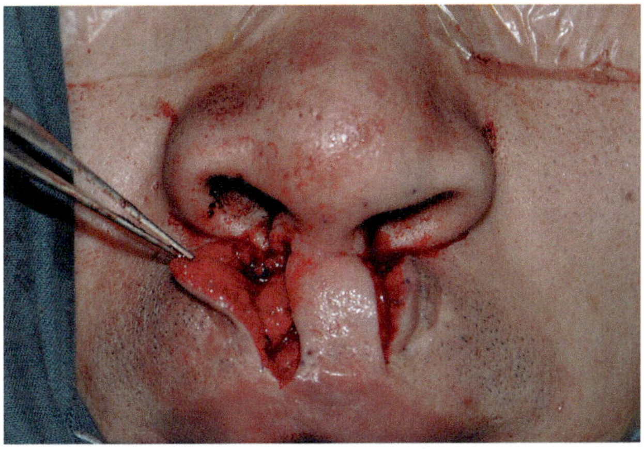

Fig. 9.36 Lifting up the orbicularis oris muscle

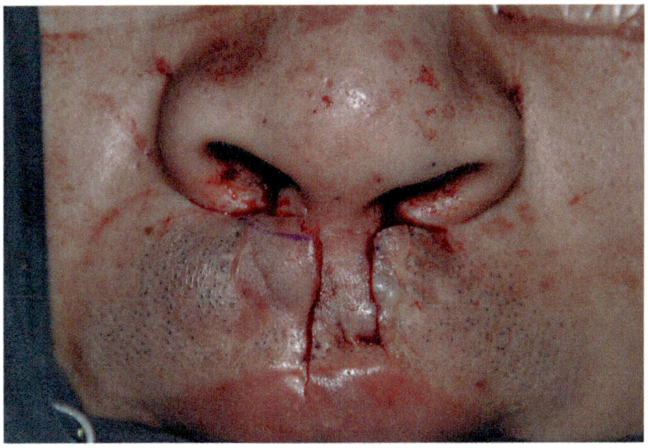

Fig. 9.37 Cutaway the excess muscle and skin

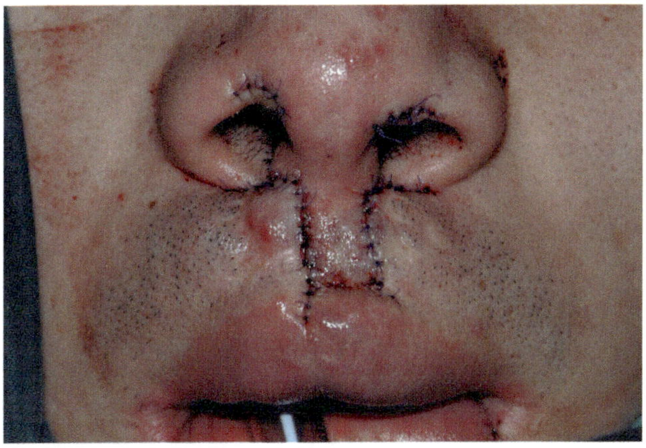

Fig. 9.38 Surgery completed

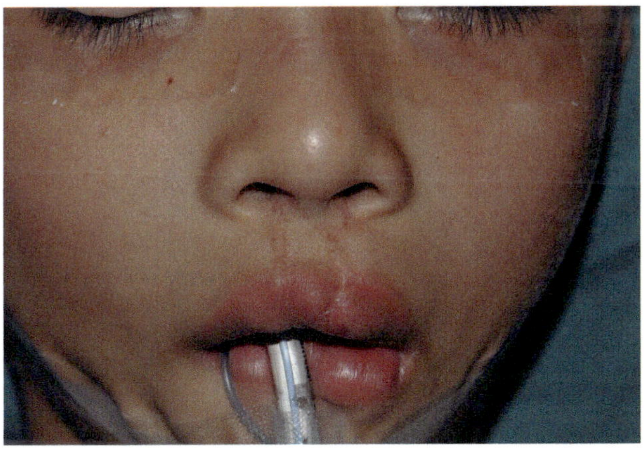

Fig. 9.39 Whistle deformity, prominent scars on the philtrum ridges, and long lateral lip on the left side

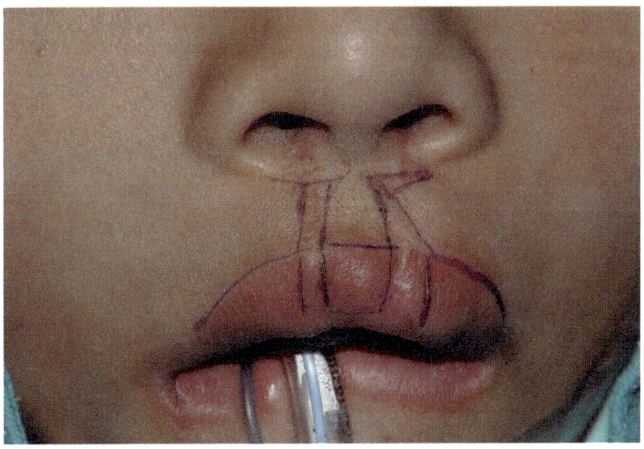

Fig. 9.40 Excise away the scars. Cut the orbicularis oris muscle on the left side and re-adjust its position

3. Points to Note:
   (i) The palatal incisions should extend from the alveolar crest to the apical end of the cleft to ensure complete closure of the defect. The rotation point of the N-flaps should not be at the most apical point of the cleft.
   (ii) Sequence of alveolar bone grafting and cleft closure: Closure of the palatal side → closure of the nasal floor → closure of the alveolar bone cleft → closure of the buccal side. The nasal floor must be closed completely to prevent complications from the extrusion of graft materials into the nasal cavity.

(iii) Compression of the bone graft material should be done laterally and not vertically. The latter can lead to the extrusion of the material.

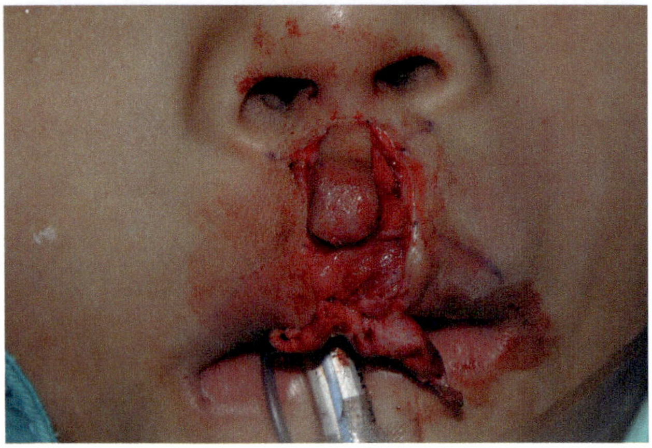

Fig. 9.41 Rotate the tissue layer underneath the scars by 90° to the lip tubercle region. Following this, lift up the orbicularis oris muscle and secure it to the anterior nasal spine

(iv) The bone graft material should be flat against the adjacent bone. Overfilling can lead to excessive tension of the mucosa.

(v) In patients with bilateral alveolar cleft, the incisions on the premaxilla should not meet nor involve the labial frenulum.

9.7 Management of Severe Upper Lip Retrusion Secondary to an Underdeveloped Maxilla

The maxilla tends to develop poorly after the repair of the cleft lip and palate. This becomes more obvious as the patient grows. The maxilla will appear hypoplastic, and the lips will be retruded. The prognosis will be poor if the surgery is performed on an upper lip that is constricted. There is usually a need for the patient to first undergo alveolar bone grafting, orthodontic therapy, or even orthognathic surgery.

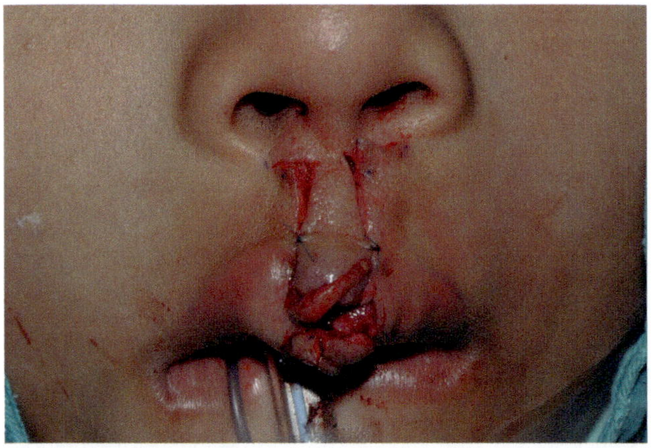

Fig. 9.42 Cut away the excess skin and match the peaks of the Cupid's bow

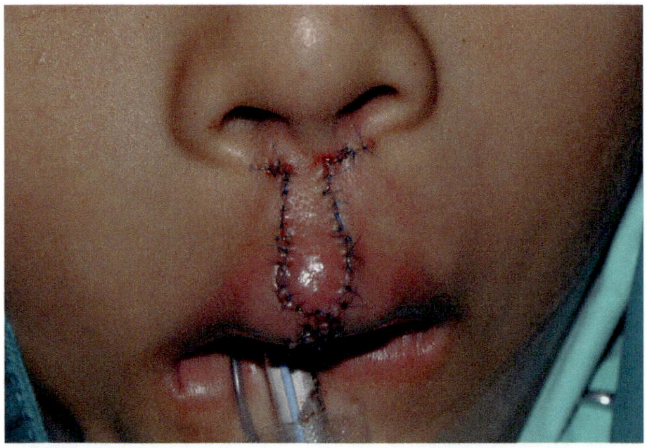

Fig. 9.43 Surgery completed

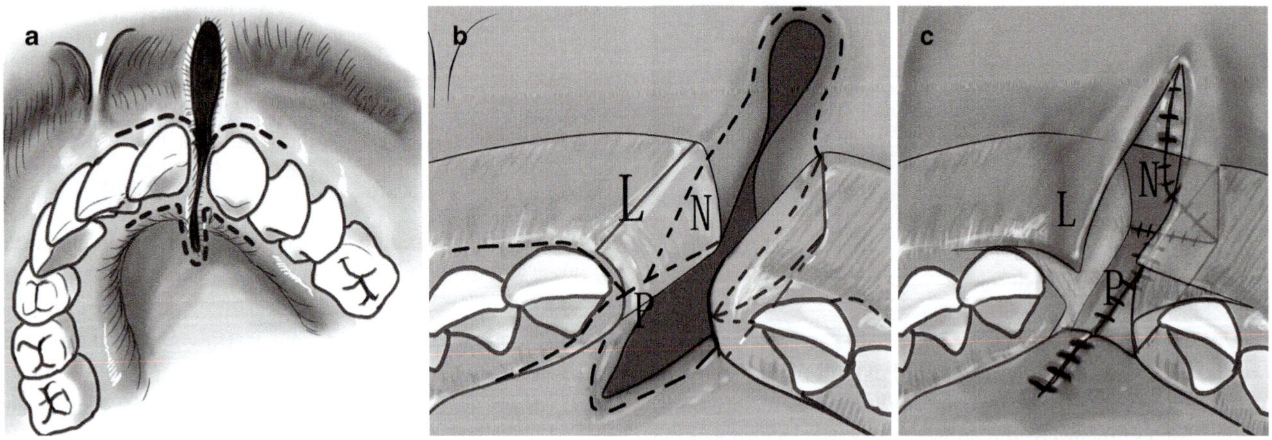

Fig. 9.44 (**a**, **b**, and **c**) Schematic diagram of the surgical incisions

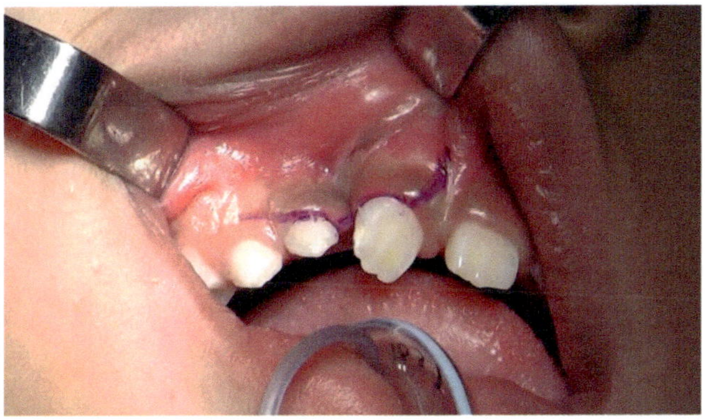

Fig. 9.45 Incision on the buccal surface

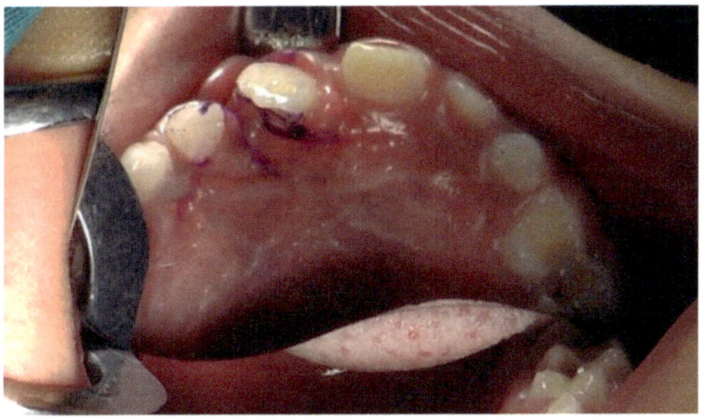

Fig. 9.46 Incision on the palatal surface

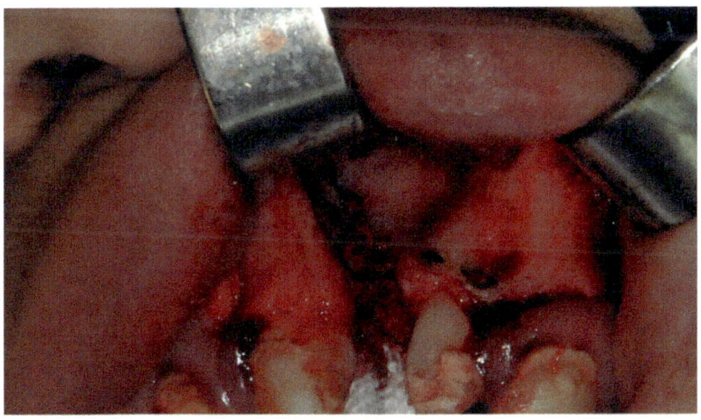

Fig. 9.47 Exposure of the recipient site

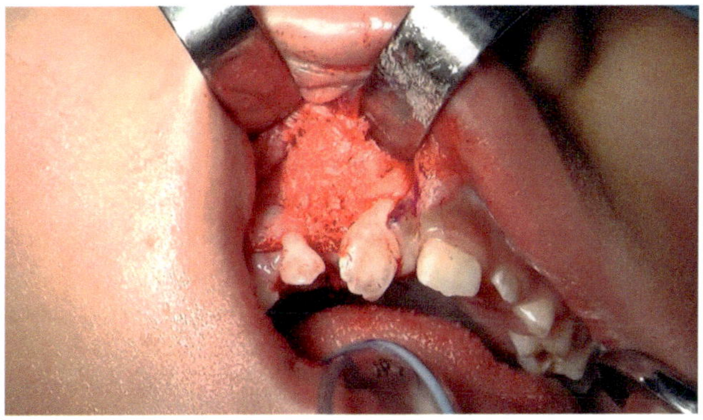

Fig. 9.48 Cancellous bone graft

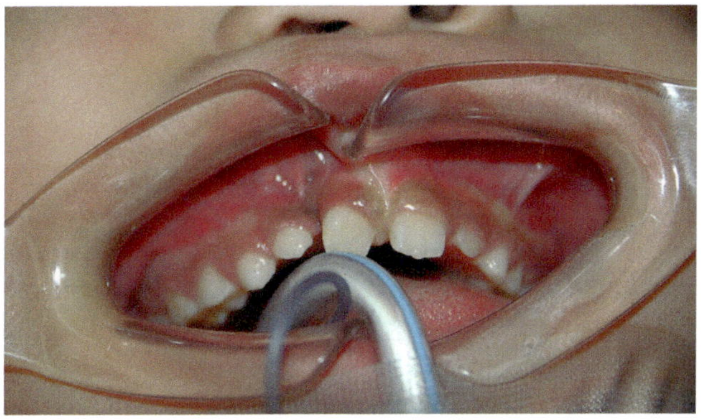

Fig. 9.49 Pre-operative condition

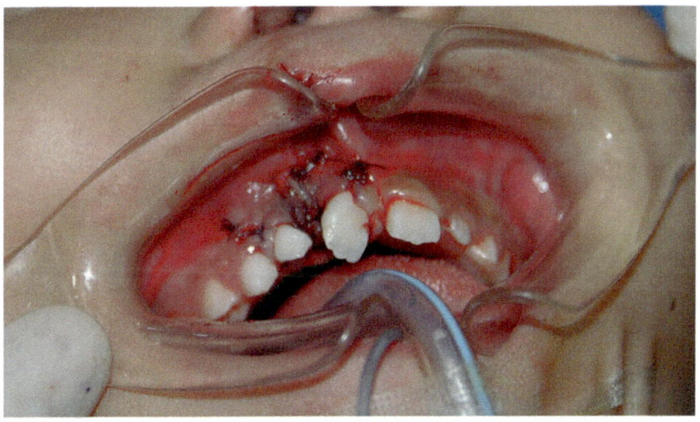

Fig. 9.50 Post-operative condition

1. Indications
   - (i) Patients that have reached skeletal maturity (at least 18 years old).
   - (ii) Post-alveolar bone graft patients.
   - (iii) Patients that have undergone orthodontic treatment in which the teeth of the maxillary arch has been realigned.
   - (iv) Absence of systemic diseases.
2. Surgical Methods and Technique:
   - (i) Pre-Operative Preparation:

     The management of upper lip and maxillary retrusion requires a multidisciplinary team, including an orthognathic surgeon, orthodontist, plastic surgeon, etc. The first phase of treatment involves arch expansion and teeth alignment by the orthodontist. Pre-operative Virtual Surgical Planning (VSP) should be used to determine the direction and degree of surgical movements.

(ii) Operative Procedure:

(1) Maxillary Le Fort I Osteotomy: The osteotomy is performed according to the pattern of a Le Fort I fracture. A horizontal sub-apical osteotomy is made across the maxilla and nasal septum. The teeth bearing part of the maxilla is then moved into its new position. The vascular supply is provided by the palatal mucoperiosteum.

(2) Sagittal Split Ramus Osteotomy: The occlusion will be altered upon the movement of the maxilla. Therefore, it is necessary to move the mandibular dentition to regain proper occlusal relationship. The mandibular ramus is separated in the sagittal plane, forming a distal segment and a proximal segment. The former carries the dentition and the inferior alveolar nerve, while the latter carries the condyle and coronoid process. Using a pre-fabricated occlusal wafer, the mandible can be moved anteriorly, posteriorly, or even rotated to regain proper occlusion with the maxilla.

Classic Example (Figs. 9.54, 9.55, 9.56, 9.57):

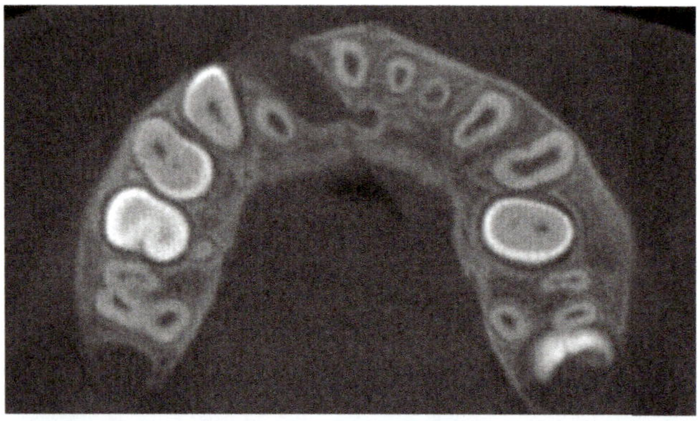

Fig. 9.51 Pre-operative CBCT

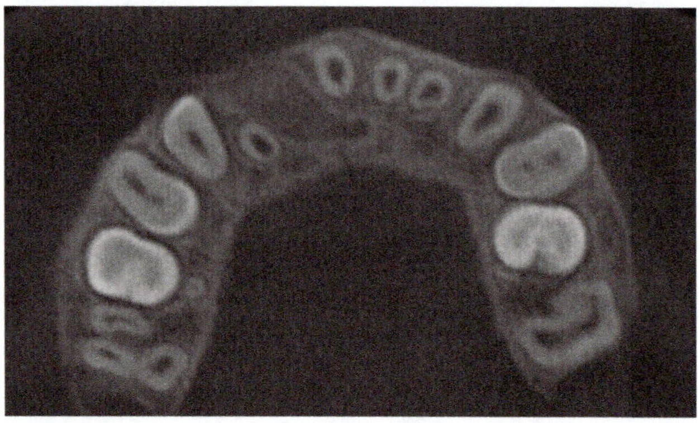

Fig. 9.52 Post-operative CBCT

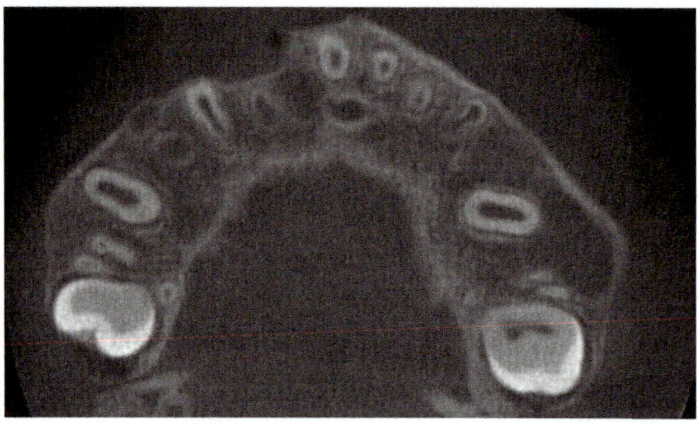

Fig. 9.53 CBCT taken after 1 year

3. Points to Note:

(i) Orthognathic surgery is a technically difficult and risky procedure. It is recommended for an experienced surgeon to perform the surgery. This is to avoid undesired complications and sequelae.

(ii) Hypotensive anesthesia is required during the maxillary osteotomy to reduce intra-operative bleeding. The upper and lower limit of the blood pressure should be 80–90 mmHg and 50–60 mmHg, respectively.

(iii) Post-operative monitoring at the ICU is recommended for the first 24 h. Prior to the transfer of patients to a general ward, at least an hour of observation is required post-extubation [3].

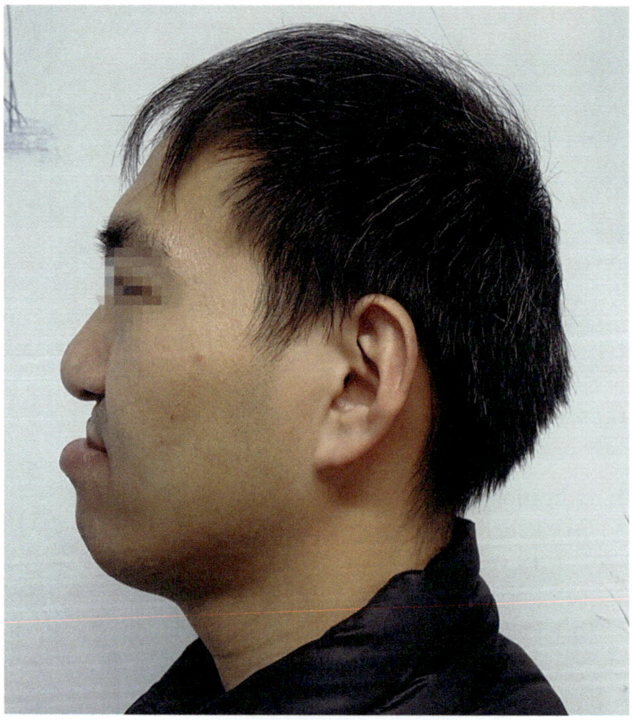

Fig. 9.54 Pre-operative profile view

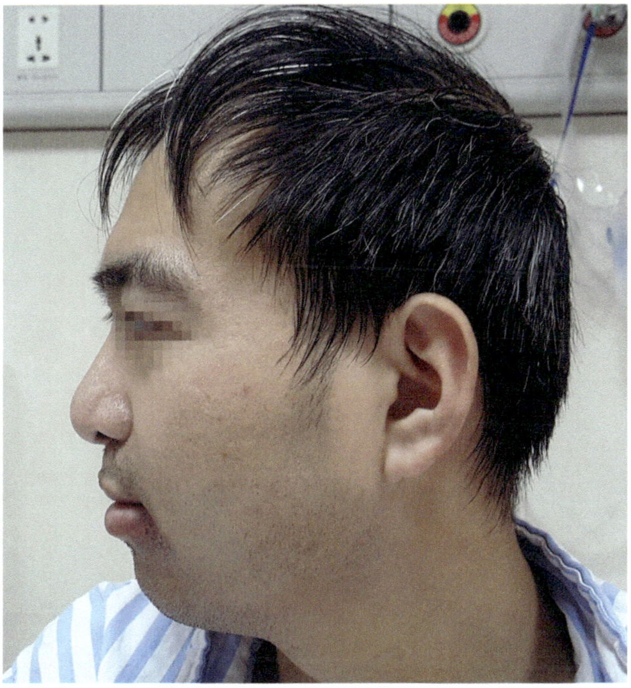

Fig. 9.55 Post-operative profile view

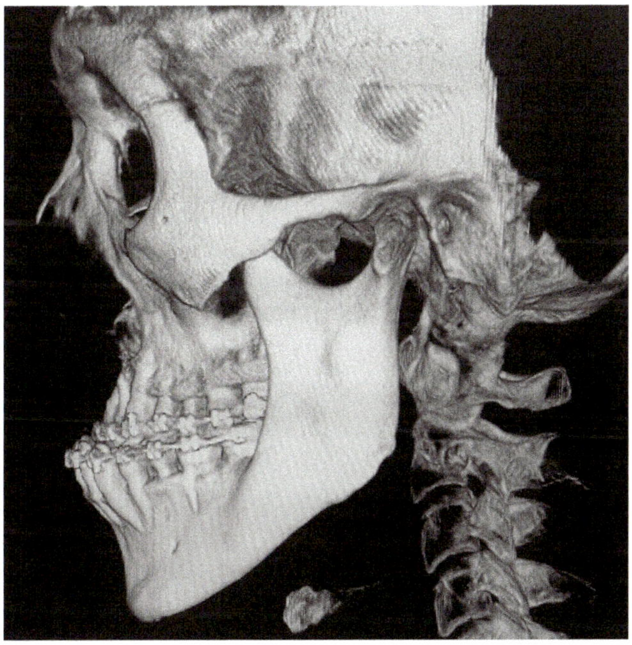

Fig. 9.56 Pre-operative CBCT

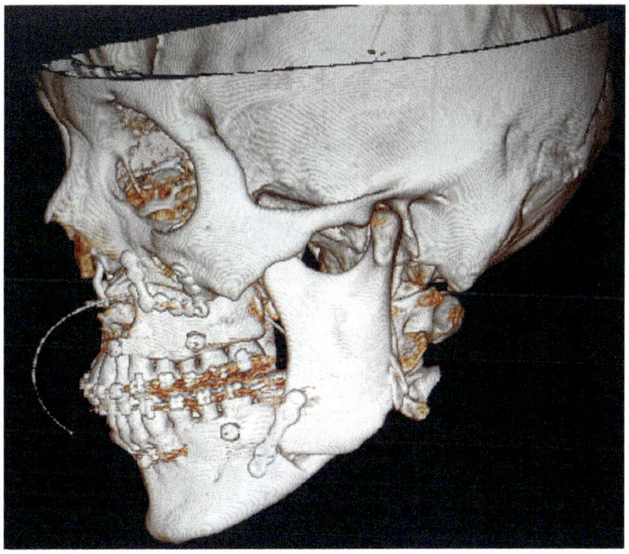

Fig. 9.57 Post-operative CT

References

1. Wang Y, Cheng-hao L. Plastic surgery of cleft lip and palate (in Chinese). Military Science Publishing House; 2015.
2. Ming Z. McCarthy's modern plastic surgery (in Chinese). People's Medical Publishing House; 2007.
3. Mahmoud AAA, Fouad AZ, Mansour MA, et al. A novel intubation technique in bilateral cleft palate pediatric patients: hard gum shield-aided intubate. Pediatr Anesth. 2013;23(4):349–54.

Correction of Secondary Nasal Deformities of Unilateral Cleft Lip Repair

10

Wang Zheng and Qian Zheng

10.1 Internal Fixation of the Nasal Alar Cartilage

1. Indications
   (i) Patients of 15 years old and above: Repaired unilateral cleft lip but with a slightly collapsed alar.
   (ii) Patients ranging from 2 to 15 years old: Repaired unilateral cleft lip with a collapsed alar.
2. Surgical Methods and Procedures
   1. On the cleft side make a C-shaped incision around the skin of the nasal base, columella, and alar. This is to allow the nostril to rotate upwards and outwards as a whole. Dissect and separate the skin away from the alar cartilage, and then suture the alar cartilage to the lateral nasal cartilage.

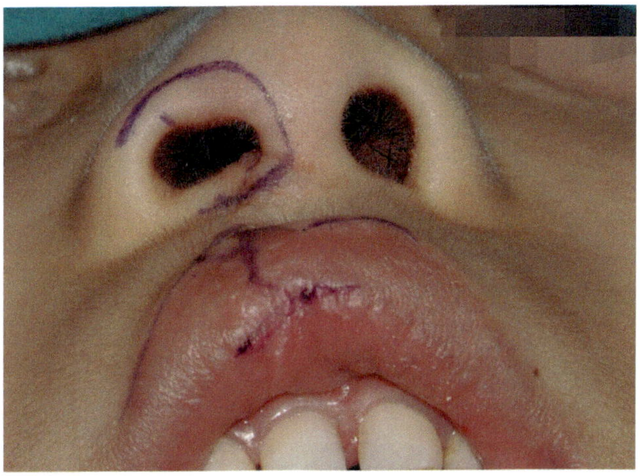

Fig. 10.1 Alar-Columella-Base of nose "C" shaped incision

An Example of the Surgical Procedure:

On the cleft side make a curved incision around the nostril, starting from the alar to the columella. Extend the incision horizontally along the base of the nose towards the cleft side. The total length of the nasal base on the cleft side and the columella determines the length of the horizontal incision. The design of the incision should be C-shaped (Fig. 10.1).

Incise the skin and subcutaneous layer, and dissect the superficial surface of the alar cartilage. After which, deglove the skin over the nasal base, columella, and alar, to expose medial and lateral crus of the alar cartilage. Separate the attachments between the alar cartilage and the lateral nasal cartilage, and cut the connective tissue attachments to the cartilage. Keep the width of alar cartilage between 8 and 10 mm. Up to 2–3 mm of cartilage can be excised if required (Fig. 10.2).

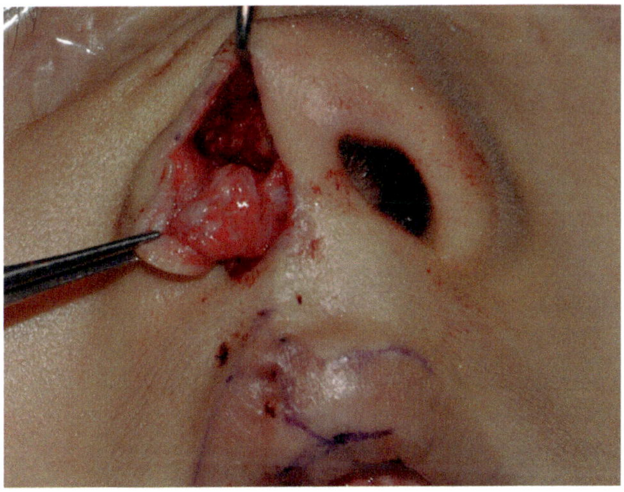

Fig. 10.2 Dissect and exposure the alar cartilage

After freeing the alar cartilage adequately on the cleft side, suture the middle third of the alar cartilage to the lateral nasal cartilage. Next, suture the bilateral medial crus of the alar together at their highest point (Fig. 10.3).

The deep muscle layers of the affected alar can be sutured to the periosteum of the anterior nasal spine, to adduct and

W. Zheng · Q. Zheng (✉)
Department of Cleft Lip and Palate Surgery, West China Stomatology Hospital, Sichuan University, Chengdu, China

J. Liu, B. Shi (eds.), *Atlas of Lip and Nose Plastic and Cosmetic Surgery*, https://doi.org/10.1007/978-981-16-1911-3_10

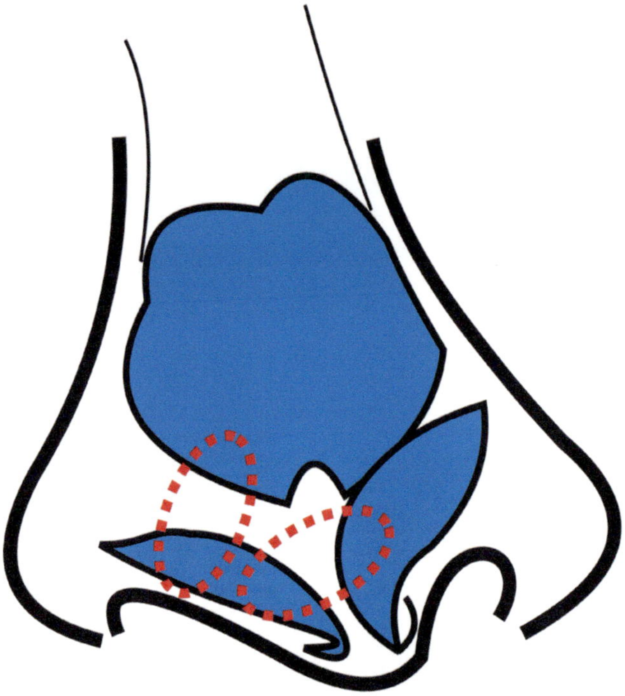

Fig. 10.3 Fixate the alar cartilage to the lateral nasal cartilage

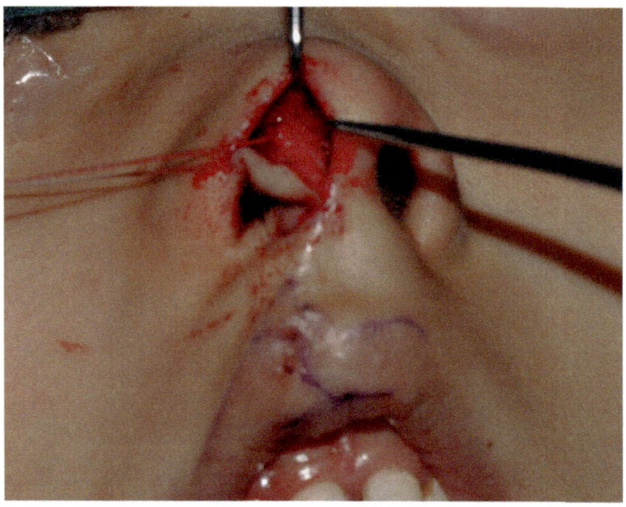

Fig. 10.4 Adduct the flared alar base and close the incisions

suspend the alar. If there are excess tissues after closure, it can be excised by extending the incision from the base of the columella towards the philtrum. The nasal mucosa can be sutured to the skin to eliminate any protrusion of the nasal mucosa tissues (Figs. 10.4 and 10.5).

Classic Example (Figs. 10.6, 10.7, 10.8):

3. Points to Note:
   (i) The alar cartilage on the cleft side must be adequately dissected and anchored tightly to a higher position on the lateral nasal cartilage.

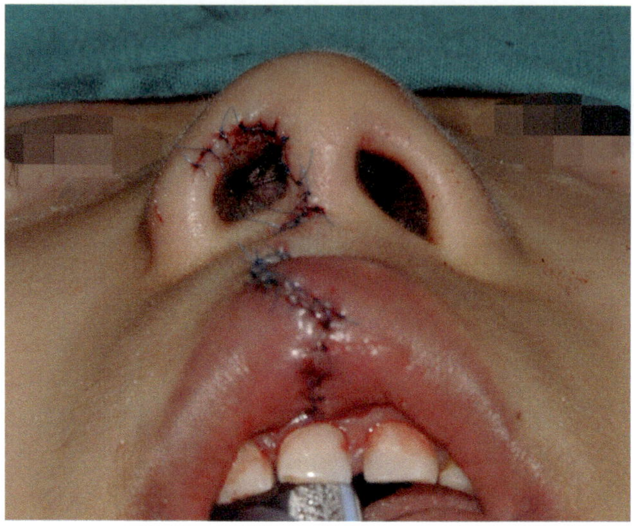

Fig. 10.5 Surgery completed

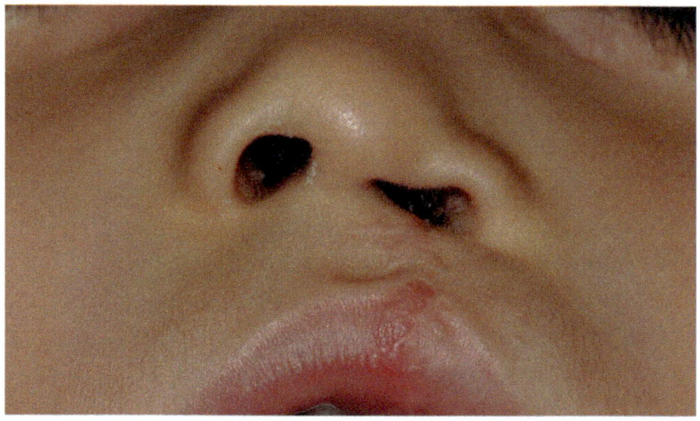

Fig. 10.6 Alar collapse in a patient with repaired left cleft lip

10.2 Reconstruction of the Alar Cartilage with Septal Cartilage Graft

1. Indications
   (i) Patients 15 years old and above: Moderately severe collapsed alar on a repaired unilateral cleft lip.
   (ii) Persistent collapse of the alar despite corrective surgery.
2. Surgical Methods and Procedures
   (i) Dissect and loosen the alar cartilage on the cleft side. Harvest part of the septal cartilage and shape it into strips. Anchor the lateral end of the alar cartilage to the septal cartilage deep to the columella (across the nasal cavity). Make use of the elasticity of the septal cartilage to suspend the alar cartilage to reconstruct the shape of the alar.

An Example of the Surgical Procedure:

On the cleft side, make a curved incision around the nostril starting from the alar to the center of the columella.

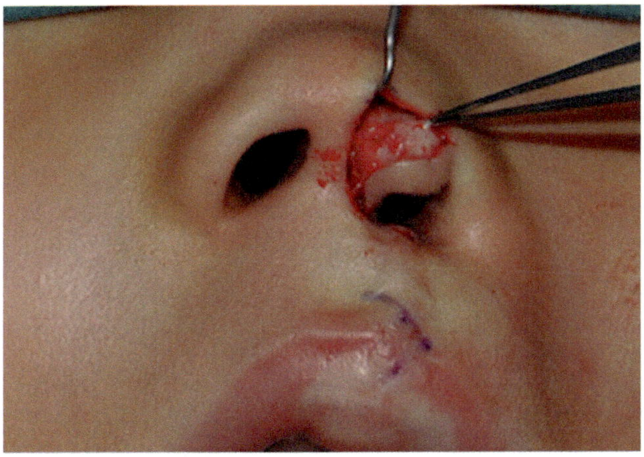

Fig. 10.7 Dissection of the alar cartilage

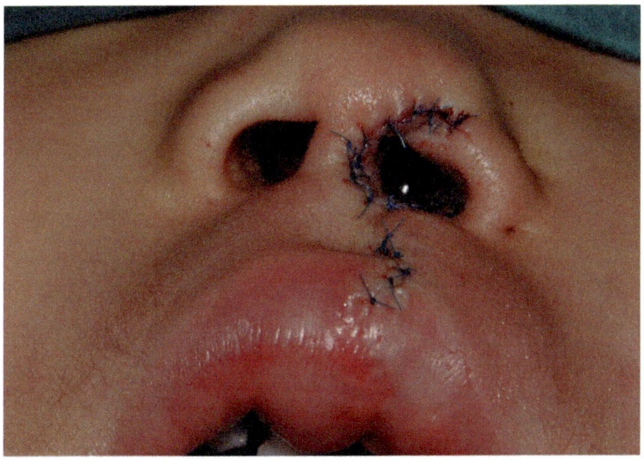

Fig. 10.8 Surgery completed

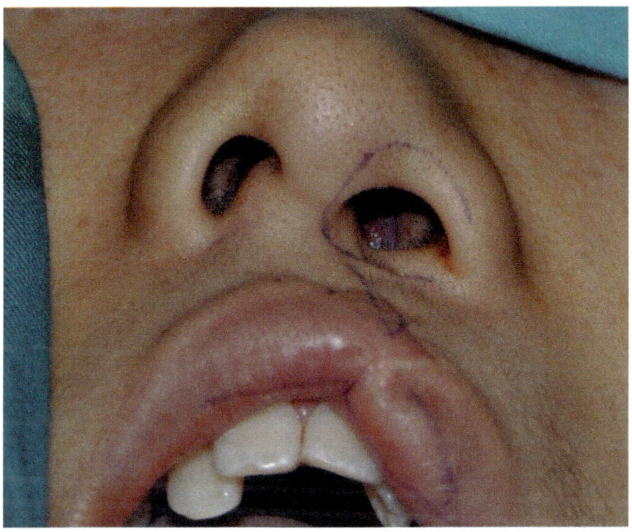

Fig. 10.9 C-shaped incision involving the alar, columella, and the base of the nose

Extend the incision horizontally along the base of the nose towards the cleft side. The total length of the nasal base on the cleft side and the columella determines the length of the horizontal incision. The design of the incision should be C-shaped (Fig. 10.9).

Incise the skin and subcutaneous layer according to the line drawn. Raise the skin layer over the nasal base, columella, and alar region. Expose the medial and lateral crus of the alar cartilage, and cut away the attachments between the medial alar cartilage and lateral nasal cartilage. Keep the width of alar cartilage between 8–10 mm. Up to 2–3 mm of cartilage can be excised if required (Fig. 10.10).

Separate the medial crus of the alar and the lateral nasal cartilage on the cleft from the septal cartilage. Make an incision on the anterior nasal spine, enter the subchondral plane, and strip the perichondral layer beyond the septal cartilage. There may be some difficulty at the junction between the cartilaginous and osseous septum. Keep the perichondral layer intact. Harvest a portion of the septal cartilage, leaving at least 7 mm of the L-shaped cartilage scaffold at the upper and frontal margin (Fig. 10.11).

Cut the harvested septal cartilage into long strips 5 mm in width, and connect the strips together to increase the length. While the septal cartilage in the Chinese population is often not long enough, the width is usually sufficient. There should be enough cartilage to form a long strip 4 cm in length. Scratches or incisions on the cartilage are to be avoided (Fig. 10.12).

Insert the cartilage strips into the previously created nasal alar cavity. The cartilage should suspend from the columella base, through the whole columella, and make an arch over to the alar on the cleft side. The elasticity of the cartilage will help form the natural shape of the alar. The cartilage strips are secured in the following manner: First, tie the end of the cartilage strip with either the anterior nasal spine or the short end of the L-shaped cartilage scaffold. Then secure the grafted cartilage together with the pre-existing alar cartilage. Tie the two ends of the bilateral medial crus to the cartilage graft. Lastly, tie the upper margin of the cartilage strip with the lateral nasal cartilage (Fig. 10.13).

In cases with a deviated columella, the L-shaped cartilage scaffold must be detached from the anterior nasal spine prior to the cartilage graft. This will help to correct the deviation.

Suture the skin layer to its new position after the cartilage graft. Cutaway excess skin of the alar as required. Depending on the degree of the alar flare and the droop, the muscles of the alar can be tied to the periosteum of the anterior nasal spine to adduct and suspend the alar base (Fig. 10.14).

If there are excess tissues after closure, it can be excised by extending the incision from the base of the columella towards the philtrum. The nasal mucosa can be sutured to the skin to eliminate any protrusion of the nasal mucosa tissues (Fig. 10.15).

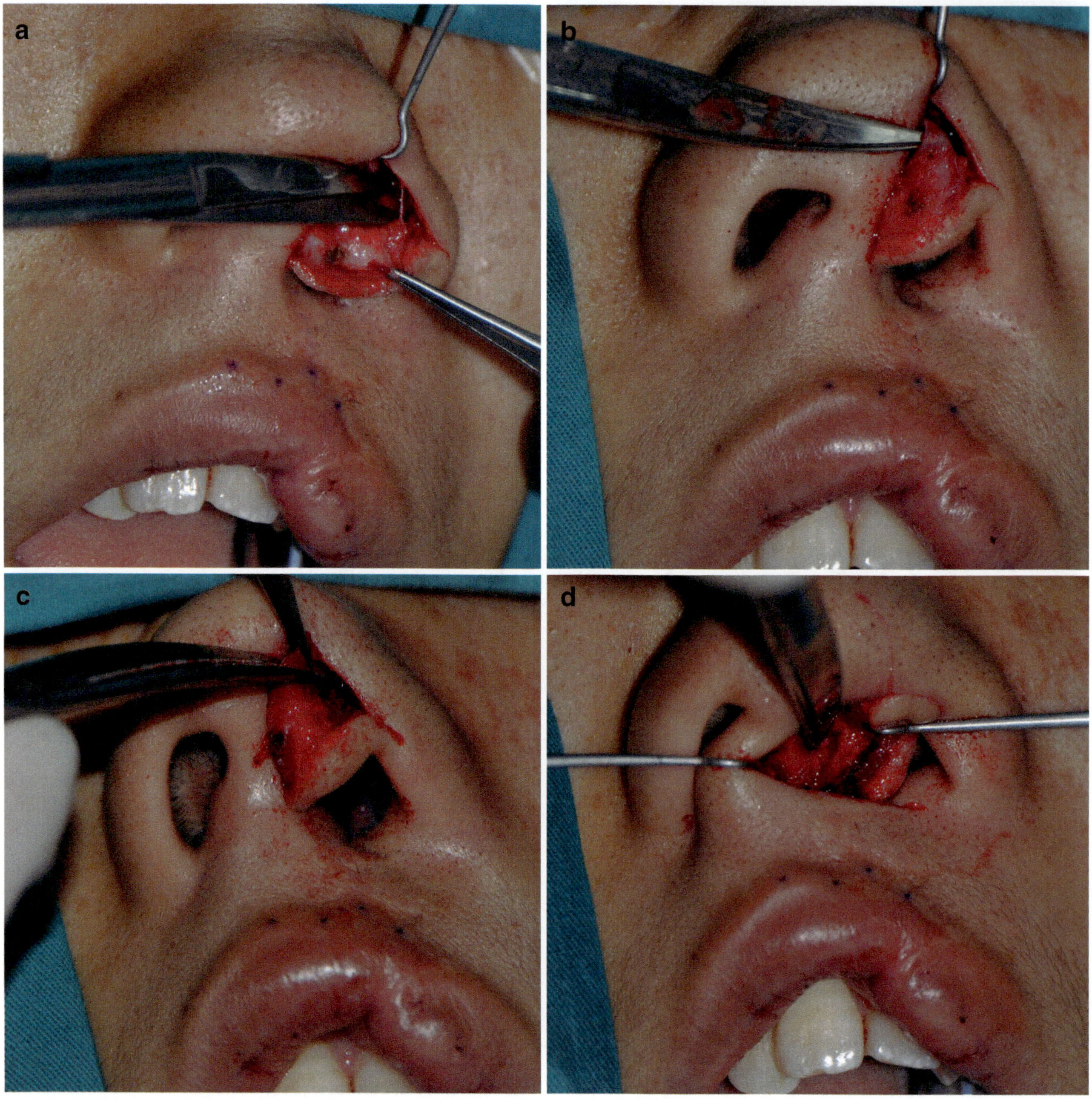

Fig. 10.10 (**a**, **b**, **c**, and **d**) Reconstruction of the alar cartilage

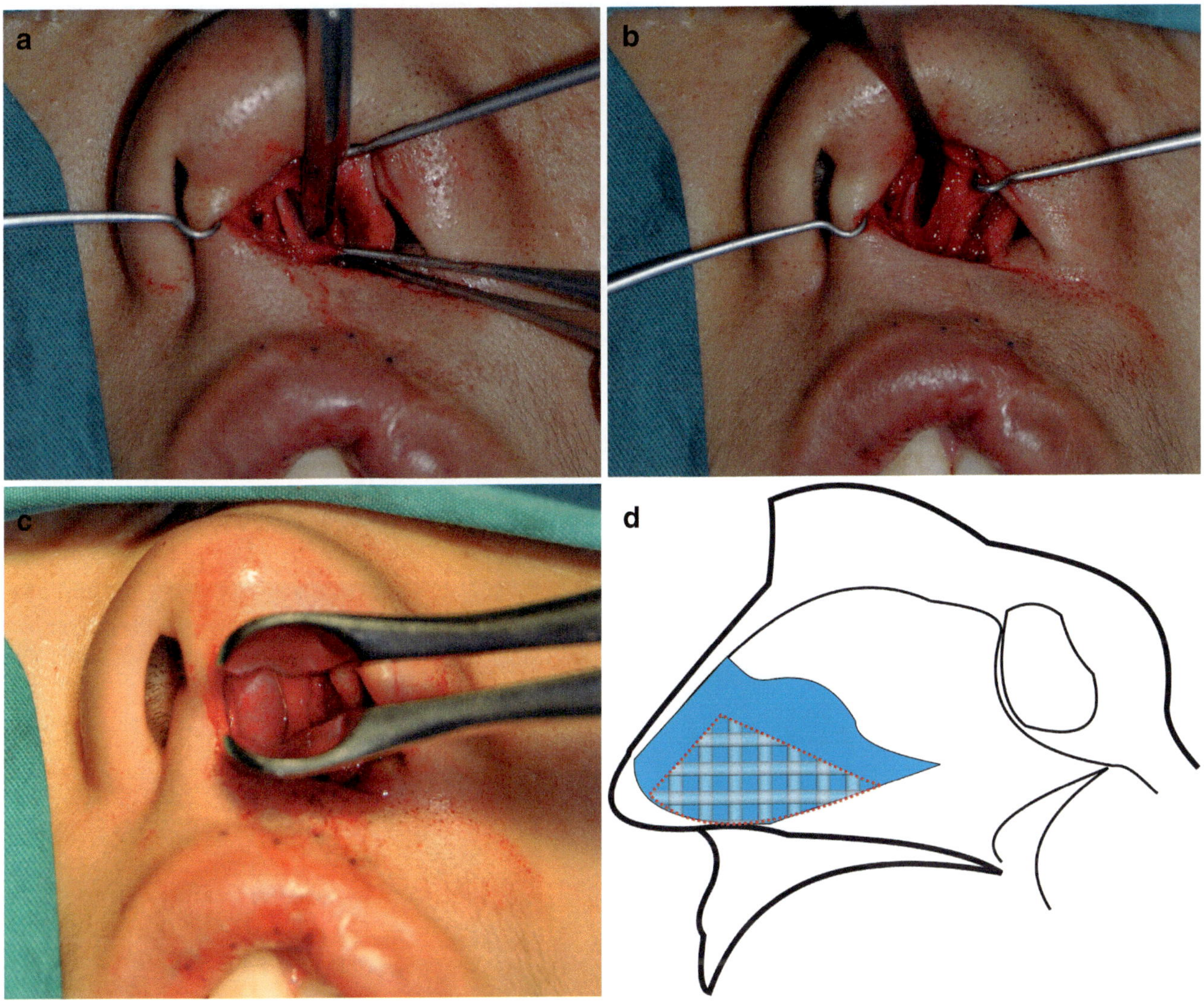

Fig. 10.11 (**a**, **b**, **c**, and **d**) Expose and harvest a part of the septal cartilage

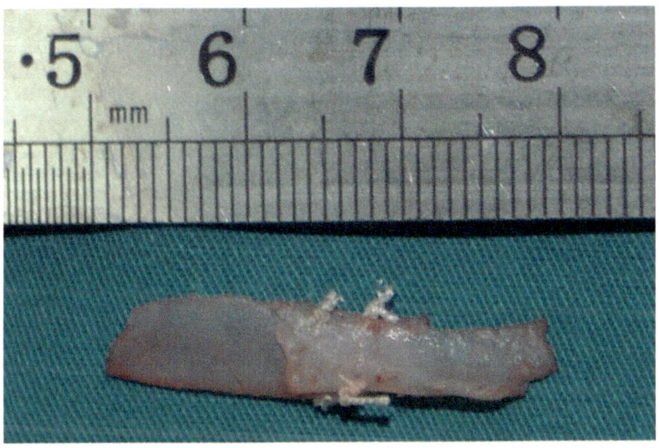

Fig. 10.12 Chondroplasty

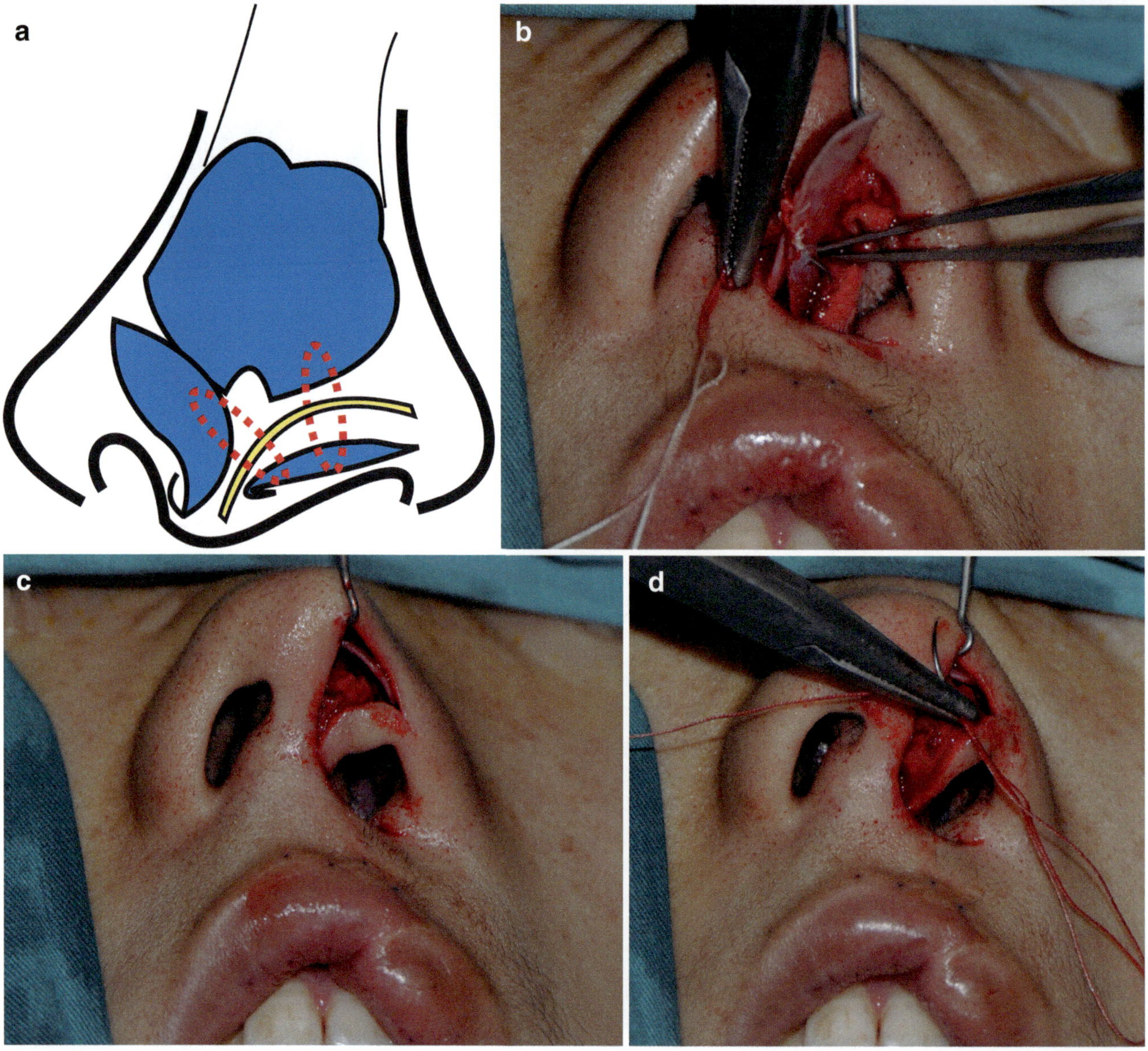

Fig. 10.13 (**a**, **b**, **c**, and **d**) Grafting of cartilage

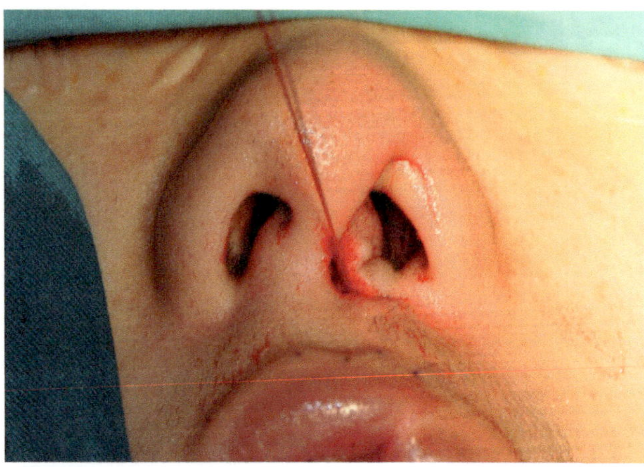

Fig. 10.14 Adduction of the nasal base on the cleft side

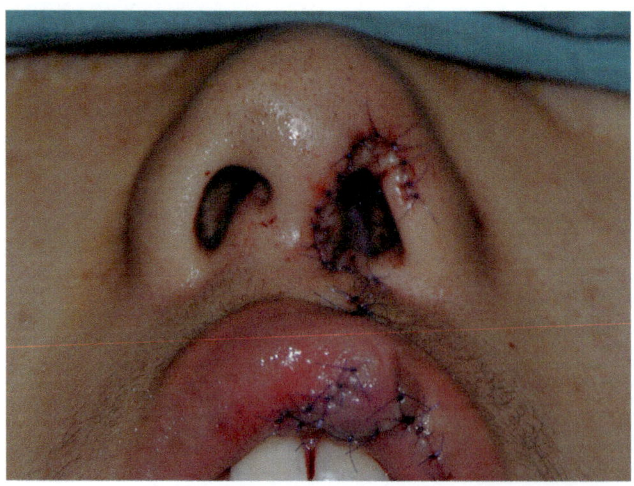

Fig. 10.15 Closure of the skin layer

Classic Example (Figs. 10.16, 10.17, 10.18):

3. Points to Note
   (i) Failure to preserve the L-shaped cartilage scaffold can lead to a saddle nose deformity.
   (ii) The nasal septum cartilage is usually divided into two parts parallel to the vomer. The hardness of the cartilage varies, with the part nearer to the vomer being harder. Therefore, that portion should be used to support the nasal columella. The cartilage away from the vomer has more elasticity and should be used to reconstruct the alar cartilage.

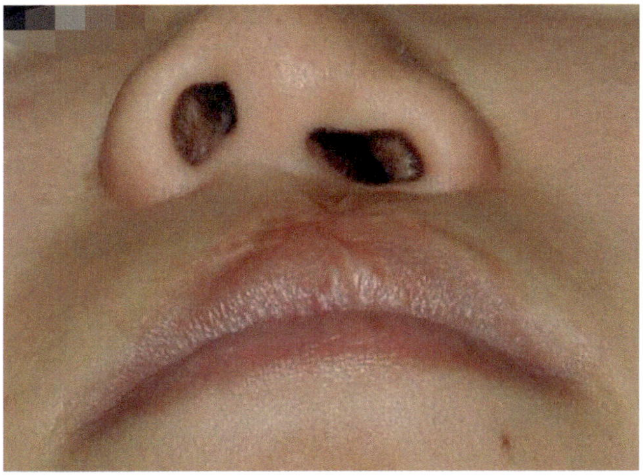

Fig. 10.16 Pre-operative appearance

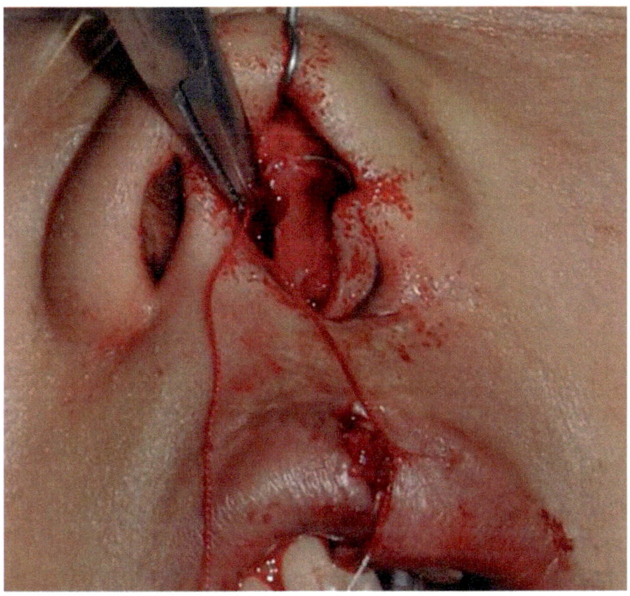

Fig. 10.17 Grafting of cartilage from the nasal septum

10.3 Correction of Constricted Nostrils

10.3.1 Auricular Composite Tissue Transfer

1. Indications
   (i) Patients 15 years old and above: Atresia or a constricted nostril after unilateral cleft lip repair.
2. Surgical Methods and Procedures
   (i) The incision can be made either through the scar or at concealed locations such as the alar base. Make the cuts through the skin, cartilage, and mucosa. Enlarge the nostril until it is the same diameter as the unaffected alar. Finally, the auricular composite tissue flap is used to repair the defect.

An Example of the Surgical Procedure (Figs. 10.19, 10.20, 10.21, 10.22, 10.23, 10.24, 10.25, 10.26):

3. Points to Note:
   (i) Eric gauze can be stuffed in the nasal cavity during the operation to reduce wound contamination. Cold compression can be applied after the operation to reduce the metabolism of the transplanted tissue, which allows for better graft survival. A nasal mold can be used to prop up the nasal tissues for a year to reduce tissue contraction.
   (ii) The main objective of the first phase of tissue grafting is to increase the amount of soft tissue. The remaining deformities can be reconstructed in the second phase.

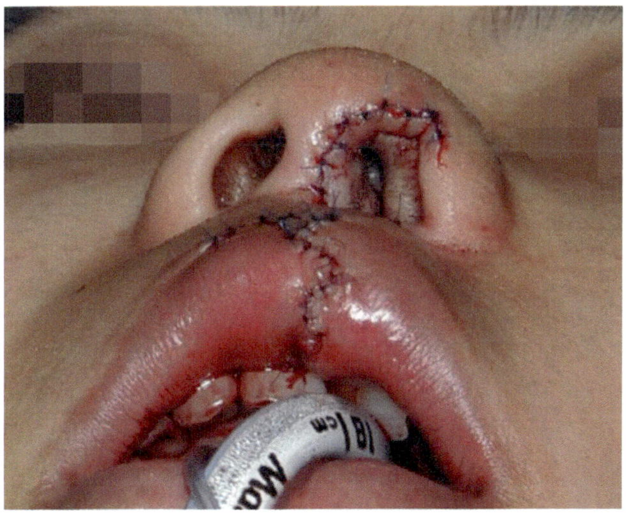

Fig. 10.18 Post-operative appearance

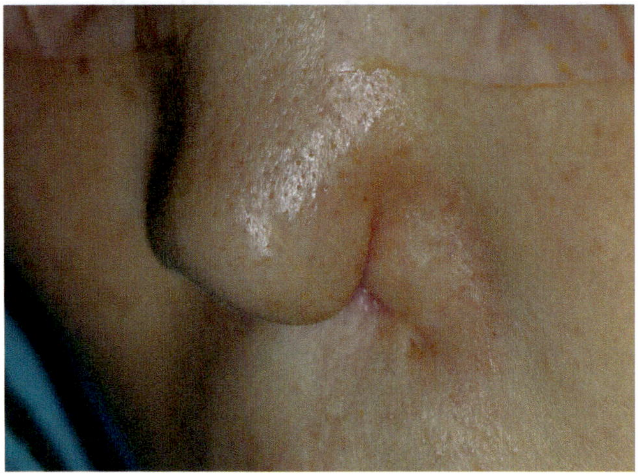

Fig. 10.19 Pre-operative appearance of the nose

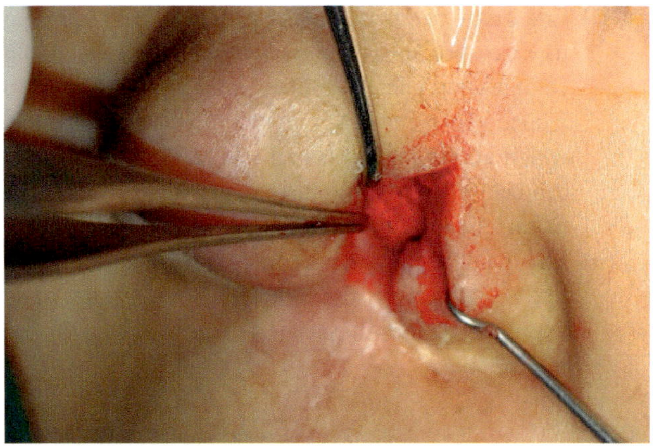

Fig. 10.20 Full thickness cut along the scar

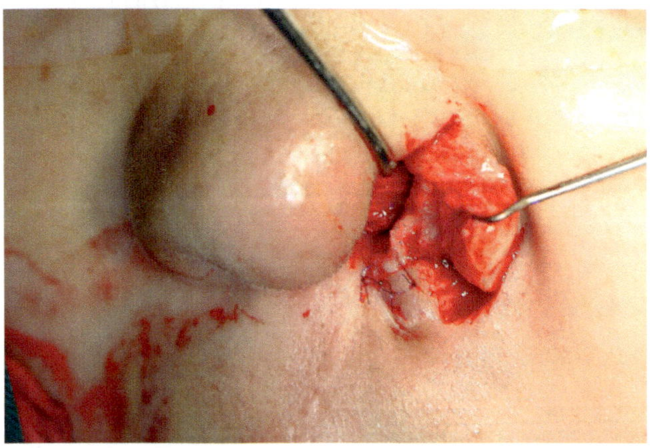

Fig. 10.21 Cut along the alar base and adjust the size of the nostril

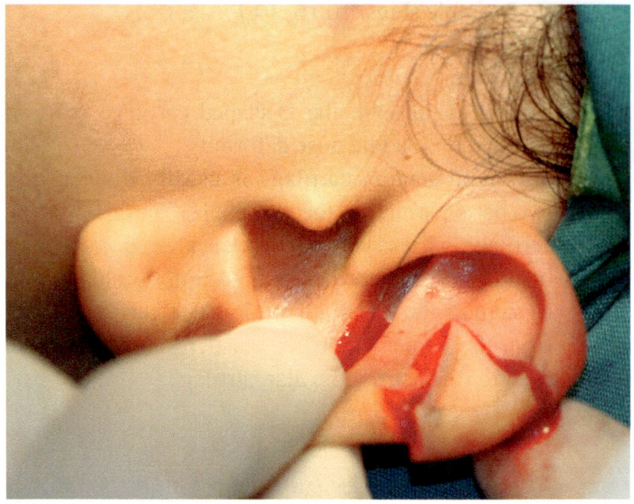

Fig. 10.22 Auricular composite tissue flap

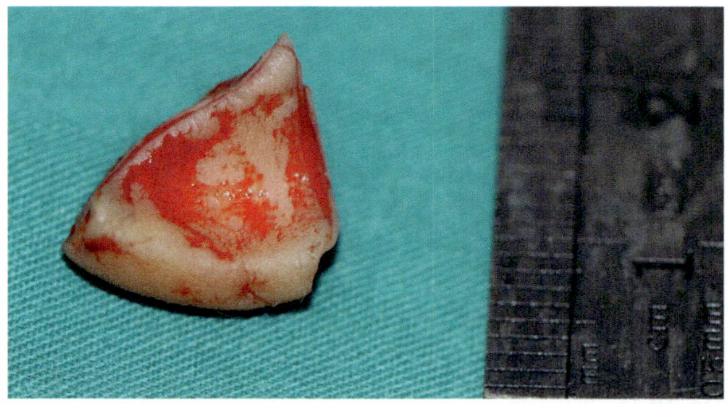

Fig. 10.23 Auricular composite tissue flap

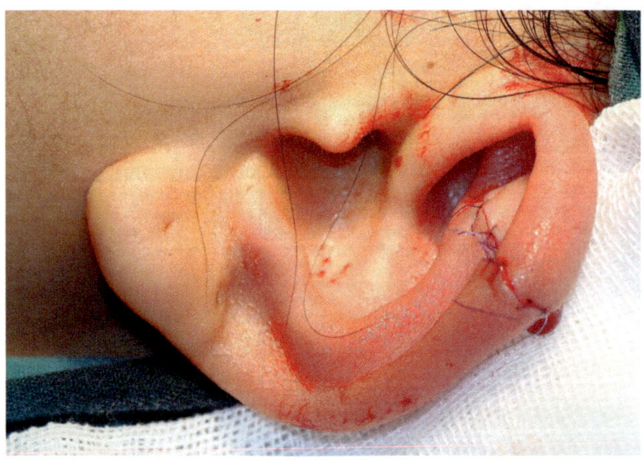

Fig. 10.24 Primary closure of the auricle

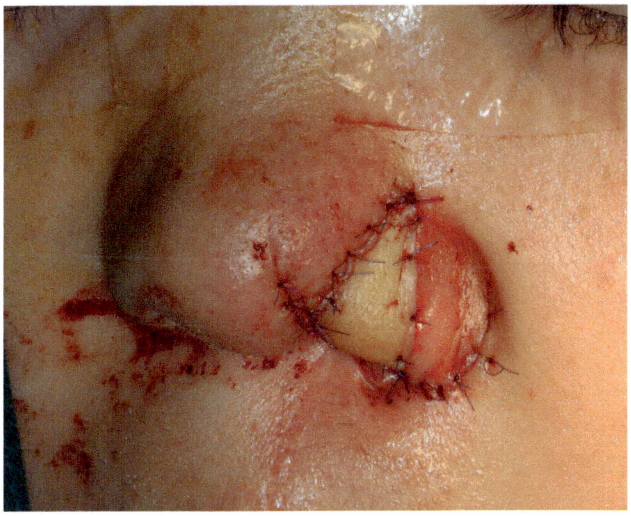

Fig. 10.25 Graft the auricular composite tissue flap into the defect

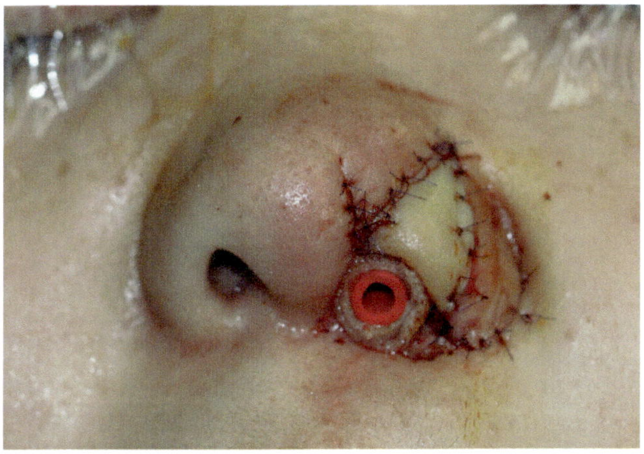

Fig. 10.26 Post-operative appearance of the nose

10.3.2 Rhinoplasty

1. Indications:
   (i) Alar collapse and a constricted nostril after unilateral cleft lip repair.
2. Surgical Methods and Procedures:
   (i) The alar will be lifted, and the nostril will be enlarged after the shape and position of the alar cartilage is fixed. Make an incision along the alar and pull the skin tissues inwards into the nasal cavity. The peri-alar skin will slide inwards to fill up the resultant defect. As a result, the diameter of the nostril will be enlarged.

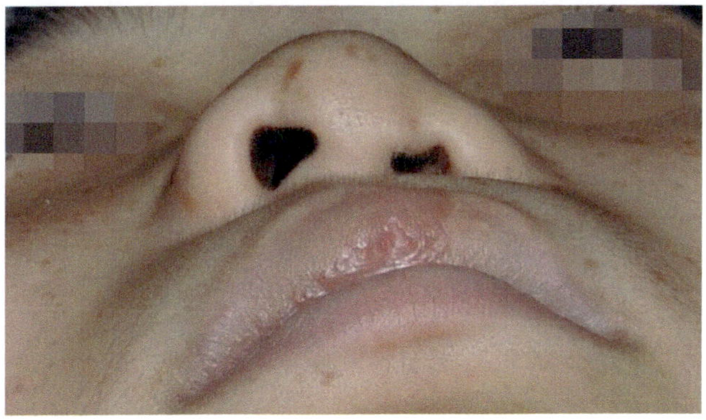

Fig. 10.27 Pre-operative appearance

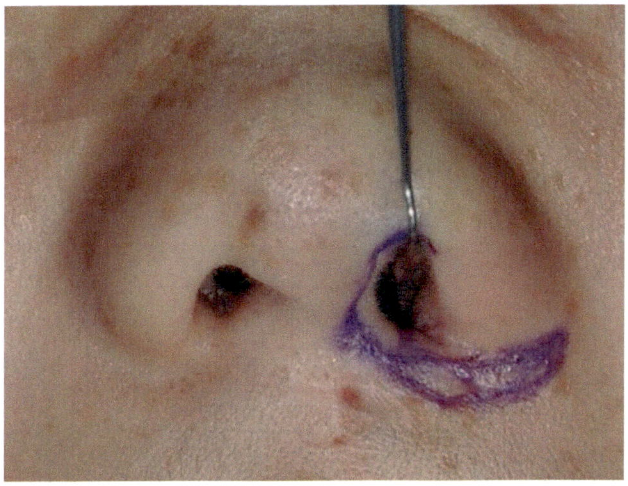

Fig. 10.28 Design of the surgical incisions

An Example of the Surgical Procedure (Figs. 10.27 and 10.28):

Make a C-shaped incision along the alar, columella, and nasal base.

First, incise through the skin and dissect the alar cartilage. Next, expose and harvest the septal cartilage (Fig. 10.29).

Insert the cartilage graft to reconstruct the columella and alar cartilage (Figs. 10.30, 10.31, 10.32).

Classic Example (Figs. 10.33 and 10.34):

3. Points to Note:
   (i) The choice between internal fixation or chondroplasty of the alar cartilage for the reconstruction of the alar depends on the age of the patient and the degree of alar collapse [1, 2].

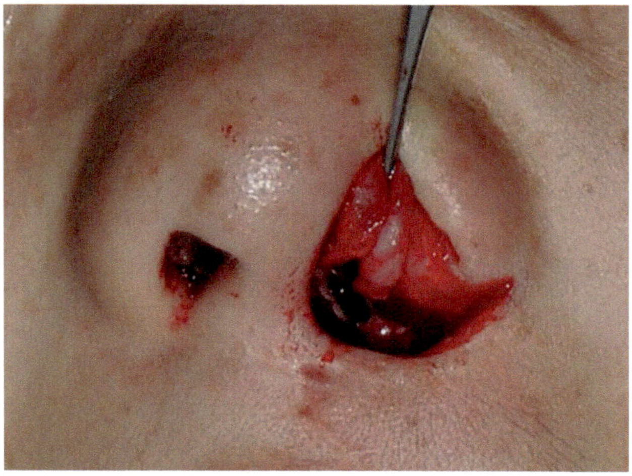

Fig. 10.29 Harvest of septal cartilage

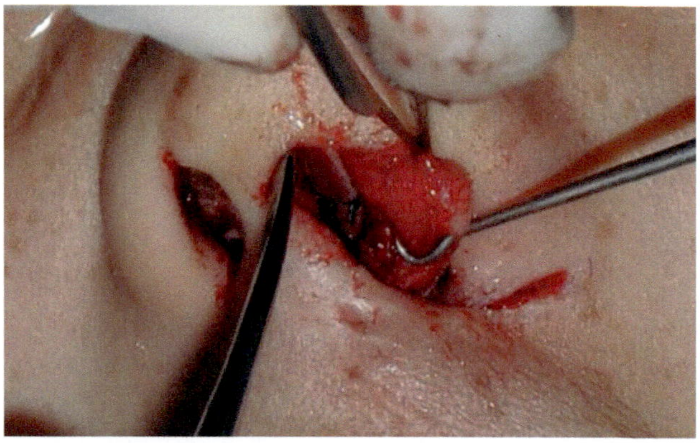

Fig. 10.30 Cartilage graft

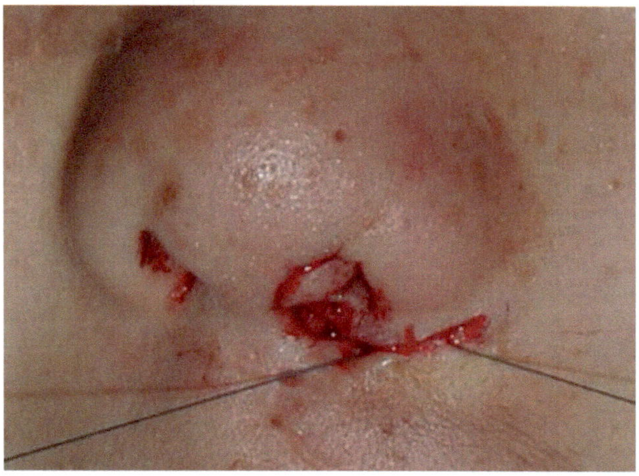

Fig. 10.31 Repositioning of the alar base

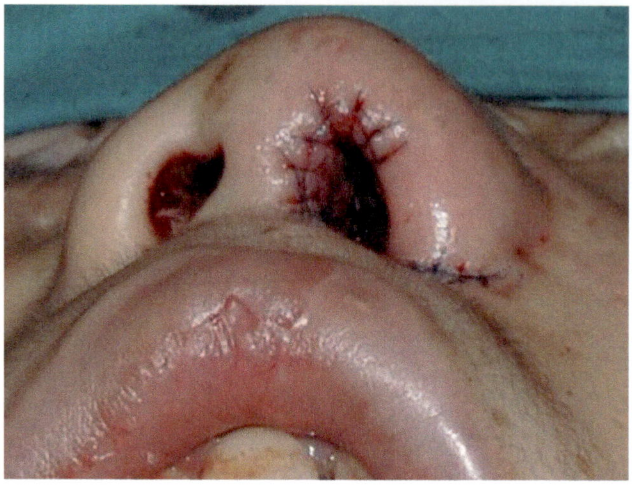

Fig. 10.32 Post-operative appearance

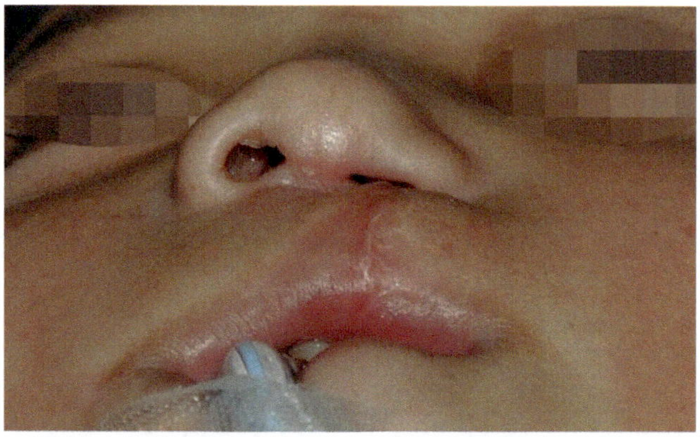

Fig. 10.33 Pre-operative appearance of the nose

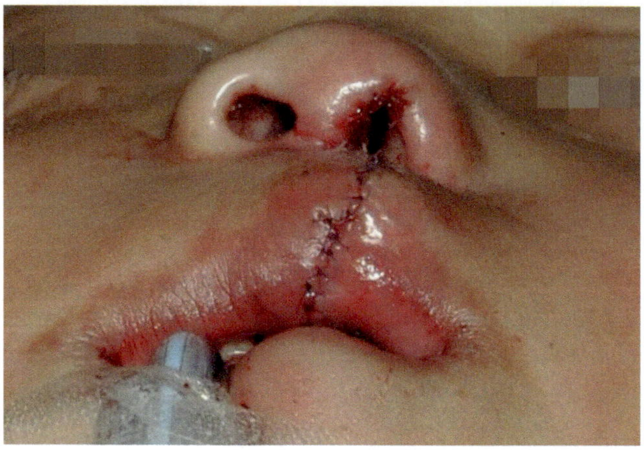

Fig. 10.34 Post-operative appearance of the nose

References

1. Lu S. Composite treatment of cleft lip and palate (in Chinese). People's Medical Publishing House; 2011.
2. Shi B. Cleft lip and palate primary repair. Springer and Zhejiang University Press; 2013.

Correction of Secondary Nasal Deformities of Bilateral Cleft Lip Repair

11

Qian Zheng

11.1 Lengthening of the Nasal Columella

1. Indications
   (i) An acceptable upper lip shape but with a short columella and a nasal tip that droops downwards.
   (ii) The philtrum has an adequate length but is too wide.
   (iii) Growing children (under the age of 15) are not suitable as they may not tolerate the combination of having upper lip flaps to lengthen the columella and lower lip Abbe flap tissue transfer.
2. Surgical Methods and Procedures
   (i) Make a reverse V incision along the base of the nose and the columella. Pull the tissues towards the nasal tip and perform a V–Y closure of the columella. This will simultaneously lift the nasal tip and reduce the alar flare.

An Example of the Surgical Procedure:

Make a horizontal incision starting from the lateral ends of the alar base on each side towards the columella. At this point, turn the incisions vertically and converge the incisions at the base of the columella. Continue the incision for a short distance towards the nasal tip (Fig. 11.1).

Raise the tissues of the columella and nasal base. Following this, dissect the tissues attached to the alar base (Fig. 11.2).

Pull the tissues from the nasal base inwards and upwards to the nasal tip. Suture the tissues together in the midline (Fig. 11.3).

Close up the wound along the base of the nose (Fig. 11.4).

Classic Example 1 (Fig. 11.5):

Classic Example 2 (Fig. 11.6):

3. Points to Note

Q. Zheng (✉)
Department of Cleft Lip and Palate Surgery, West China Stomatology Hospital, Sichuan University, Chengdu, China

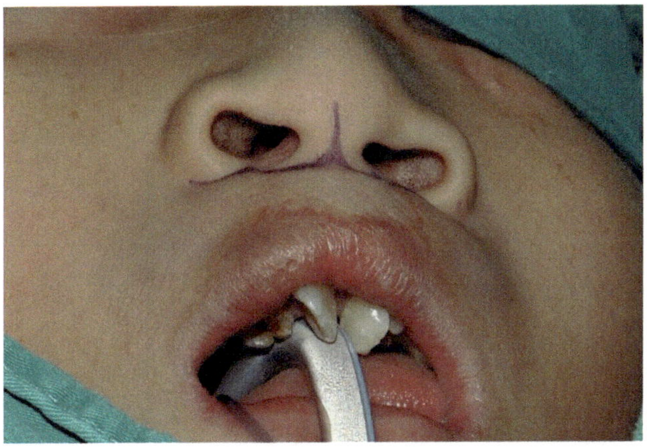

Fig. 11.1 Design of the surgical incisions

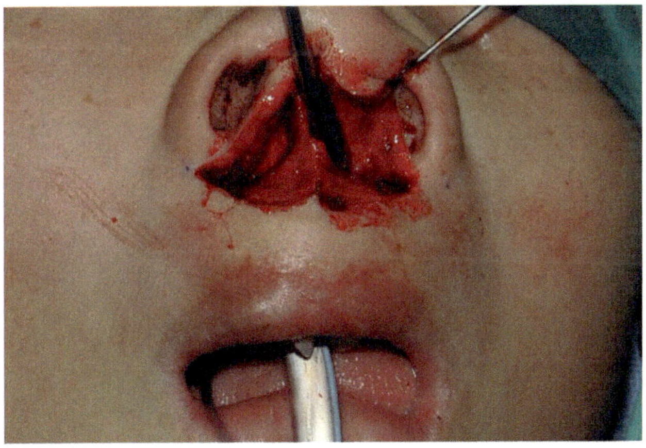

Fig. 11.2 Nasal base raised

   (i) Release the tissues of the alar base from the piriform aperture and anterior nasal spine. If necessary, parallel incisions can be made in the nasal vestibule to further lengthen the columella. Adduct the alar base to reduce the likelihood of recurrence.
   (ii) There may be excess tissues along the horizontal incision after the lengthening of the columella and

J. Liu, B. Shi (eds.), *Atlas of Lip and Nose Plastic and Cosmetic Surgery*, https://doi.org/10.1007/978-981-16-1911-3_11

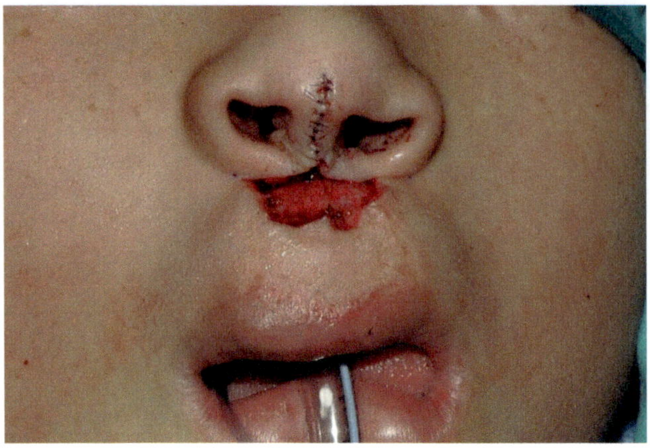

Fig. 11.3 Adduction of the alar base and lengthening of the columella

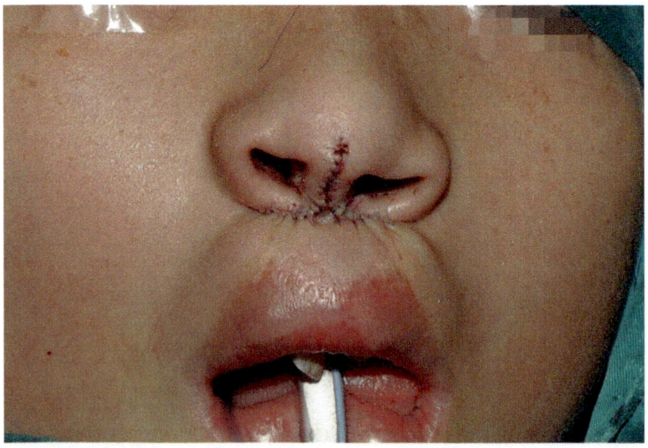

Fig. 11.4 Surgery completed

adduction of the alar base. A V-shaped incision can be made along the pre-existing scars to remove the excess tissues.

(iii) A non-resorbable suture should be used to anchor the deep tissues of the alar base to the midline. The point at which the tissues of the alar are to be sutured depends on the amount of adduction needed. The resultant alar base width should be equal to the inter-canthal distance.

11.2 Reconstruction of the Nasal Tip with Costal Cartilage

1. Indications
   (i) Severely short columella with a flat nasal tip that droops downwards. Poorly developed alar cartilages with thick overlying soft tissue.
   (ii) Collapsed nasal bridge.
   (iii) Patients 15 years old or above: When the peak growth period has passed.
2. Surgical Methods and Procedures
   (i) Harvest the straightest part of the eighth costal cartilage and reshape it with a scalpel. The harvested cartilage will be used to create both a columella and a nasal bridge graft. The dimensions depend on the degree of deficiency.
   (ii) Create a tunnel on the nasal dorsum as per the standard rhinoplasty technique. Pull the tissues from the nasal base and upper lip upwards to lengthen the columella and prop up the nasal tip. Insert the nasal bridge graft into the dorsum tunnel and the columella graft in front of the nasal septum. Adjust the carti-

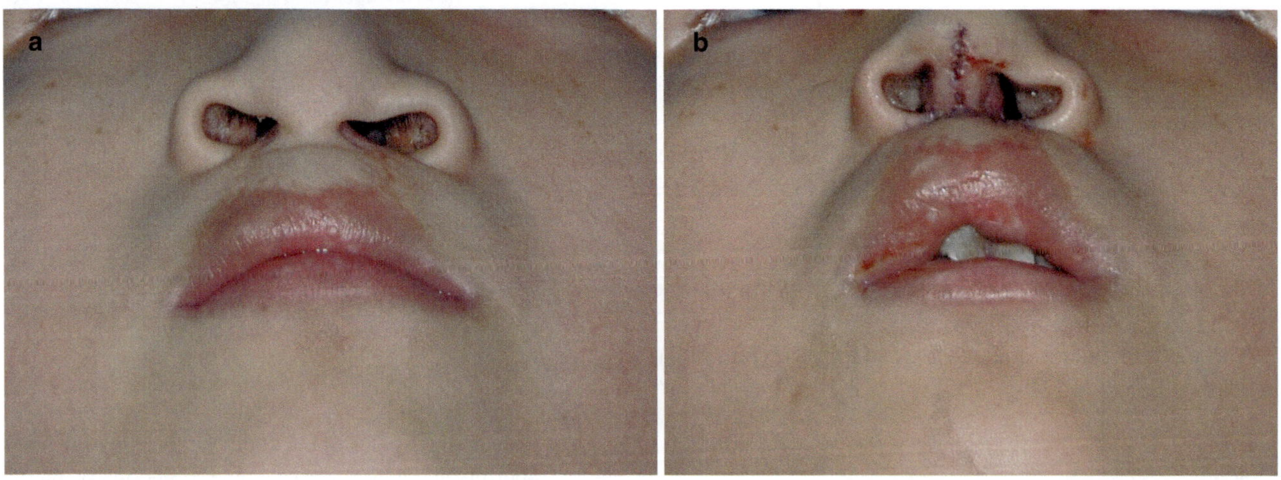

Fig. 11.5 (**a** and **b**) Pre-operative and post-operative comparison

lages until an acceptable outcome is achieved. Secure the position of the cartilage with non-resorbable silk or nylon sutures. Finally, suture the columella graft with the anterior margin of the nasal septum and cover it with the skin from the upper lip.

An Example of the Surgical Procedure:

The shape, length, and width of the graft are determined by the appearance of the patient's nose and face. Removal of the scar on the upper lip skin can facilitate the lengthening of the columella (Fig. 11.7).

Harvest the cartilage from either one of the left seventh, eighth, or ninth rib. The eighth rib cartilage is preferred as it is easier to obtain a long and straight graft (Fig. 11.8).

Make an incision according to the lines drawn and elevate the tissues adjacent to the scar and columella. Pull the nasal tip high up and expose the anterior margin of the nasal septum. Make a tunnel above the upper edge of the nasal septum (Fig. 11.9).

Pull the lateral lips together until they are in intimate contact with the philtrum, and ensure that the peaks of the Cupid's bow are aligned (Fig. 11.10).

The upper edge of the columella graft must be flat to fit suitably the nasal bridge graft (Fig. 11.11).

Through the tunnel created previously, insert the nasal bridge and columella graft into the nasal dorsum and the anterior portion of the nasal septum, respectively. Using either silk or nylon sutures, tie the lower edge of the nasal bridge graft with the upper edge of the columella graft. Lastly, anchor the columella graft with the anterior edge of the nasal septum (Fig. 11.12).

Advance the upper lip skin flap towards the columella to cover the columella graft. Close the skin flaps in this new position (Fig. 11.13).

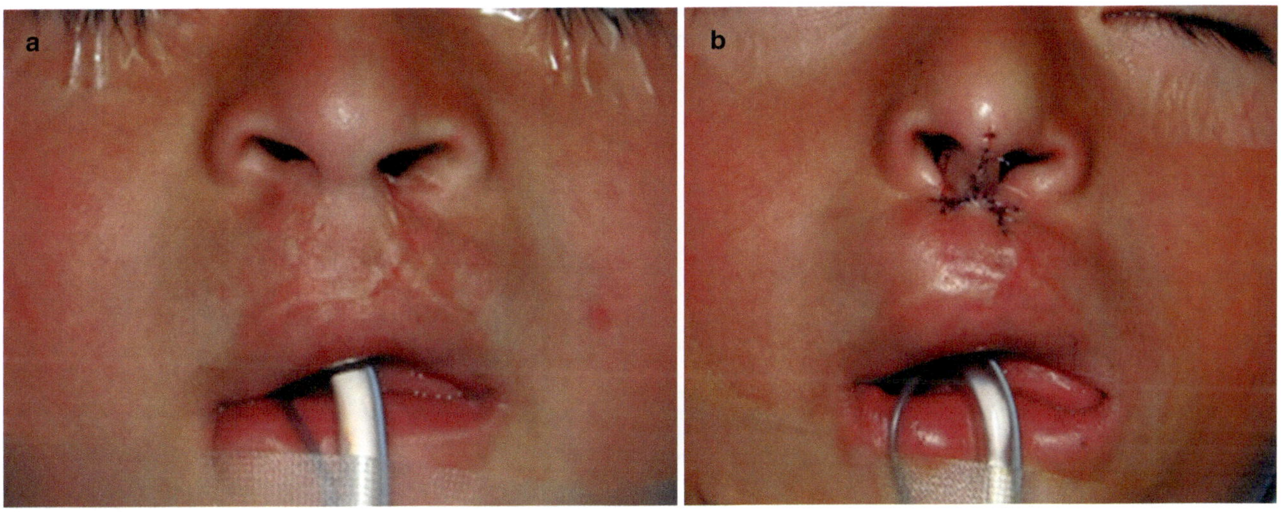

Fig. 11.6 (**a** and **b**) Pre-operative and post-operative comparison

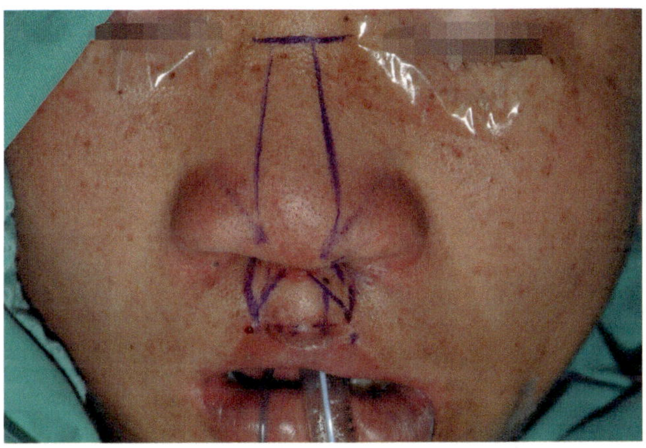

Fig. 11.7 Planned location of the nasal bridge graft and design of the surgical incisions

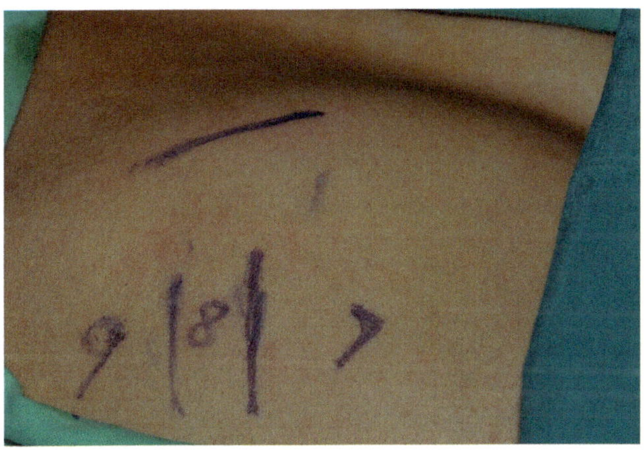

Fig. 11.8 Site of costal cartilage harvest

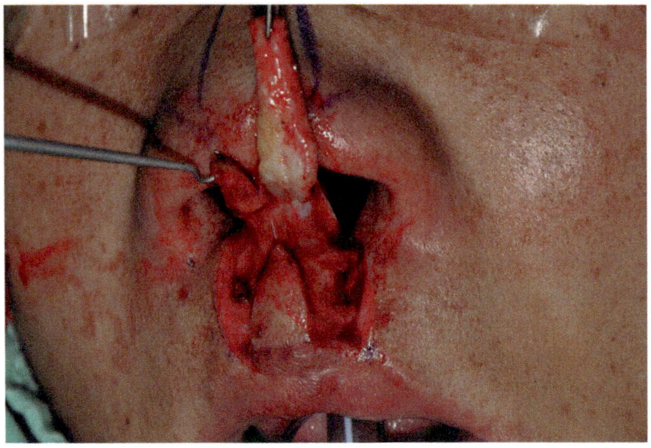

Fig. 11.9 Incision and exposure

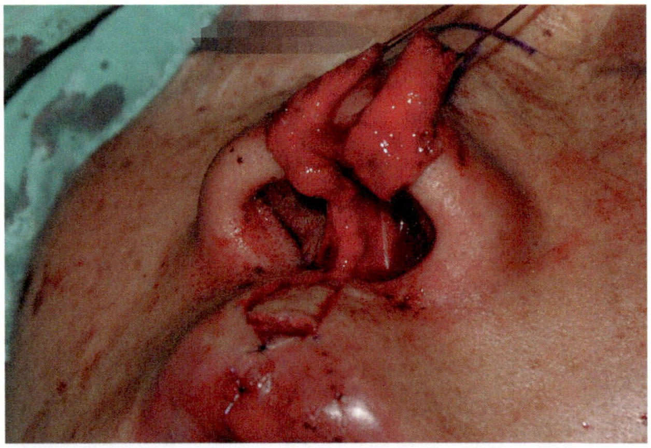

Fig. 11.10 Adduct the alar base and align the peaks of the Cupid's bow

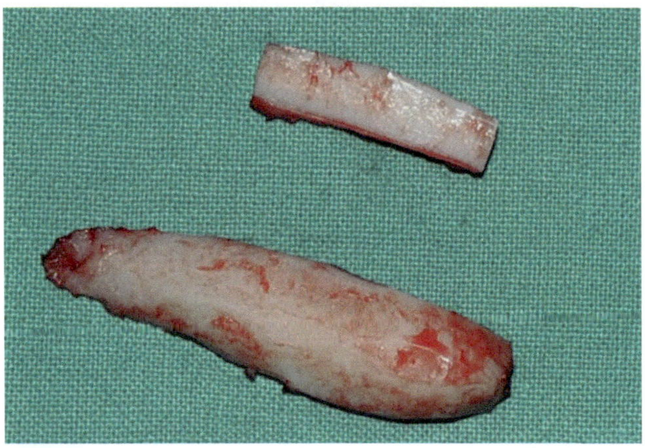

Fig. 11.11 Preparation of the columella and nasal bridge graft

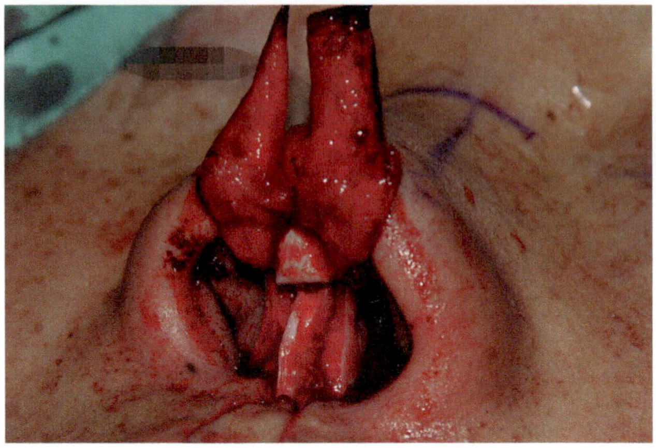

Fig. 11.12 Insertion of the columella and nasal bridge graft

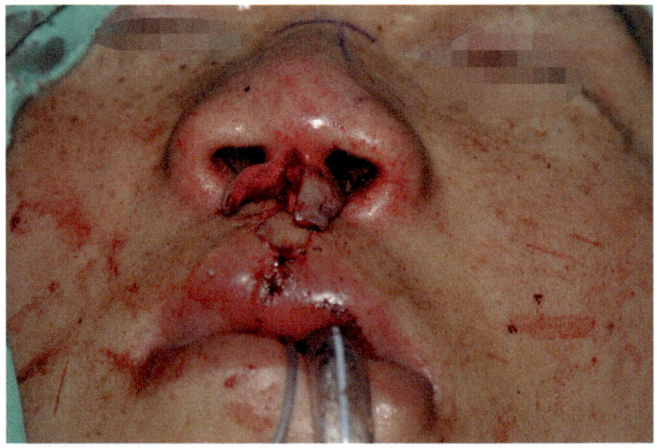

Fig. 11.13 Closure of the skin flaps

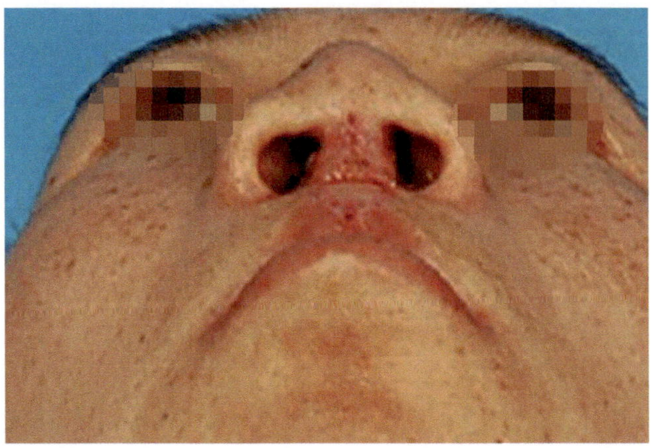

Fig. 11.14 Surgery completed

The columella is lengthened, and the nasal tip is raised (Fig. 11.14).

3. Points to Note
   (i) Preparation of the Nasal Bridge Graft: As their shapes are drastically different, the harvested rib cartilage must be fashioned prior to its use as a nasal bridge graft. The size, length, height, and curvature of the graft must be harmonious with the patient's facial appearance. The surface and edges of the nasal bridge graft must be smoothened after the shaping process.

(ii) Preparation of the Tunnel in the Nasal Dorsum: With one finger guiding, use a nasal periosteum stripper to dissect sub-periosteal towards the root of the nose. The lateral dissection must be beyond the nasal bones.

(iii) Position of the Nasal Tip: The tip of the nose must not be too sharp or lifted too high as it can induce excessive tension. The inserted graft may break through the high tension area and become exposed, leading to graft failure.

(iv) Shape of the Nose Tip: The shape of the nose tip is affected by contact between the lower edge of the nasal bridge graft and the upper edge of the columella graft.

(v) Fixation of the Nasal Columella: Elevate the tissue superficial to the anterior nasal spine and envelope the lower edge of the columella graft in the soft tissue pocket. Suture the lower edge of the columella graft to the periosteum of the anterior nasal spine. The middle portion of the graft is to be secured with the nasal septum, while the upper portion is secured to the nasal bridge graft [1, 2].

References

1. Kim SW, Oh M, Park JL, et al. Functional reconstruction of the philtral ridge and dimple in the repaired cleft lip. J Craniofacial Surg. 2007;18(6):1343–8.
2. Ming Z. McCarthy's modern plastic surgery (in Chinese). People's Medical Publishing House; 2007.

Plastic Surgery of Facial Cleft

12

Wang Zheng and Qian Zheng

12.1 Horizontal Facial Cleft Repair

1. Indications
   (i) Unilateral or bilateral horizontal facial clefts.
2. Surgical Methods and Procedures

   The surgery can usually be performed when the patient is as young as 3 months old.

   (i) The following methods can be used to determine the corners of the upper lip:
1. The distance from the intended corner of the lip to the peak of the Cupid's bow on the cleft side is equal to that of the unaffected side.
2. The corner of the lip should coincide with a vertical line drawn from the inner one-third of the eye.
3. The border of the lip mucosa where there is an obvious change in color can help to determine the new lip corner.

   (ii) The following methods can be used to determine the corners of the lower lip:
1. From the mandibular labial frenulum, make a straight line perpendicular to the lower lip. The distance between the corners of the lips on each side to the straight line should be equal.
2. The distance between the corners of the lower lip should be double the distance between the peak of the Cupid's bow and lip corner.
3. The border of the lip mucosa where there is an obvious change in color can help to determine the new lip corner.

   (iii) Raise a lip mucosal flap 5 mm in length and 4 mm in width at the corner of the upper lip. The free end of the flap should face the distal side. The flap is inserted to a corresponding site on the lower lip, and a segment of it is curled to form the new oral commissure. Avoid contact of the upper and lower lip margins at the corner. If the closure is at the corner of the mouth, movements during function may cause the sutures to open up and shift the position of the oral commissure. The orbicularis oris muscle from both sides of the cleft should also be reconstructed. By crossing triangular flaps from the skin at both sides of the cleft, we may create an upward angle of the commissure and prevent linear scar contraction [1].

Mark point 3 as the intended corner of the upper lip and point 2 as the intended corner of the lower lip. Point 1 is located on the vermillion border at about 5 mm distal to point 3, while point 4 is on the vermillion border 5 mm medial to point 2. Draw a 4 mm line from point 1 to point 5 on the lip mucosa (Line 1–5). Similarly, draw a 4 mm line from point 4 to point 6 on the lip mucosa (Line 4–6). Draw a continuous line along the vermillion border from points 3 and 4 to the corner of the cleft (Point A) (Fig. 12.1).

After the excision of the excess tissues, raise a rectangular mucosal flap on the upper lip. Pull the flap at such points 1 and 4 meet. Fold the flap around point 3 to create the new oral commissure (Figs. 12.2 and 12.3).

An Example of the Surgical Procedure (Figs. 12.4, 12.5, 12.6, 12.7, 12.8):

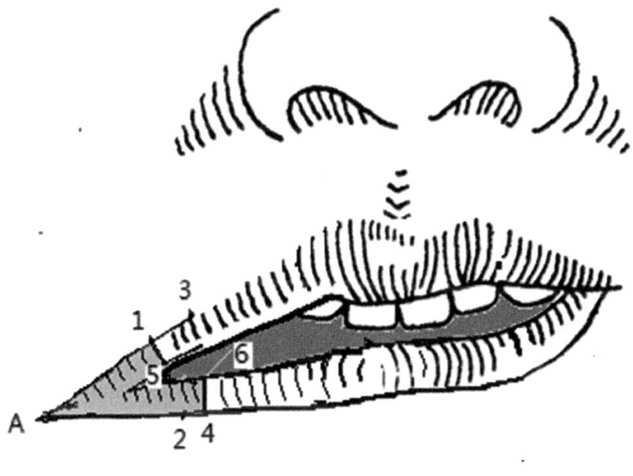

Fig. 12.1 Schematic diagram of the surgical design

W. Zheng · Q. Zheng (✉)
Department of Cleft Lip and Palate Surgery, West China Stomatology Hospital, Sichuan University, Chengdu, China

J. Liu, B. Shi (eds.), *Atlas of Lip and Nose Plastic and Cosmetic Surgery*, https://doi.org/10.1007/978-981-16-1911-3_12

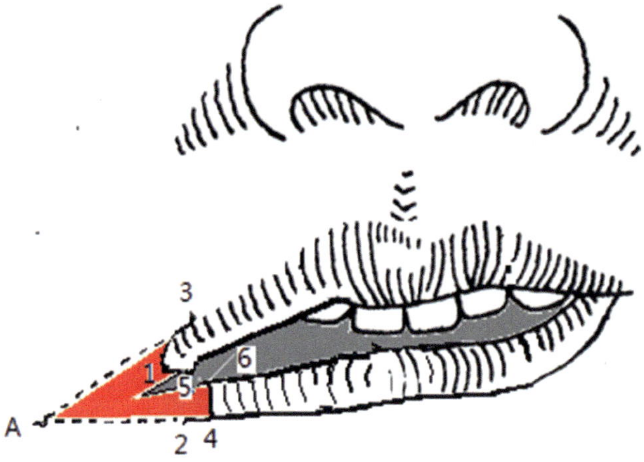

Fig. 12.2 Design of the surgical incisions

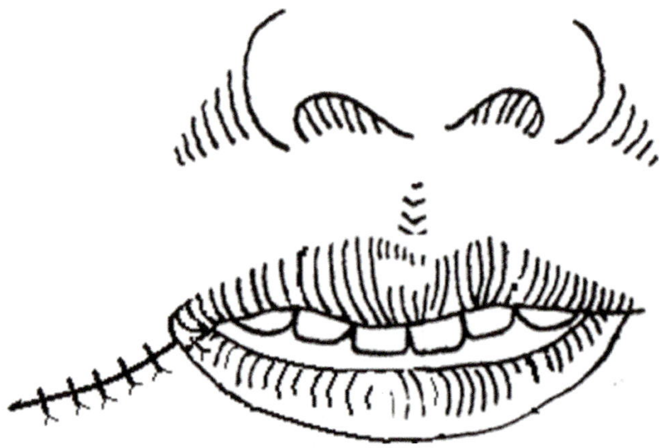

Fig. 12.3 Schematic diagram of the post-operative appearance

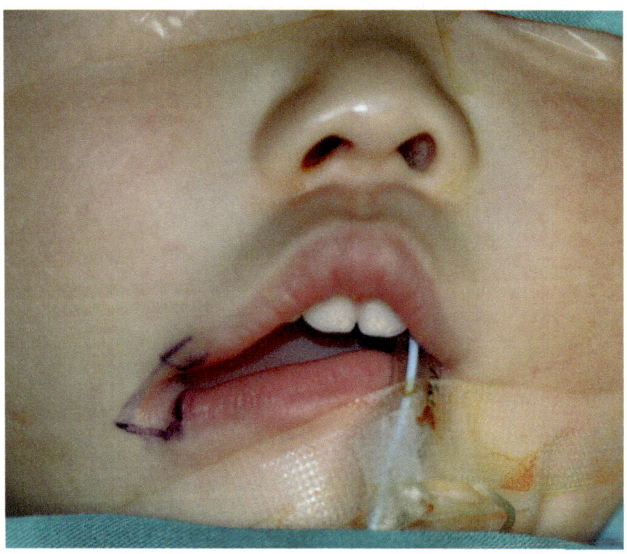

Fig. 12.4 Design of the surgical incisions

Place an anchoring suture in the submucosal tissues of the upper lip at the location of the new oral commissure. This will further highlight the form of the oral commissure.

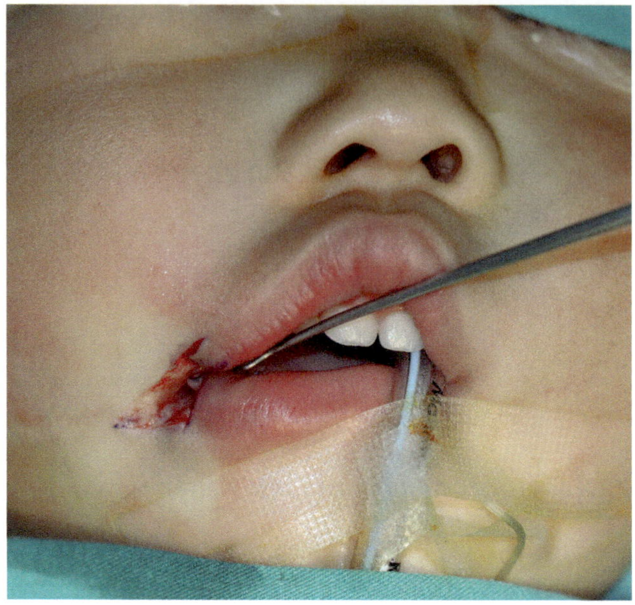

Fig. 12.5 Make the incisions into the skin and mucosa according to the lines drawn, and raise a rectangular mucosal flap

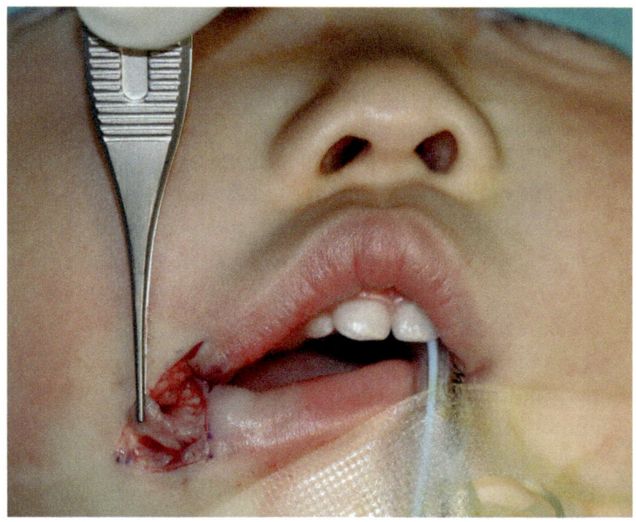

Fig. 12.6 Dissect the orbicularis oris muscle above and below the cleft, and suture them together

In this example, the skin can be closed in a straight line as the cleft is short. Generally, if the skin incision is within 1 cm, the wound can be closed in a straight line. Any incisions greater than 1 cm should be closed in a Z-shape to prevent contraction (Fig. 12.9).

Classic Example 1 (Fig. 12.10)

Classic Example 2 (Fig. 12.11)

3. Points to Note:
   (i) The upper and lower lips may become distorted during surgery due to the anesthesia intubation tubes. Therefore, if the patient is co-operative, determine the locations of the corners of the mouth before the opera-

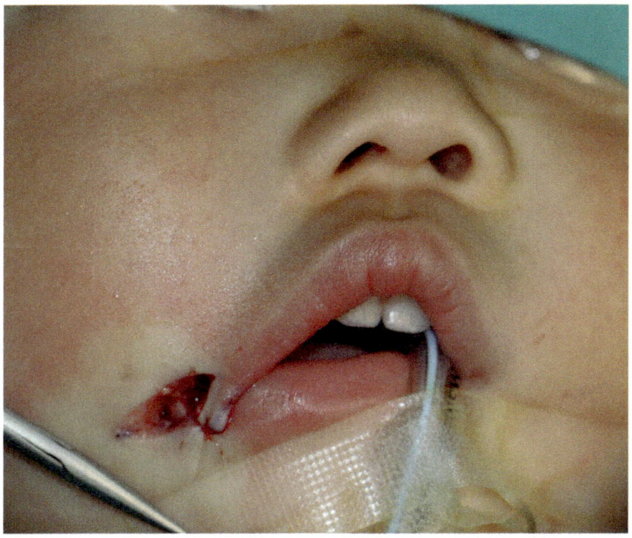

Fig. 12.7 Turn the upper lip mucosal flap downwards to the lower lip

tion. If the patient is not co-operative, determine the corners of the mouth before the endotracheal intubation so as to reduce the deviation in measurements caused by tissue distortions [2].

12.2 Median Facial Cleft Repair

1. Indications:
   (i) Median facial cleft that involves mainly the nose and lip region.
2. Surgical Methods and Procedures:
   (i) Excise away the excess tissues between each alar, and achieve a normal alar width. Close the mucosal, muscle, and skin layers. Opposing triangular flaps can be used to reconstruct the skin and mucosal layers.

Mark point 1 and 2 as the right and left peak of Cupid's bow, respectively. Point 3 is located on the vermillion border 3 mm

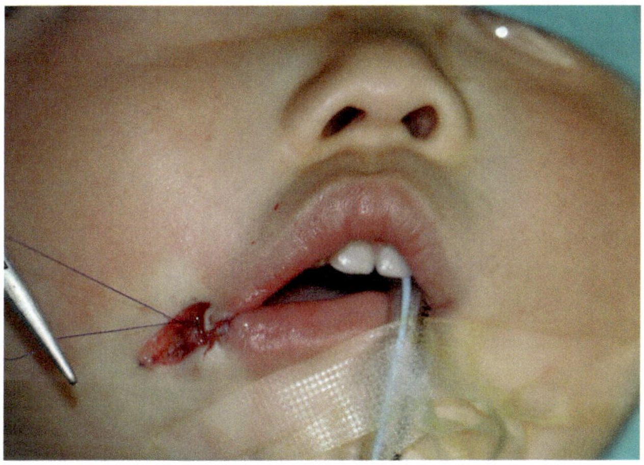

Fig. 12.8 Submucosal fixation of the oral commissure

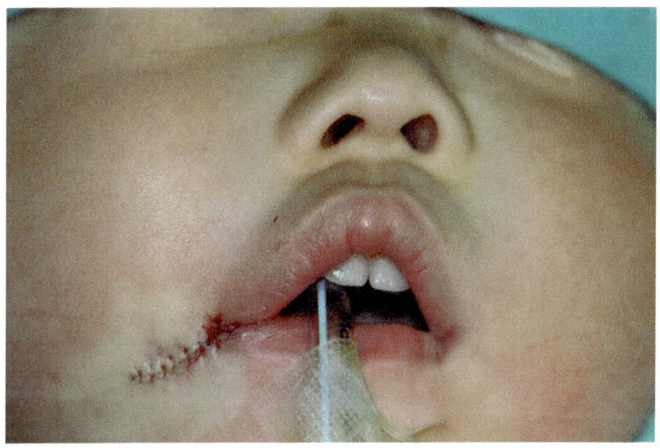

Fig. 12.9 Closure of the skin and mucosa

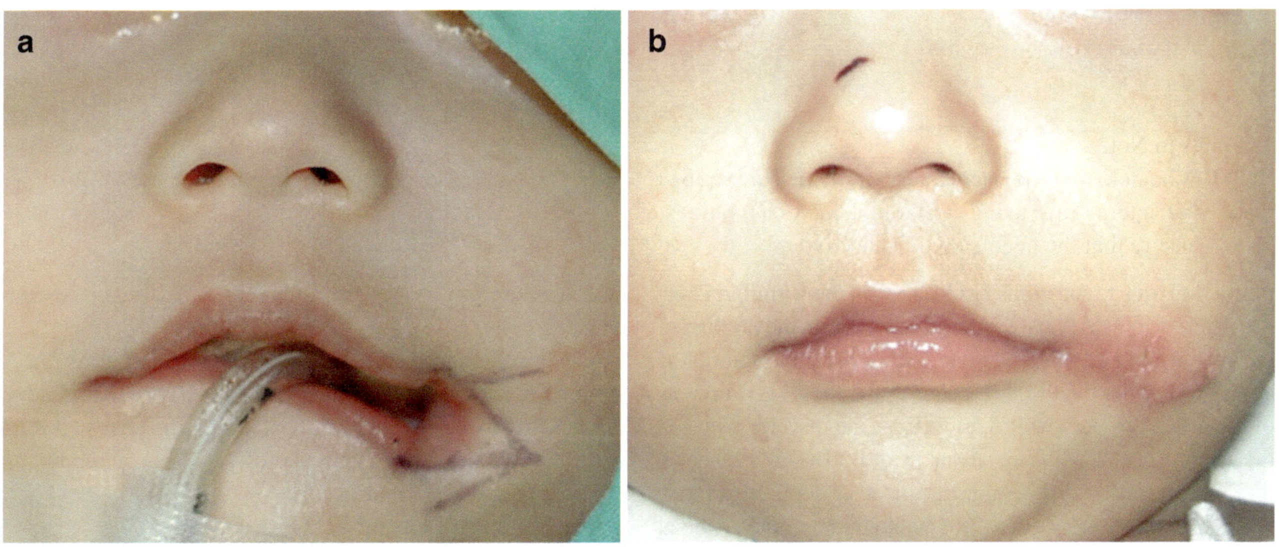

Fig. 12.10 (**a** and **b**) Before and after surgery. **a**: Pre-operative surgical design, **b**: Post-operative

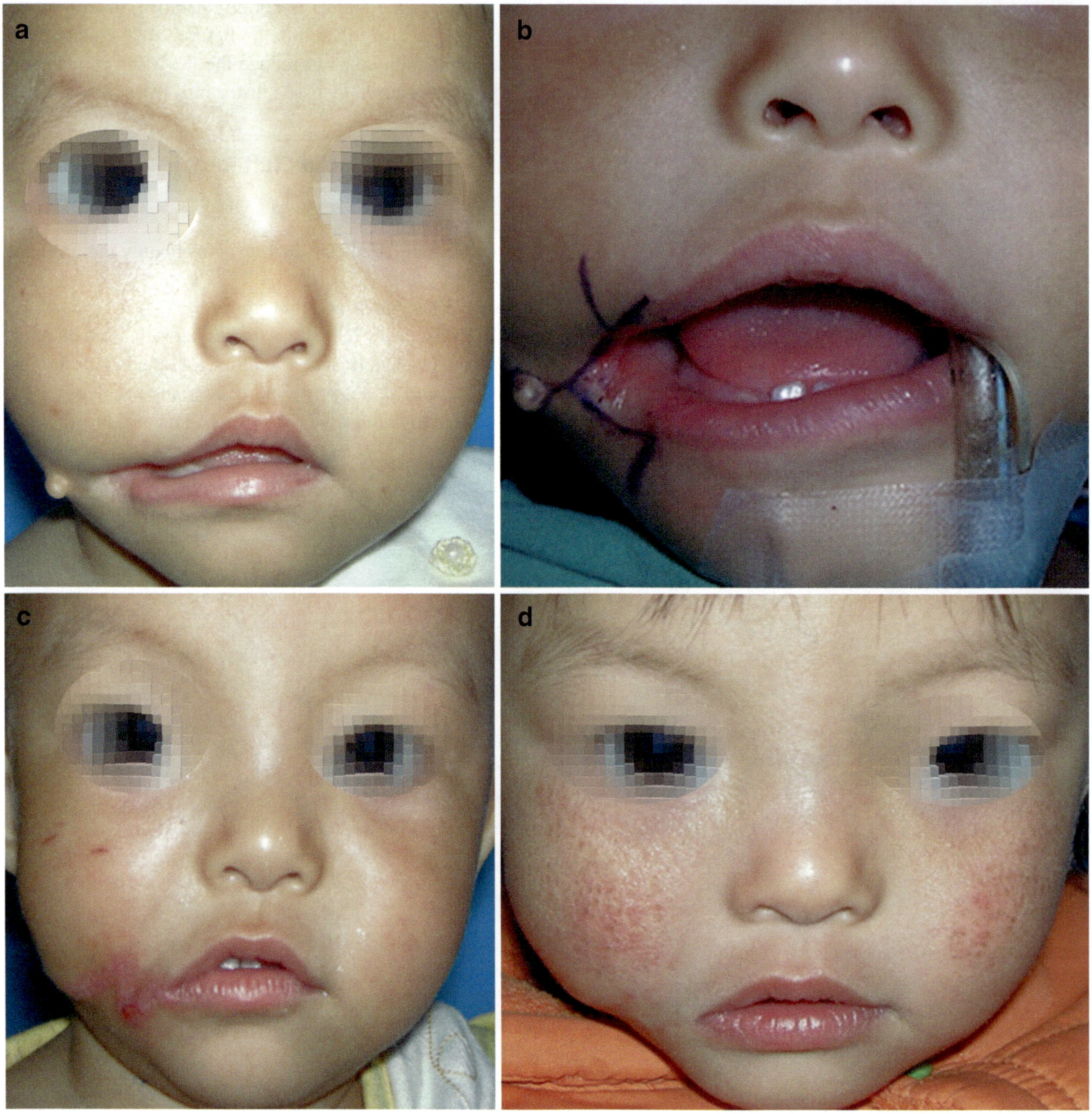

Fig. 12.11 (**a**, **b**, **c**, and **d**) Before and after surgery, **a**: Pre-operative appearance, **b**: Surgical design, **c**: Post-operative appearance, **d**: Two years after surgery

medial to point 1, and point 4 is located on the vermillion border 3 mm medial to point 2. Point 5 is located in the midline of the root of the nose. Points 6 and 7 are lateral and inferior to point 5. Measure the distance between the most lateral points of the alar (Alar flare width), as well as, the distance between the medial canthus (inner canthal width). The difference in their length is used to determine the distance between points 6 and 7. (Points 6–7 = Alar flare width minus inner canthal width). Connect points 5–6–3 and 5–7–4 (Fig. 12.12).

Excise excess tissues from the alar and around the cleft (Fig. 12.13).

Design Z-shaped incisions on the nose to prevent a straight scar contraction. Make a horizontal incision along the base of the nose, and adduct the nostril. Lastly, design triangular flaps on the lip mucosal to create a plump lip tubercle (Figs. 12.14 and 12.15).

An Example of the Surgical Procedure:

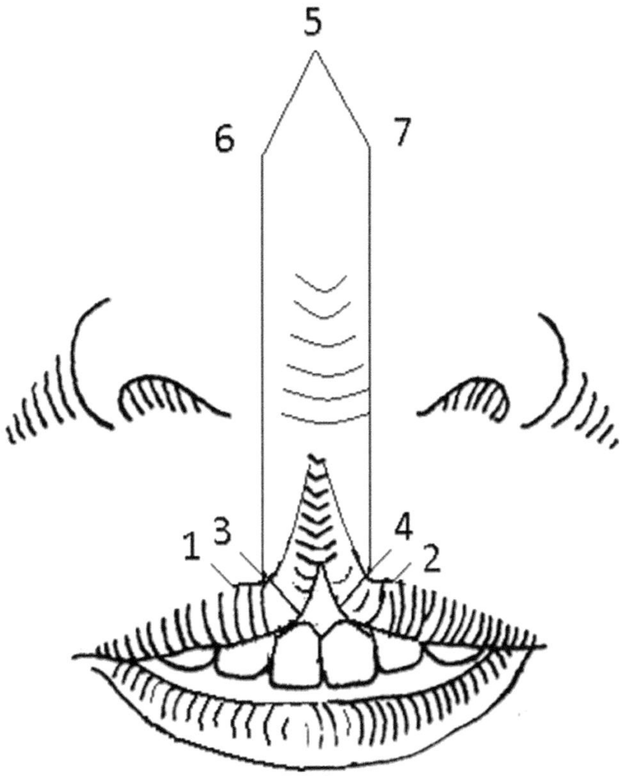

Fig. 12.12 Before and after surgery

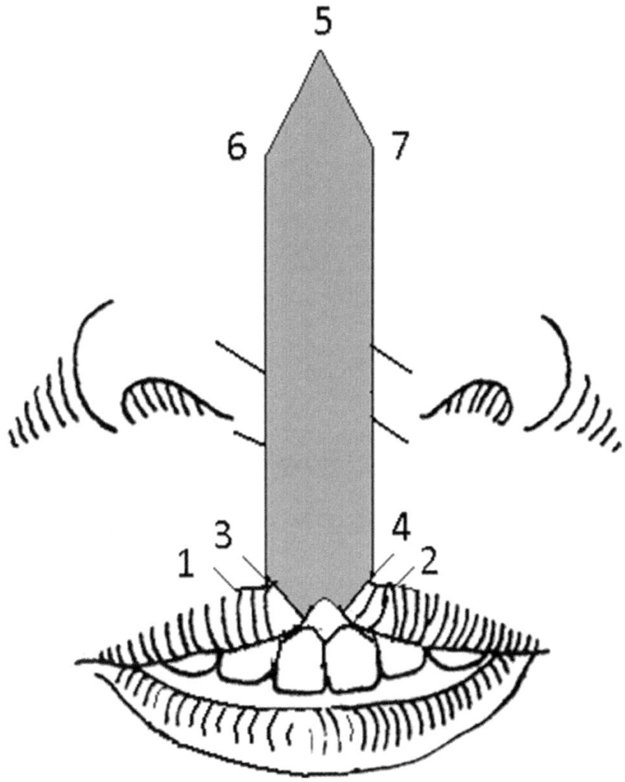

Fig. 12.14 Schematic diagram of the surgical design

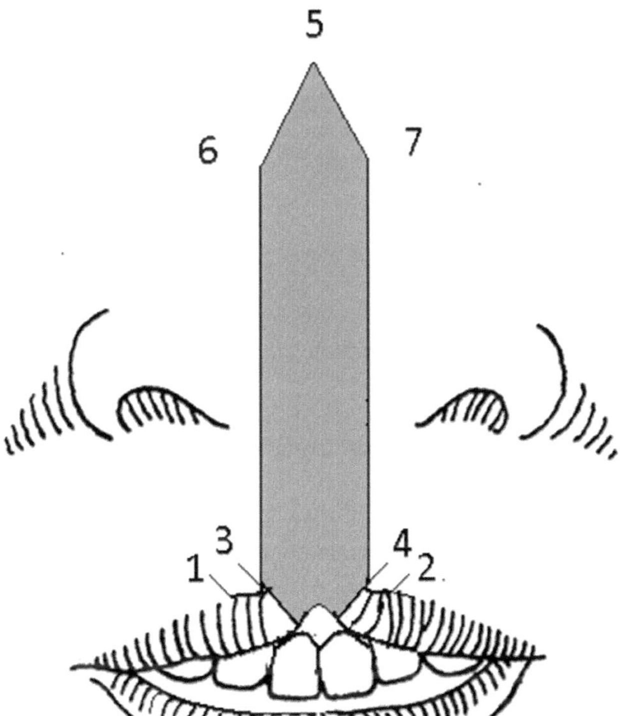

Fig. 12.13 Schematic diagram of the surgical design

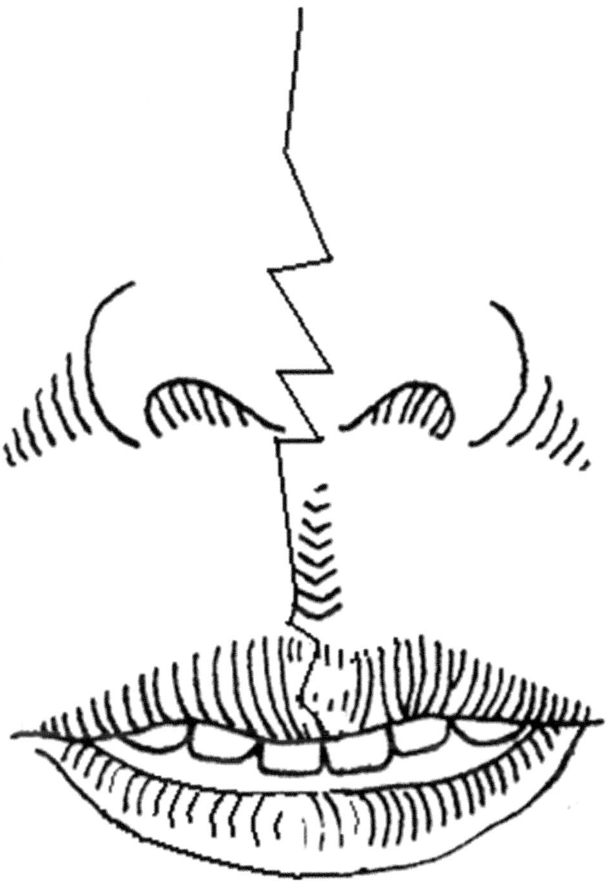

Fig. 12.15 Schematic diagram of the completed surgery

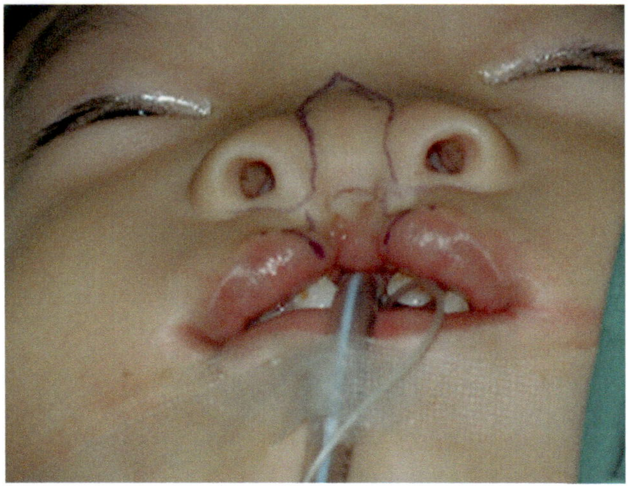

Fig. 12.16 Design of the surgical incisions

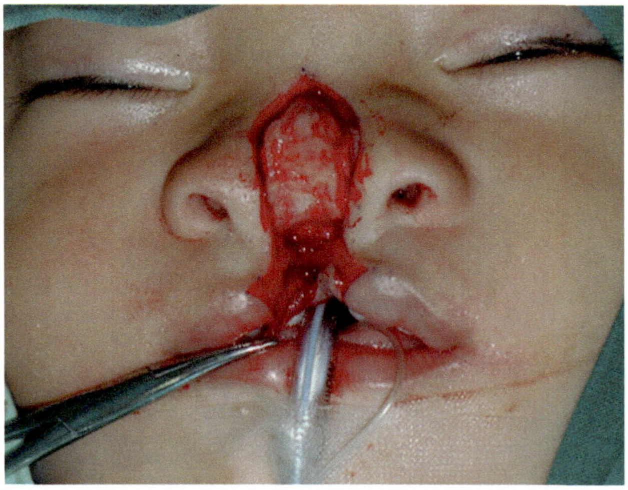

Fig. 12.17 Removal of excess tissues

This patient has a median facial cleft that extends from the upper lip, columella, and the tip and dorsum of the nose. It is accompanied by telecanthus. Design the incisions within the cleft region and remove a width of tissue equivalent to the alar flare width minus the inner canthal distance. That is to say, the post-operative nasal width should be equal to the distance between the medial canthus (Figs. 12.16 and 12.17).

On the nasal dorsum, design opposing triangular flaps to lengthen the skin and allow the nose tip to be lowered (Fig. 12.18).

Appose and close the skin of the dorsum, upper lip, and lip mucosa (Fig. 12.19).

3. Points to Note:
   (i) Patients with median facial fissure may also present with a meningocele. Pre-operative investigations, such as an X-ray or CT examination, should be conducted. Consult a neurosurgeon should there be evidence of cranial pathology.

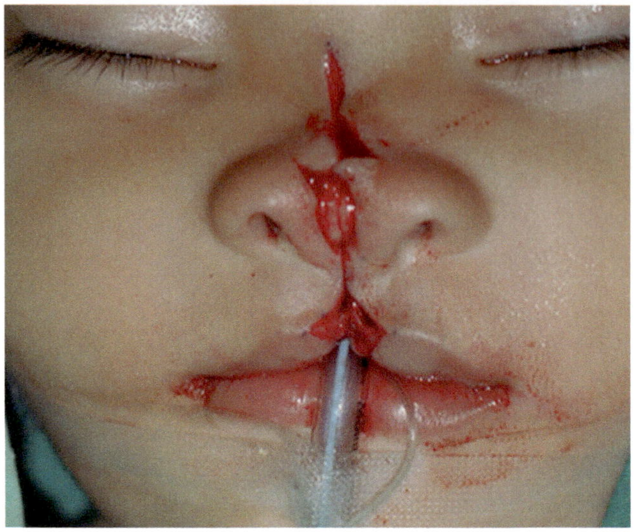

Fig. 12.18 Design opposing triangular flaps on the nasal dorsum

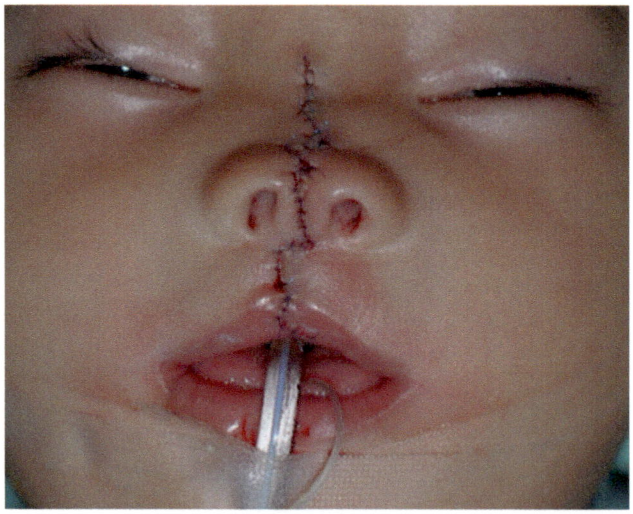

Fig. 12.19 Post-operative appearance

12.3 Oblique Facial Cleft Repair

1. Indications:
   (i) Unilateral or bilateral oblique facial clefts.
2. Surgical Methods and Procedures:
   (i) Oblique facial clefts are often accompanied by bony tissue clefts.
   (ii) Early extensive surgeries on an infant will hinder the development of the jaw, therefore, surgery is usually performed 6–12 months after birth, once the facial landmarks are more obvious. Local skin flaps are

recommended for the repair of soft tissue defects. Bony tissue reconstruction is as important as soft tissue repair. Autogenous rib cartilage or iliac cancellous bone can be used to repair bony defects.

(iii) For infant patients, the soft tissue defects can be repaired first, while the repair of craniofacial bone defects may be deferred until after the end of puberty. For adult patients, both the soft tissue and bony tissue defects can be repaired simultaneously.

(iv) An Ophthalmologist should be consulted if oculoplastic surgery is required. The orbicularis oculi muscle and orbicularis oris muscle should be reconstructed to restore normal sphincter activity. Preserve as much tissue as possible during the first stage of surgery, and leave the remaining deformities to be corrected in the second stage.

An Example of the Surgical Procedure:

Design a rectangular flap to bring down the cleft of the upper lip. A corresponding flap should be made on the lateral side of the cleft to fill the defect created after shifting the upper lip inferiorly. It is vital to suture the orbicularis oris muscle from both sides of the cleft to reconstruct the muscle (Figs. 12.20, 12.21, 12.22).

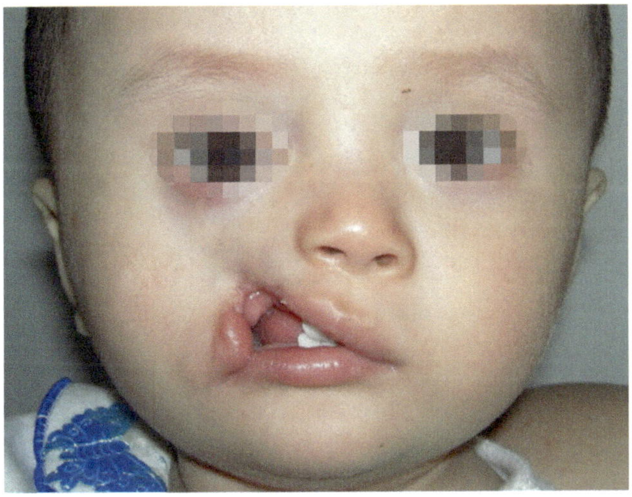

Fig. 12.20 Pre-operative appearance

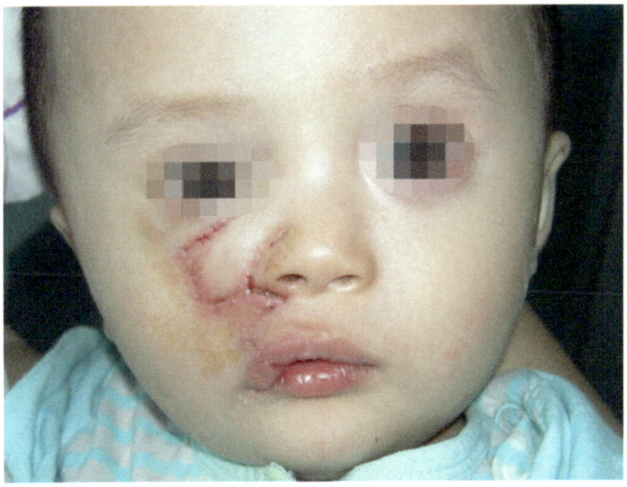

Fig. 12.21 Appearance at 7 days after surgery

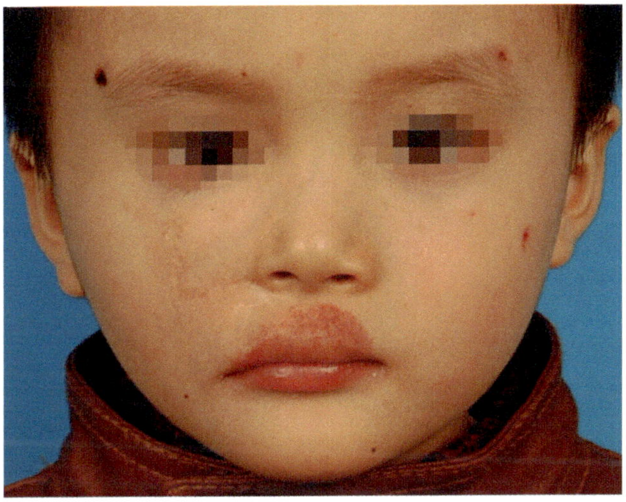

Fig. 12.22 Appearance at 3 years after the surgery

3. Points to Note:

In patients where the cleft extends to the orbital floor, the surgeon must be careful to avoid damaging the orbital contents during the operation. Consult an ophthalmologist if the surgery involves the orbital floor or reconstruction of the nasolacrimal duct.

References

1. Cutting CB, Dayan JH. Lip height and lip width after extended Mohler unilateral cleft lip repair. Plast Reconstr Surg. 2003;111(1):17–23.
2. Molendijk J, Pendleton C, Rachwalski M, et al. Harvey Cushing's contributions to plastic surgery: bilateral cleft lip repair. Cleft Palate Craniofac J. 2014;51(1):105–9.

Part IV

Acquired Nasolabial Deformities and Plastic Reconstruction

Essentials of Surgical Design for Acquired Lip Defect

13

Jianhua Liu

13.1 Safety Margin of Labial Tumor Resection

Most of the labial deformities are due to lip tumor resection, with a small number of cases secondary to trauma. Majority of the labial tumor involve the lower lip, with a minority involving the upper lip.

Most of the labial tumors involving the lower lip are moderately and well-differentiated squamous cell carcinomas and its surgical prognosis is relatively good. If the biopsy results showed moderately to well-differentiated squamous cell carcinoma, and the clinical presentation appears exophytic with well-demarcated borders, the safety resection margin can be less than 1 cm (foreign studies reported 0.3–0.7 cm). We feel that the safety resection margin should not be less than 0.5 cm and need not necessarily extend up to 1 cm. This is to preserve as much soft tissue of the lower lip as possible, which allows better restoration of function and esthetics after reconstruction.

Majority of the upper lip tumors are ulcerative or endophytic, and the safety resection margin should be larger (about 1.0 cm) to minimize the risk of recurrence. Unless the tumor is exophytic, with distinct tumor borders, a 0.5 cm margin can be chosen.

13.2 Geometry Study of Safety Margin of Tumor Resection

Most of the labial tumors are associated with the vermillion border, and its outline can be represented using a circle. Majority of the surgical resection of malignant labial tumor can utilize a V-shaped or rectangular-shaped excision along the safety resection margin. A small defect, from a V-shaped excision, can be closed primarily. A larger defect would require an advancement flap or a cross-lip flap for closure. The amount of defect from surgical resection of the labial tumor is not only dependent on the tumor size and safety resection margin, but also on the angle of the V-shaped excision. Till date, the relationship between the amount of surgical resection needed and the angle of the V-shaped excision still lacks mathematical research. We used mathematical deduction and computer analysis to establish this relationship, and this can serve as a guide for the calculation of similar flap in the future [1].

For mathematical inference and analysis purposes, we used a straight line to represent the vermillion border, and the tumor is represented by a circle drawn with a solid line. The safety resection margin is represented by a circle drawn with a dotted line. r represents the radius of the circle, and $R = r +$ safety surgical margin. The relationship between the length of the V-shaped excision and the safety surgical margin is shown in Fig. 13.1. Given that the thickness of the lip is represented by h, the angle of the V-shaped excision becomes an independent variable (Q), and the amount of normal soft tissue loss is then the dependent variable Y, whereby $Y = h * S(Q)$, where S represents the area of soft tissue loss excluding the tumor [2].

Derivative of the mathematical formula for the amount of normal soft tissue loss using the V-shaped excision:

A vertical line is drawn from the middle of the edges of the V-shape, dividing the V-shape into two symmetrical right-angled triangles. We used one of the right-angled triangles for analysis. The area of the right-angle triangle $S_\Delta = (A_1 * A_2)/2$. The total area of the V-shaped excision $S_v = 2 * S_\Delta = 2 * (A_1 * A_2)/2 = A_1 * A_2$. As A_1 and A_2 are unknown, they vary according to the angle of the V-shaped excision Q. Based on Sin a = opposite/ hypotenuse, we obtain $\sin a_1 = R/A_1$, $\sin a_2 = R/A_2$, and hence $A_1 = R/\sin a_1$, $A_2 = R/\sin a_2$.

J. Liu (✉)
Department of Oral and Maxillo-facial Surgery, First Affiliated Hospital, Zhejiang University School of Medicine, Hangzhou, China

J. Liu, B. Shi (eds.), *Atlas of Lip and Nose Plastic and Cosmetic Surgery*, https://doi.org/10.1007/978-981-16-1911-3_13

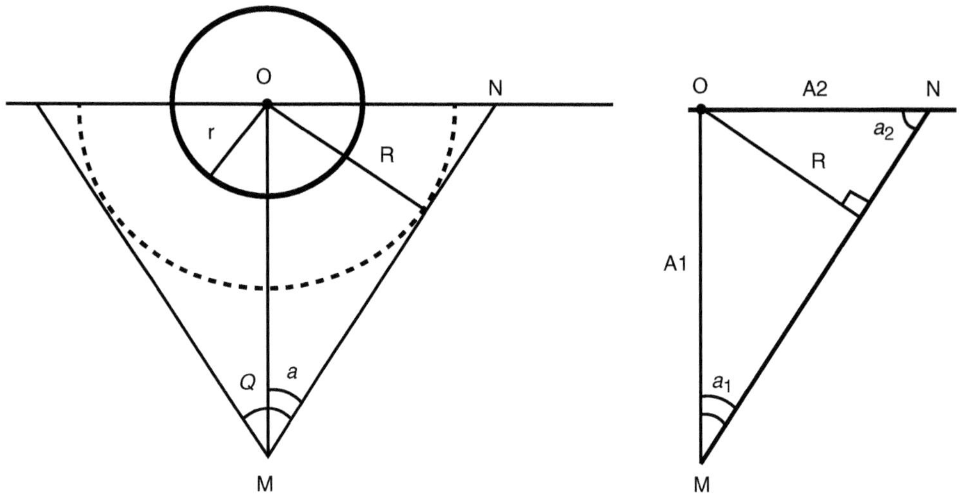

Fig. 13.1 Analysis of normal soft tissue loss following "V"-shaped excision

Table 13.1 The relationship between the angle of the V-shaped excision (*Q*) and the amount of soft tissue loss (*Y*)

Q =	0	2	6	10	14	18	22	26
Y =	∝	227.6589	74.9634	44.4994	31.4977	24.3177	19.7849	16.6786
Q =	30	34	38	42	46	50	54	58
Y =	14.4292	12.7355	11.4234	10.3850	9.5505	8.8725	8.3177	7.8626
Q =	62	66	70	74	78	82	86	90
Y =	7.4898	7.1863	6.9426	6.7516	6.6079	6.5078	6.4487	6.4292
Q =	94	98	102	106	110	114	118	122
Y =	6.4487	6.5078	6.6079	6.7516	6.9426	7.1863	7.4898	7.8626
Q =	126	130	134	138	142	146	150	154
Y =	8.3177	8.8725	9.5505	10.3850	11.4234	12.7355	14.4292	16.6786
Q =	158	162	166	170	174	178	180	
Y =	19.7849	24.3177	31.4977	44.4994	74.9634	227.6589	∝	

Note:
1. *Q* represents the V-shaped excision angle, with a unit of degree
2. *Y* represents the ratio of soft tissue loss; The larger the ratio, the larger amount of soft tissue loss

Using the area of V-shaped excision S_V to subtract the area of the semicircle demarcated by the dotted line, then multiply by the thickness of the lip (*h*), we get $Y = h*[(A_1*A_2)-\pi r^2/2]$, which gives us $Y = h*[(R/\text{Sin } a_1)*(R/\text{Sin } a_2)-\pi r^2/2]$. And because $a_1 + a_2 = 90°$ (Pythagoras theorem), $a_2 = 90°-a_1$, therefore $Y = h*[(R/\text{Sin } a_1)*(R/\text{Sin } 90°-a_1)-\pi r^2/2]$.

Mathematical deduction and computer analysis of V-shaped excision:

Using an independent variable *a* as one and half of the angle of the V-shaped excision, the normal soft tissue loss becomes a dependent variable *Y*, whereby $Y = h*[(R/\text{Sin } a_1)*(R/\text{Sin } 90°-a_1)-\pi r^2/2]$. At the same time, we allow a constant of $h = 1$ and program using the MATLAB programming language. When the step variable for *a* is 2, the V-shaped excision angle $Q(Q = 2a)$ and the corresponding value of *Y* is observed in Table 13.1. When the step variable *a* is 0.1, the corresponding functional curve is seen in Fig. 13.2.

According to the quantitative calculation results (Table 13.1), when the V-shaped excision angle $Q = 90°$, the smallest amount of soft tissue loss *Y* is 6.4292. When *Q* is smaller or larger than 90°, the value of *Y* becomes larger. When *Q* is smaller than 20° or larger than 160°, the value of *Y* becomes exponentially larger. The calculated functional curve (Fig. 13.2) is similar to a U-shaped parabolic curve. When the independent variable $Q = 90°$, the value of *Y* is the smallest. When *Q* approaches 0° or 180°, *Y* tends to infinity. The range of *Q* whereby *Y* is covered by not more than 50% of the minimum value is between 45° – 135° (i.e., 90° ± 45°), as seen in the shaded region in Fig. 13.2.

According to the above-mentioned research results, the amount of soft tissue loss during the V-shaped excision is not only dependent on the tumor size and its safety surgical margin, but also is related to the size of the V-shaped excision angle. The relationship between the V-shaped excision angle and the amount of soft tissue loss lacks quantitative analysis. Most of the flap designs rely on clinical judgment. If the quantitative calculation results can be integrated, it would benefit the design of the flap and possibly minimize the amount of normal soft tissue loss.

From Table 13.1 or the functional curve in Fig. 13.2, when the angle becomes 90°, the amount of normal soft tissue loss is the least, and the ratio is similar to a rectangular excision. Therefore, we conclude that: When choosing between the V-shaped or rectangular excision for a lip tumor, the rectangular excision should be preferred. This is because apart from the need for the calculation of the best excision angle, other excision angles would result in more normal soft tissue loss than the rectangular excision.

If the lip tumor is small, and the predicted defect after excision is around one-third of the width of the lip, then the V-shaped excision can be closed primarily, which is easy and convenient and does not result in much functional deficit. According to the theoretical analysis, when the V-shaped excision angle is 90°, the amount of normal soft tissue loss is the least. However, when the V-shaped excision angle is larger than 60°, this easily results in a "dog-ear" effect. From Fig. 13.2, when the angle is between 45° – 135°, the functional curve plateaus, and implies that the change in the amount of soft tissue loss is minimal. In order to avoid creating a "dog-ear" effect and at the same time minimize the amount of soft tissue loss, the V-shaped excision angle is best chosen to be between 45° – 60°. However, a 90° angle would be suitable in the case of a cross-lip flap, because the contralateral transfer of lip flap is around 45°, and the V-shaped excision would just require opposing of the 2 edges at 45° to close the defect, and this will not result in a "dog-ear" effect.

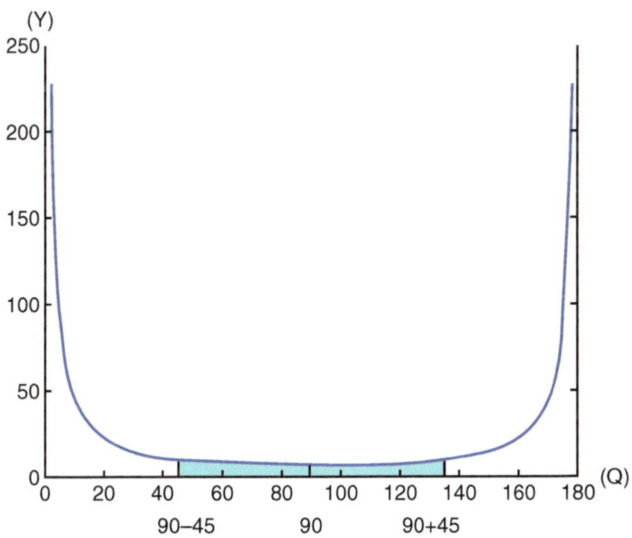

Fig. 13.2 The relationship between the "V" shape excision angle Q and the amount of soft tissue loss Y

13.3 Study on Stretchability of Labial Soft Tissue

There are many etiologies to varying degrees of lip defect, resulting in numerous reconstructive choices clinically, and most options employ the use of localized flaps for closure. Commonly, there is insufficient consideration for the amount of stretchability of normal lip tissue, primarily because of the lack of quantification analysis. We studied 200 patients from the departments of Oral and Maxillofacial Surgery, as well as Ear, Nose, and Throat departments, obtained the data of lip measurement. We analyzed the data and discussed its application to the reconstruction of the lip via various flap designs and their respective rationale [3].

Method: Four measurements are made for each patient's lip, namely the lip width in static and stretched positions, the height of the lower lip, as well as the depth of the lower lip sulcus. Measurements are made using a Vernier caliper and a spring tension meter. Measurements are recorded in centimeters. The measurement of the lip in static is done with the patient's lips relaxed, and the distance between the two corners of the mouth is measured. The measurement of the lip in the stretched state is done via two curved hooks of the spring tension meter (with sterilized rubber bands) at each of the corner of the mouth, together with an applied 0.3 kg force in opposing direction, and the distance between the two corners of the mouth is measured. The height of the lower lip is taken from the peak of the vermilion of the lower lip to the lowest border of the chin. The lower lip sulcus depth is measured from the peak of the vermillion of the lower lip to the lowest point in the lower labial sulcus.

The measurements are presented in Tables 13.2 and 13.3. There is no statistical differences between gender and among different age groups. The width of the lips in static and stretched states is wider in males than females ($p < 0.05$), and there is no statistical difference between males and females in terms of ratio (B/A). In addition, the height of the lower lip and the lower sulcus depth is larger in males than females ($p < 0.05$). When the stretchability of the lower lip among different age groups are compared (Table 13.3), there is no statistical difference ($p < 0.05$) in terms of ratio (B/A).

Table 13.2 Comparison of lip measurements between males and females (Unit:cm)

Gender	Age	No. of Cases	Static lip (A)	Stretched lip (B)	B/A	Height of lower lip	Lower sulcus depth
Male	45.4	125	4.97 ± 0.46	9.55 ± 0.87	1.92	4.59 ± 0.44	2.55 ± 0.24
Female	44.9*	75	4.45 ± 0.51**	8.91 ± 0.90**	2.00	4.34 ± 0.48**	2.24 ± 0.26**
Total	45.3	200	4.77 ± 0.47	9.31 ± 0.88	1.95	4.50 ± 0.45	2.44 ± 0.25

Note: Comparison between males and females, T-test: *$p > 0.05$, **$p < 0.05$

Table 13.3 Comparison of lip stretchability among different age groups (Unit:cm)

Age group	20 – 29	30 – 39	40 – 49	50 – 59	60 – 69	70 – 79	Total
No. of cases	46	30	35	29	36	24	200
Width of static lip (*A*)	4.37	4.53	4.89	4.94	4.96	5.10	4.77
Width of stretched lip (*B*)	8.44	9.15	9.54	9.46	9.80	9.88	9.31
B/*A*	1.93	2.02	1.95	1.91	1.98	1.94	1.95

Note: No statistical differences among different age groups B/A ($F = 2.18$, $p > 0.05$)

However, as age increases, the measurement of the lower lip in both static and stretched states has variable increases.

With regards to the tolerance level of lip stretching in an average population, there is none in the literature for adaptation. We, therefore, experimented with the amount of force needed on volunteers. The lip feels tight when the range of force is between 0.3–0.5 kg. When the amount of force is larger than 0.5 kg, there is pain at the lip. In addition, there is no significant increase in lip width when the amount of force increases from 0.3 kg to 0.5 kg. Therefore, we chose 0.3 kg as amount of force applied during measurement. None of the patients reported discomfort during measurement.

The removal of malignant lip tumors often results in large defects. Various flap designs often employ the principle of the movement of two sliding flaps, which amounts to the defect size. However, the amount of stretchability of the remaining soft tissue is still unknown. Our research shows that there is a great amount of stretchability in the lip of an average person. Under tolerable forces, the lip can stretch to almost twice the width (under 0.3 kg force, $B/A = 1.95$). We modified our flap design by using the two adjacent sliding flaps to reconstruct two-third of the defect, and the remaining one-third is reconstructed via stretching of the remaining soft tissues of the lip. We achieved satisfactory clinical results. Our research results can serve as a basis to develop further thinking and theories for various flap designs and cross-lip flaps at the lip and chin region.

Even though there are no statistical differences in the ratio (B/A) between gender and among different age groups ($p < 0.05$), there is still increases in the width of the lip in static and stretched states as the age increases. This implies that as age increases, the corners of the mouth can be stretched further. Therefore, during flap design, there is a need to consider the patient's age as the difference in stretchability of a young and old patient's lip is significant.

According to our measurements, the depth of the lower lip sulcus is an average of 2.44 cm. When a malignant lip tumor extends below the vermilion border by 1 cm, and the safety surgical margin is 1 cm, the lower border of a rectangular excision to sulcus bottom will be about 0.44 cm. This will not affect the movement of the sliding flaps. However, if a malignant lip tumor extends below the vermilion border over 1.5 cm, the rectangular excision may extend beyond the bottom of the sulcus, resulting in an inability of the two adjacent sliding flaps to move. In this case, the surgical blade should be directed upwards, keeping the tip of the blade within the lower sulcus, and thus ensuring the movement of the adjacent sliding flaps.

13.4 Classification of Lip Defect

Acquired Lip Defects Can Be Classified into:

1. Upper lip defect, Lower lip defect;
   Defect at the center of the lip (Fig. 13.3), Defect at the side of the lip (Corner of mouth) (Fig. 13.4).
2. Defect at the vermillion, Skin-muscle defect, Skin-muscle-mucosa (full thickness) defect.
3. Lip and Nose defect, Lip and Chin defect.

Classification of Defects According to the Extent:

By allowing the distance between the two corners of the mouth to be the width, the extent of the defect can be classified into:

1. One-third of the lip width, one and half of the lip width, two-third of the lip width, four-fifth of the lip width (Figs. 13.5, 13.6, 13.7, 13.8).
2. Complete lower lip defect, Complete upper lip defect.

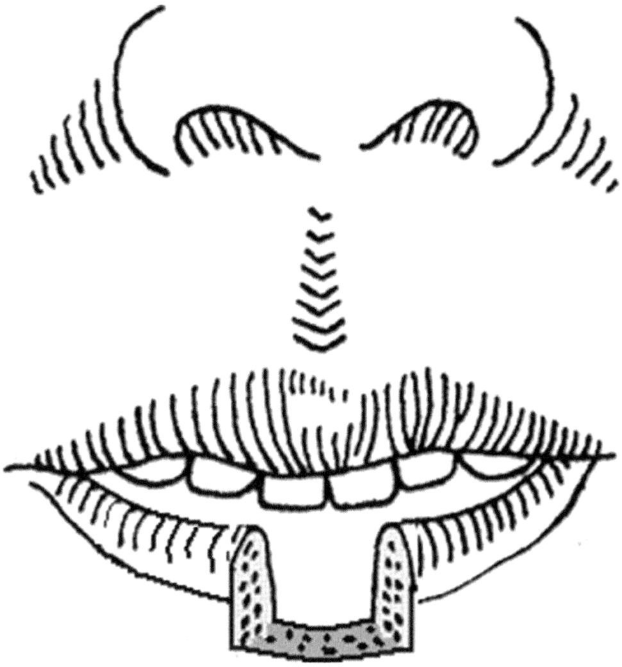

Fig. 13.3 Defect at the center of the lip

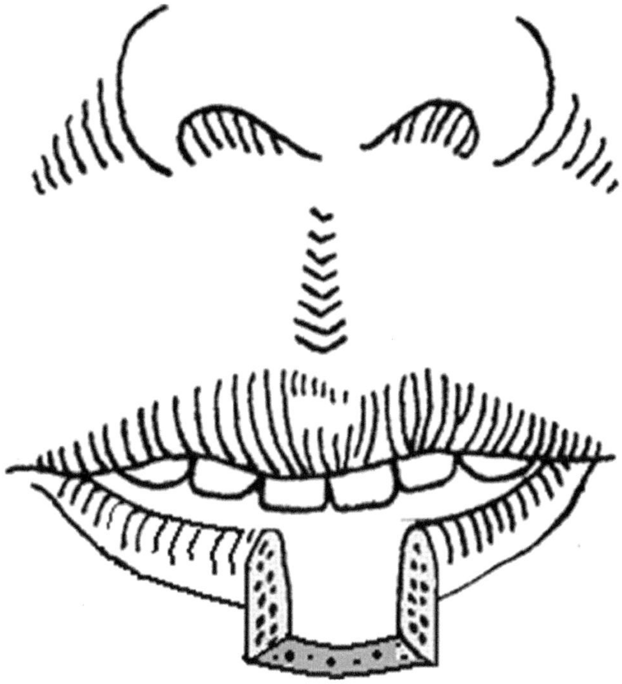

Fig. 13.5 Defect extending 1/3 of the lip width

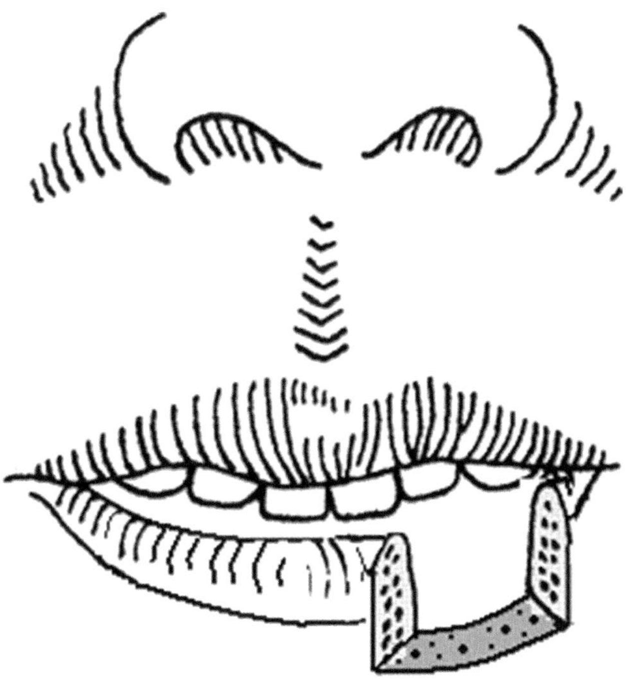

Fig. 13.4 Defect at the side of the lip (close to mouth corner)

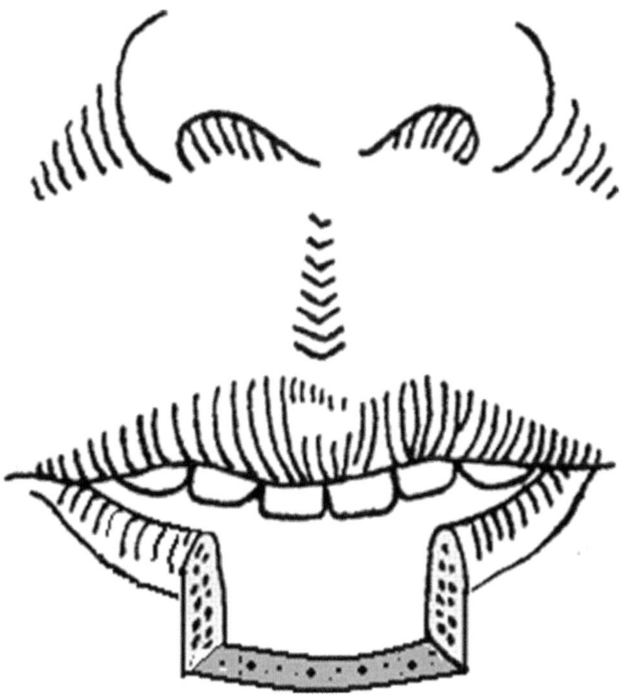

Fig. 13.6 Defect extending ½ of the lip width

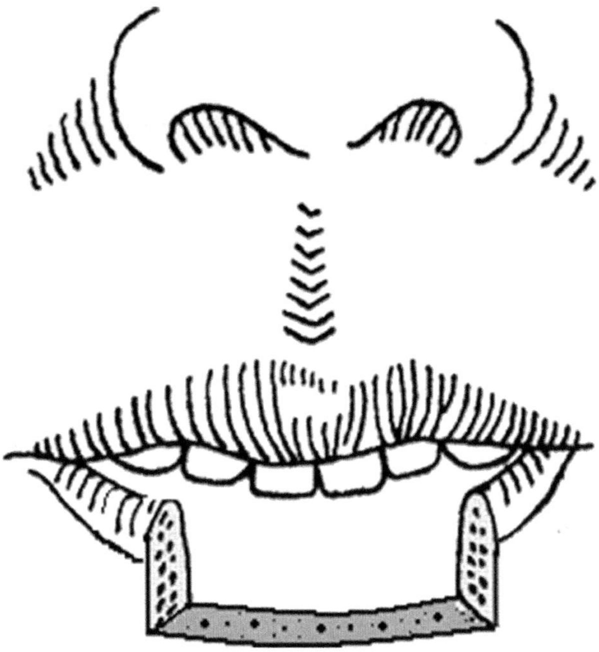

Fig. 13.7 Defect extending 2/3 of the lip width

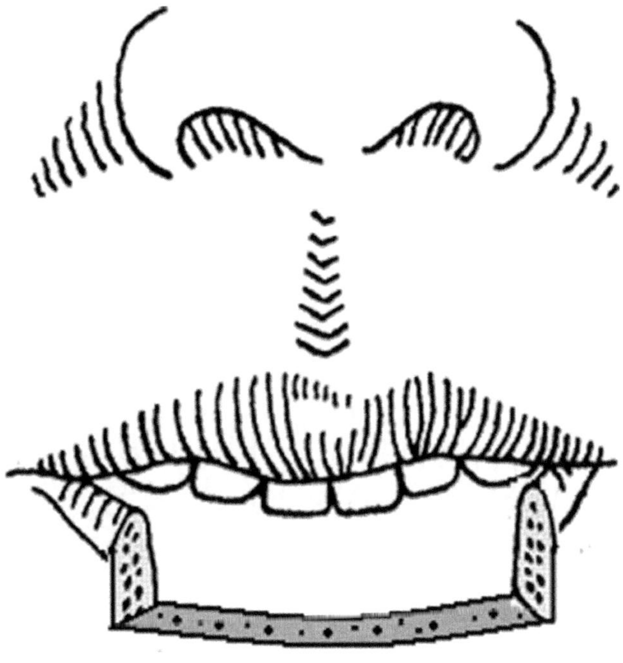

Fig. 13.8 Defect extending 4/5 of the lip width

References

1. Jian-Hua L, Wu Q-L, Zhi-Qiang C. Evaluation and geometry analysis on V-shape resection and rectangle resection of lower lip tumors (in Chinese). J Stomatol Progr. 2001;6(2):54–6.
2. Liao X-X. Handbook of modern mathematics: classical mathematics (in Chinese). 1st ed. Wuhan: Huazhong University of Science and Technology Press; 2000. p. 941.
3. Jian-Hua L, Wu Q-L. Meaning of lip extensibility on soft tissue flap design (in Chinese). J Stomatol Progr. 2002;7(1):15–6.

14 Surgical Methods of Simple Lip Defect

Jianhua Liu

14.1 Immediate Lip Repair with Defect Less Than One-Third of Lip Width

1. Indications
   (i) The lip defect is less than one-third of the lip width and not involving the corners of the mouth.
   (ii) The lip defect involves full thickness of skin, muscle, and labial mucosa.
   (iii) The simultaneous repair for the malignant lip tumor shows clear frozen margins after surgical excision.
2. Surgical Method and Procedures
   (i) For patients with a lip defect of less than one-third of the lip width, a V-shaped surgical excision is usually adopted, and this method utilizes the elasticity of the lip soft tissue. The skin, muscle, and labial mucosa layers are opposed and closed primarily.

Example of the Surgical Procedure:

The proliferative, verrucous mass is located at the upper right lip, measuring approximately 1.5 x 1 cm. It is pedunculated, foul-smelling, and bleeds spontaneously on contact. Clinical diagnosis: Squamous cell carcinoma of the upper lip (Figs. 14.1 and 14.2).

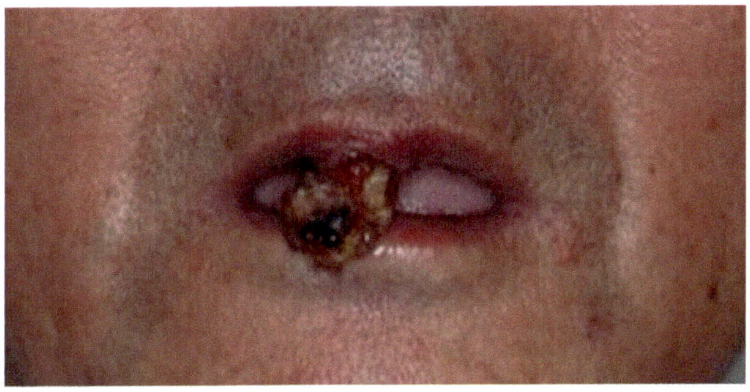

Fig. 14.1 Mass at the upper lip

3. Precautions
   (i) Most of the literature reported a safety surgical margin of 5–7 mm, with the smallest margin reported as 3 mm. If the tumor margin is clear and well-demarcated, we suggest a safety surgical margin of 5 mm. In addition, the safety surgical margin is also dependent on the type of lip tumor and its level of differentiation, as well as, whether or not the intra-operative frozen section of the surgical margin returns as positive or negative [1].
   (ii) To prevent scar contracture or tension at the lip repair site, the closure of the skin and underlying soft tissue can be modified with a Z-plasty.
   (iii) It is important to oppose the vermillion border of the lip accurately during the surgical closure.

14.2 Modified Reconstruction Design for One-Third to One and Half Lower Lip Defects

1. Indications
   (i) The lip defect secondary to trauma or tumor excision involves one-third to one and half of the lower lip width.
   (ii) The lip defect does not involve the corners of the mouth or the deepest point of the sulcus of the lower lip.

J. Liu (✉)
Department of Oral and Maxillo-facial Surgery, First Affiliated Hospital, Zhejiang University School of Medicine, Hangzhou, China

J. Liu, B. Shi (eds.), *Atlas of Lip and Nose Plastic and Cosmetic Surgery*, https://doi.org/10.1007/978-981-16-1911-3_14

(iii) The lip defect involves full thickness of skin, muscle, and labial mucosa.

(iv) The simultaneous repair for the malignant lower lip tumor shows clear frozen margins after surgical excision.

2. Surgical Method and Procedure

This surgical repair is suitable for a lower lip defect which involves one-third to one and half of the lower lip width. This is a modification of Bernard's sliding flap reconstruction (please see Sect. 4.3 for more details) [2]. Example of the Surgical Procedure (Fig. 14.3):

3. Precautions.

(i) Most of the literature reported a safety surgical margin of 5–7 mm, with the smallest margin reported as 3 mm. If the tumor margin is clear and well-demarcated, we suggest a safety surgical margin of 5 mm. In addition, the safety surgical margin is also dependent on the type of lip tumor and its level of differentiation, as well as, whether or not the intra-operative frozen section of the surgical margin returns as positive or negative.

(ii) The surgical excision margin should not extend below the deepest point of the lower lip sulcus. If the lip tumor is larger and requires the extension of the surgical margin below the deepest point of the lower lip sulcus, the surgical blade can be directed upwards into the sulcus, in order to ensure that the adjacent sliding flaps can move towards the center.

(iii) With regards to the need for neck dissection: If there are suspicious enlarged cervical lymph nodes, it would require levels I and II neck dissection. In addition, endophytic tumors have a higher risk of metastasis as compared to exophytic tumors, and hence simultaneous neck dissection should be performed. Endophytic upper lip tumors should include neck dissection of level I–III.

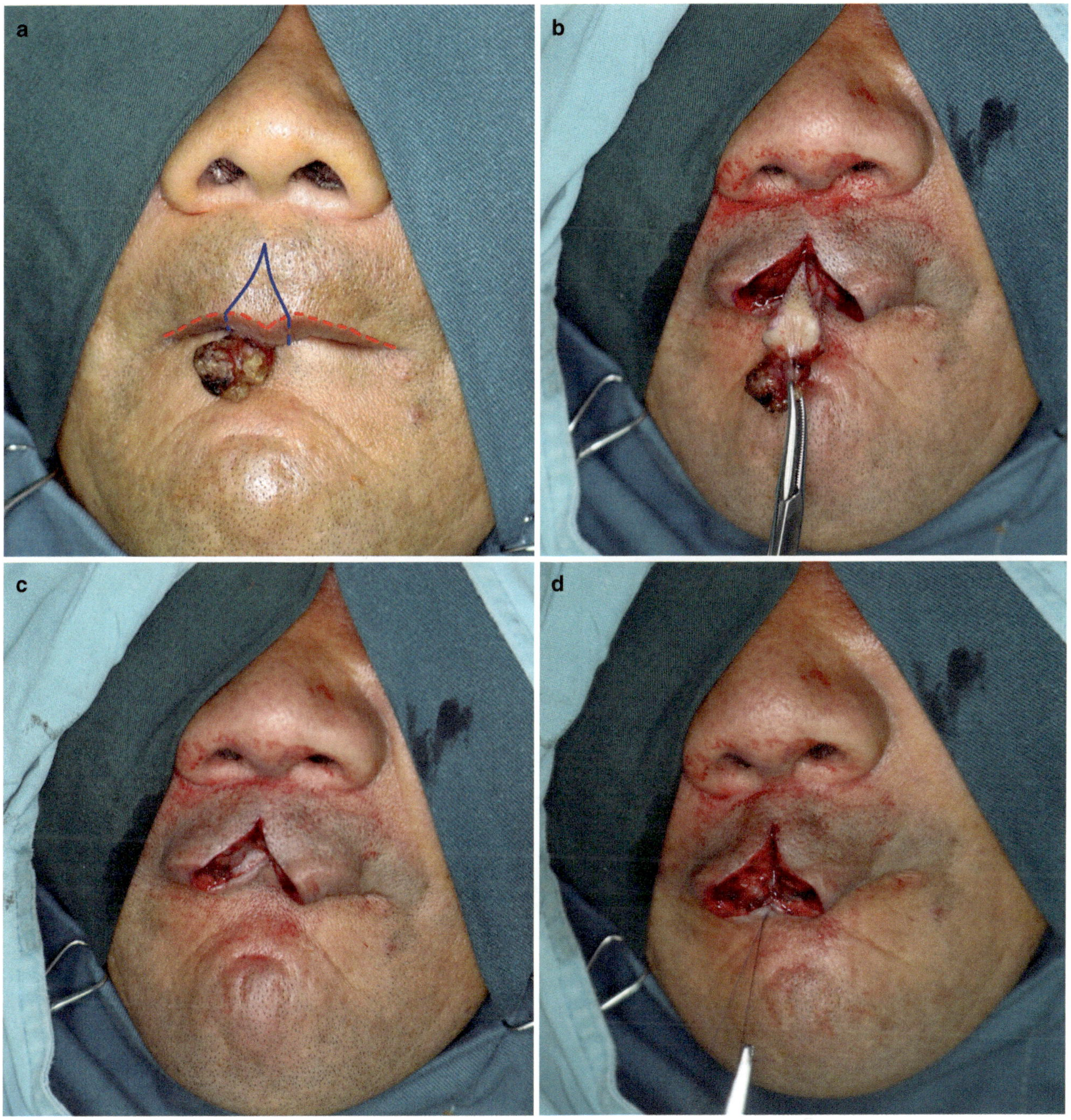

Fig. 14.2 (**a**–**f**) Surgical design and procedure. Sequence of photos: a—top left; b—top right. **a**: Surgical marking of the V-shaped excision, with its closest margin to the lip tumor at approximately 0.5 cm; **b**: Full thickness surgical excision of the upper lip; **c**: After surgical excision; **d**: Initial closure of labial mucosa layer; **e**: Closure of muscle layer; **f**: Closure of skin layer, and completion of surgery. It is important to oppose the vermillion border of the lip accurately during the surgical closure

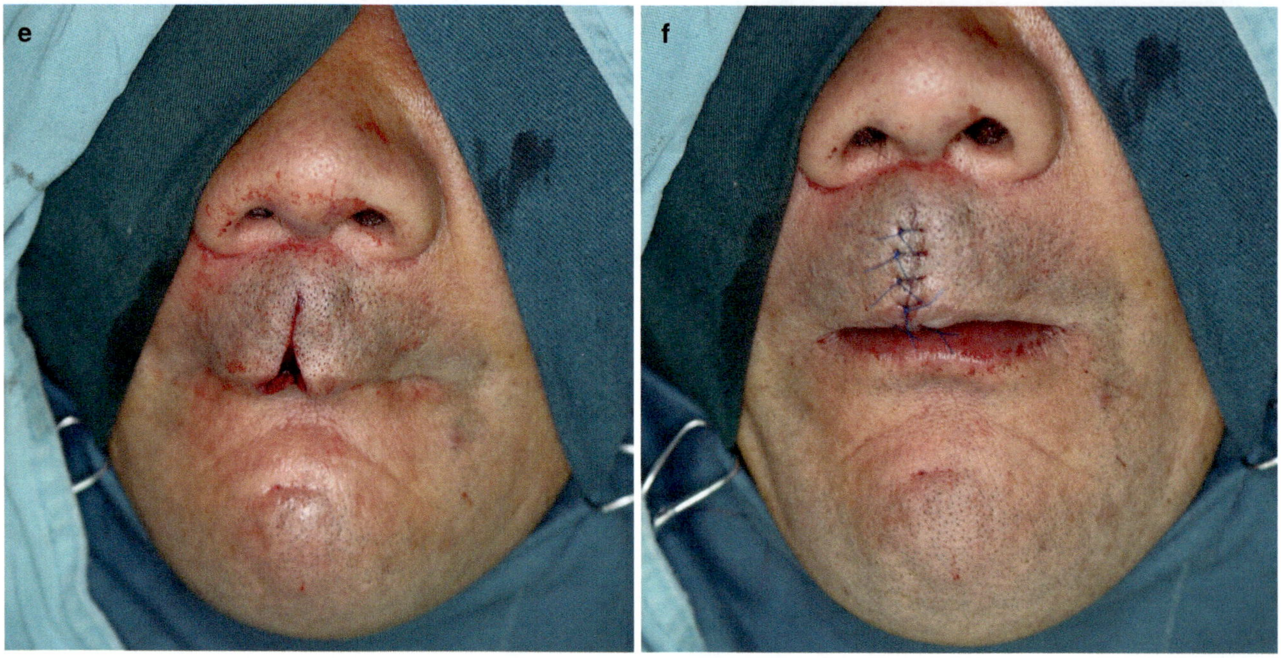

Fig. 14.2 (continued)

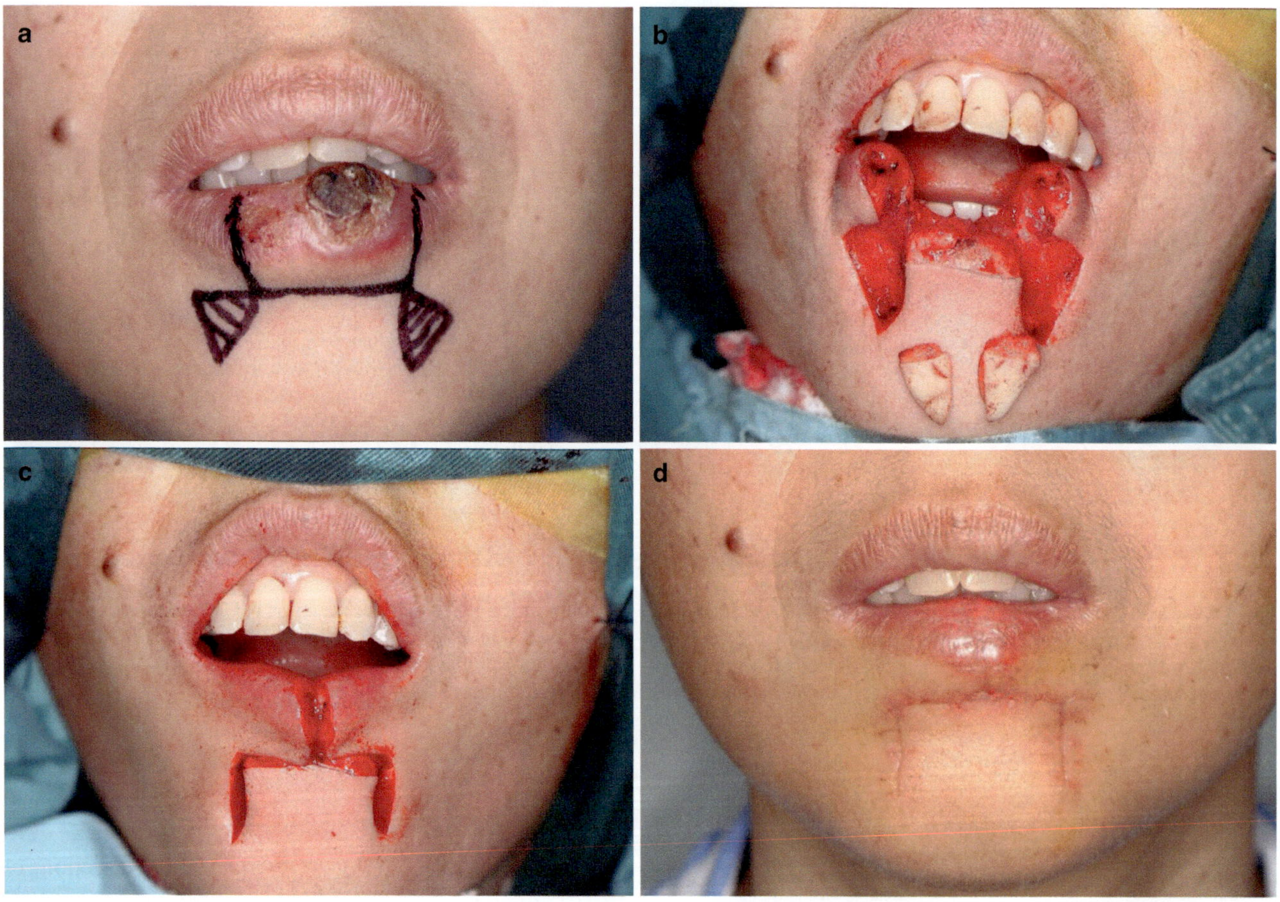

Fig. 14.3 (**a–d**) Surgical Procedure. (**a**) Surgical design of the lower lip squamous cell carcinoma excision. After including a safety surgical margin of more than 0.5 cm bilaterally, the total width of the surgical excision involves less than ½ of the lower lip width; (**b**) After the rectangular excision of the lip tumor, another triangular excision is done at the lower corners bilaterally, excising the skin and muscle layers while preserving the labial mucosa intact; (**c**) Primary closure of the lip defect by opposing the skin, muscle, and mucosa layers respectively; (**d**) Postoperative day 12, the lip repair site does not display obvious tension and is appropriate for suture removal.

References

1. Ji-Dong L, Hai-Yan Z, Zhong-Mei L. Repair of defect after lower lip tumor resection (in Chinese). Chin J Dermotol. 2013;46(10):756–7.
2. Jian-Hua L, Xin X, Zhi-Qiang C. Immediate repair of lower lip defect after cancer resection using sliding flap (in Chinese). J Oral Maxillofac Surg. 1991;1(2):46–7.

Modified Bernard's Sliding Flaps for Larger Lower Lip Defect

15

Jianhua Liu

15.1 Immediate Reconstruction of the Defect Involving One and Half of the Lower Lip

1. Indications
   (i) The lip defect secondary to trauma or tumor excision is approximately one and half of the total lip width.
   (ii) The inferior margin of the defect does not extend beyond the deepest point of the lower lip sulcus.
   (iii) The lip defect involves the full thickness of skin, muscle, and labial mucosa.
   (iv) The simultaneous repair for the malignant lip tumor shows clear frozen margins after surgical excision.
2. Surgical Method and Procedure

   This surgical repair is suitable for a lower lip defect that involves one and half of the lower lip width. This is a modification of Bernard's sliding flap reconstruction (Figs. 15.1, 15.2, 15.3).

The design of the surgical excision: The rectangular surgical excision should include the safety surgical margin. On top of that, two additional triangles (L1-C-A and L2-D-B) are included, whereby their combined width equals two-third of the rectangular width.

Illustration of the lip defect following the rectangular surgical excision.

Appearance of the lip after the opposition of the edges. The lower lip is thinner than before.

Example of the Surgical Procedure:

Following the modified Bernard's sliding flaps reconstruction (Fig. 15.4).

J. Liu (✉)
Department of Oral and Maxillo-facial Surgery, First Affiliated Hospital, Zhejiang University School of Medicine, Hangzhou, China

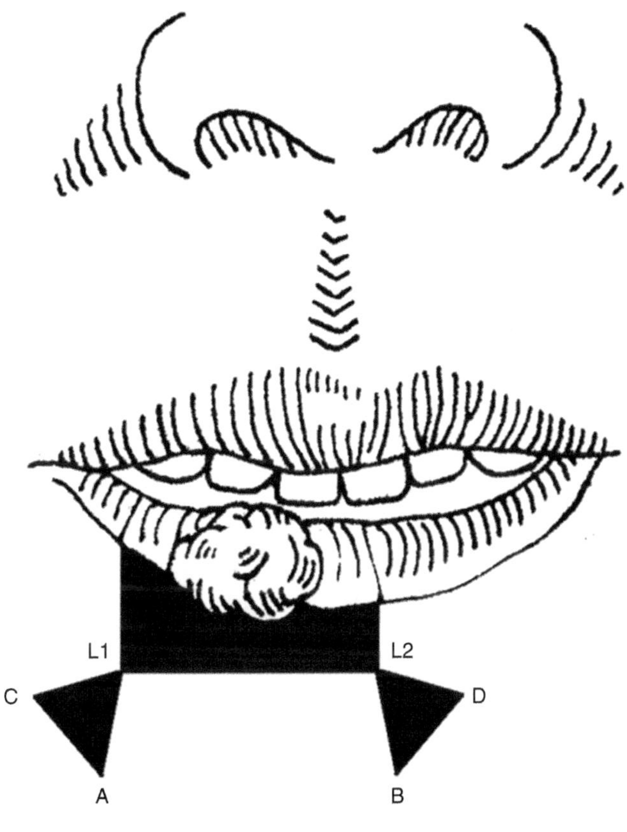

Fig. 15.1 Illustration of the surgical excision

Completion of the excision of the lip tumor, as well as the two additional triangular excisions, with hemostasis achieved (Fig. 15.5).

The labial mucosa and muscles are first sutured, followed by the accurate opposition of the vermillion of the lip (Fig. 15.6).

The mucosa and muscles layers are sutured prior to skin closure (Fig. 15.7).

The surgical excision site is fully closed, and surgery is completed (Fig. 15.8).

J. Liu, B. Shi (eds.), *Atlas of Lip and Nose Plastic and Cosmetic Surgery*, https://doi.org/10.1007/978-981-16-1911-3_15

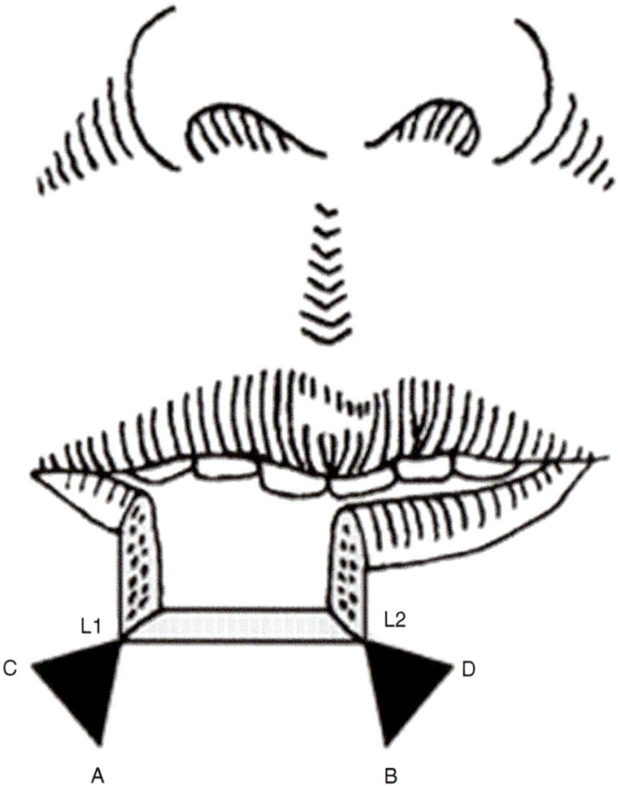

Fig. 15.2 Illustration of the surgical excision

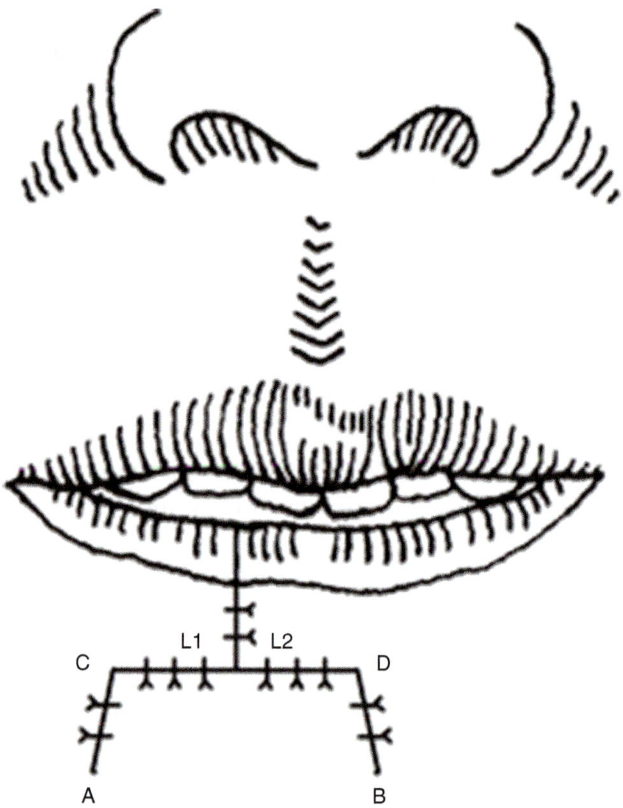

Fig. 15.3 Illustration of the surgical excision

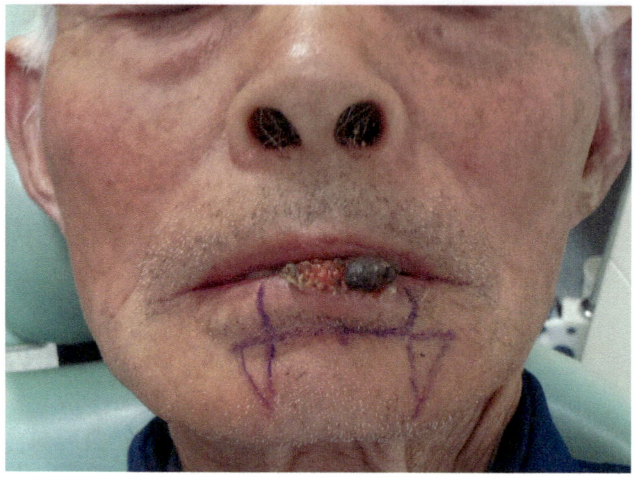

Fig. 15.4 Design of the surgical incision

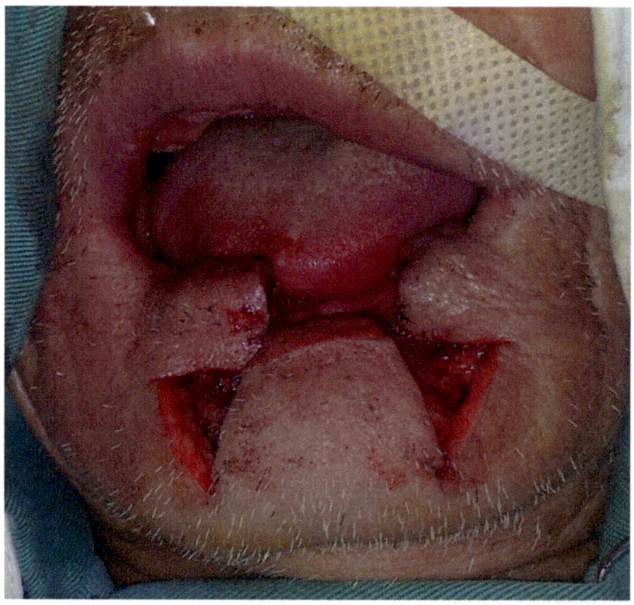

Fig. 15.5 After surgical excision of the lip tumor

Typical example 1:

Lower right lip squamous cell carcinoma pre-operatively (Fig. 15.9).

The surgical excision margin has extended to ½ the lower lip width, and the patient's soft tissues have low elasticity, therefore the two inverted triangles were made slightly larger, such that the sum of the width of the triangles equals the length of the rectangle (Fig. 15.10).

The esthetics and function of the lower lip have healed well. Note that the width and the height of the lower lip have not changed significantly, but the lower lip had become slightly thinner (Fig. 15.11).

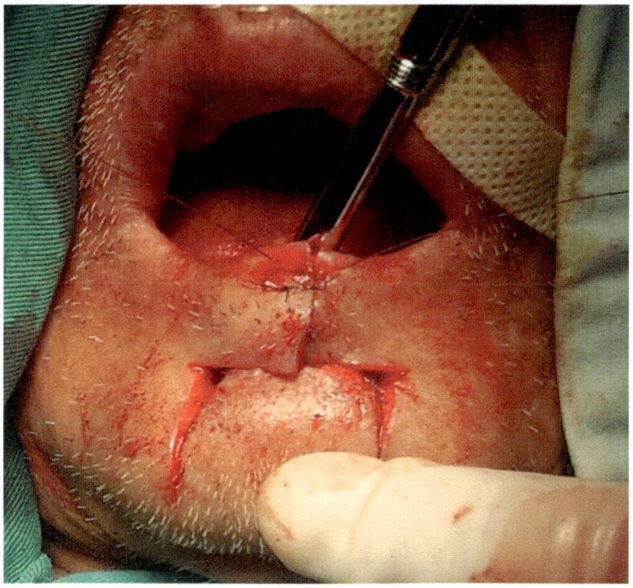

Fig. 15.6 Opposition of the respective edges

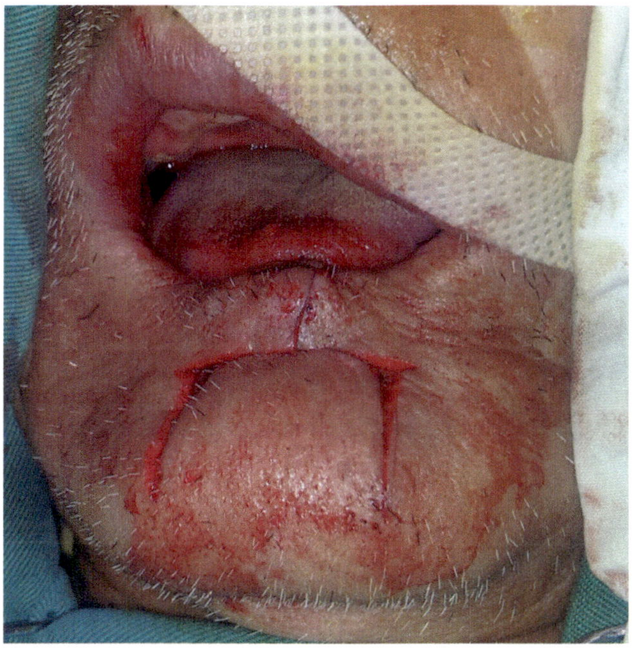

Fig. 15.7 Before skin closure

Typical Example 2:

The patient has high elasticity of the soft tissues, judging from the wrinkles of his face, and hence the sum of the width of the two triangles equals two-third of the length of the rectangle (Fig. 15.12).

At 6 months post-operative review, the esthetics of the lower lip is ideal, and there are less wrinkles at the lower half of the face, making the patient appear younger (Fig. 15.13).

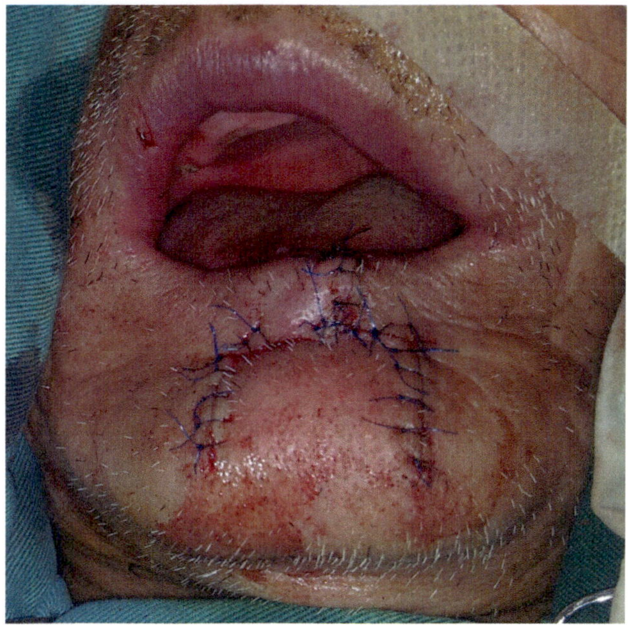

Fig. 15.8 Completion of suturing

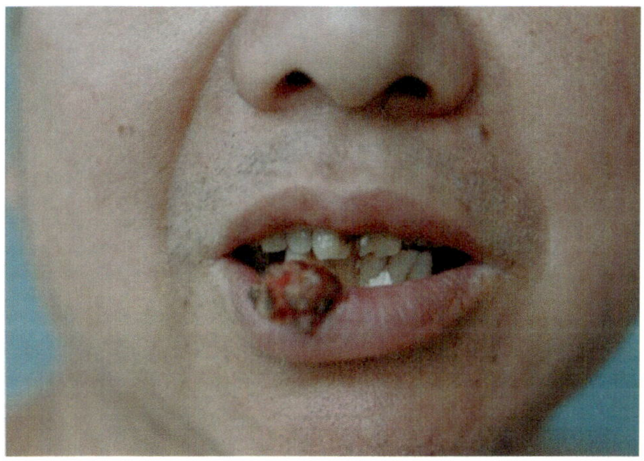

Fig. 15.9 Lower lip tumor

The post-operative function is good, and the patient has no limitation in mouth opening (Fig. 15.14).

3. Precautions
   (i) Most of the literature reported a safety surgical margin of 5–7 mm, with the smallest margin reported as 3 mm. If the tumor margin is clear and well-demarcated, we suggest a safety surgical margin of 5 mm. In addition, the safety surgical margin is also dependent on the type of lip tumor and its level of differentiation, as well as, whether or not the intra-operative frozen section of the surgical margin returns as positive or negative [1, 2].

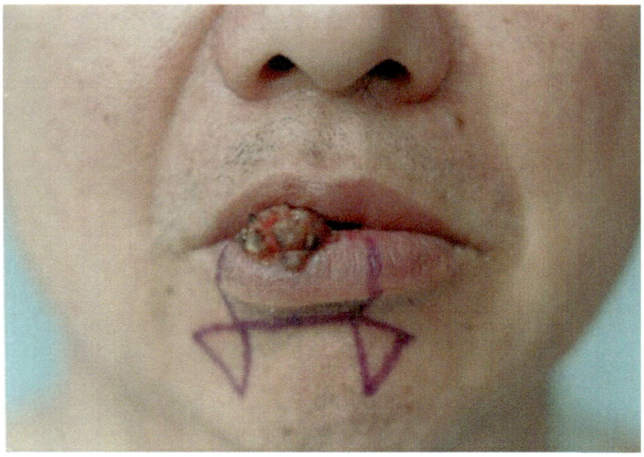

Fig. 15.10 Design of surgical incision

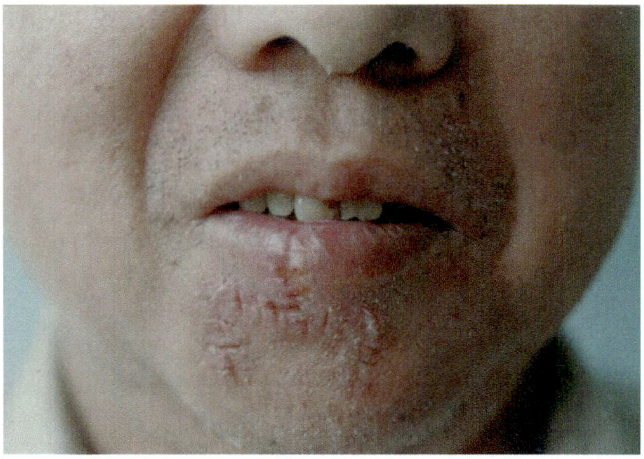

Fig. 15.11 After removal of sutures

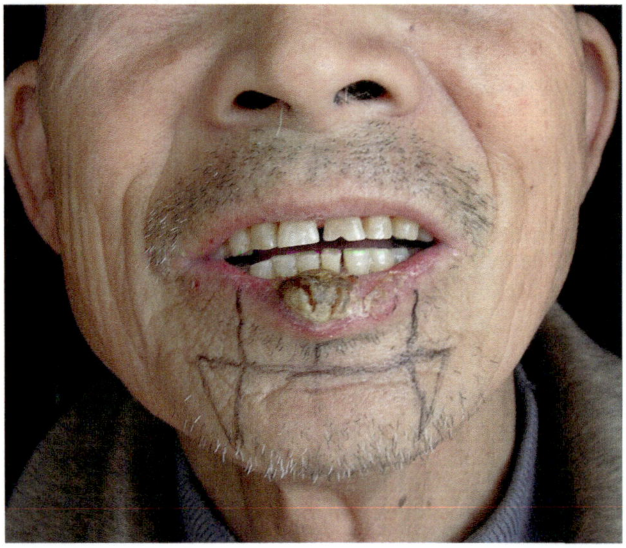

Fig. 15.12 Design of surgical excision

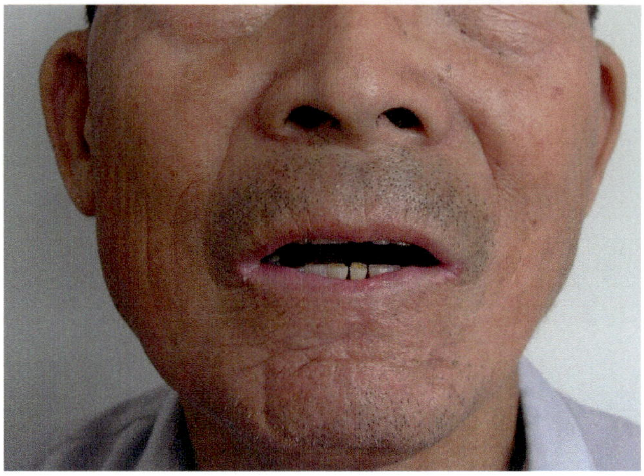

Fig. 15.13 Post-operative aesthetics

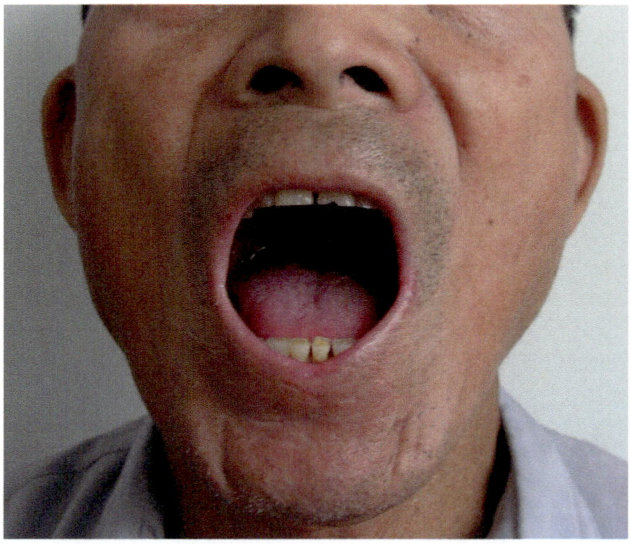

Fig. 15.14 Post-operative function

(ii) The surgical excision margin should be above the lower lip sulcus. If the lip tumor is larger and requires the extension of the surgical margin below the deepest point of the lower lip sulcus, the surgical blade can be directed upwards in order to ensure that the adjacent sliding flaps can move towards the center.

(iii) After surgical excision of the lip tumor, if there is too much tension following the primary closure of the sliding flaps, there is a need to enlarge the width of the two additional triangles. Alternatively, the immediate reconstruction of larger (two-third) lower lip defects can be considered.

15.2 Immediate Reconstruction of Large (Two-Third to Four-Fifth) Lower Lip Defect

1. Indications
   (i) The lip defect secondary to trauma or tumor excision is approximately two-third–four-fifth of the total lip width.
   (ii) The inferior margin of the defect does not extend beyond the deepest point of the lower lip sulcus.
   (iii) The lip defect involves the full thickness of skin, muscle, and labial mucosa.
   (iv) The simultaneous repair for the malignant lip tumor shows clear frozen margins after surgical excision.
2. Surgical Method and Procedure (Figs. 15.15, 15.16)
   This surgical repair is suitable for a lower lip defect that involves two-third– four-fifth of the lower lip. This is a modification of Bernard's sliding flap reconstruction [3] (see Sect. 15.1), together with two additional triangular excisions at the corners of the upper lip to improve the sliding ability of the two flaps.

The shaded areas in the figure above are areas that require excision. The upper lip M1 and M2 are approximated and sutured, similar to N2 and N1. At the surgical safety margin of the rectangular excision, L1 and L2 are approximated at the center and sutured. The sides of the triangles CA and BD are sutured to L1A and L2B, respectively. The total width of the base of the two additional triangles is equivalent to two-third of the length of the rectangle. The total width of the base of the two triangles at the nasolabial region is smaller or equivalent to two-third of the length of the rectangle.

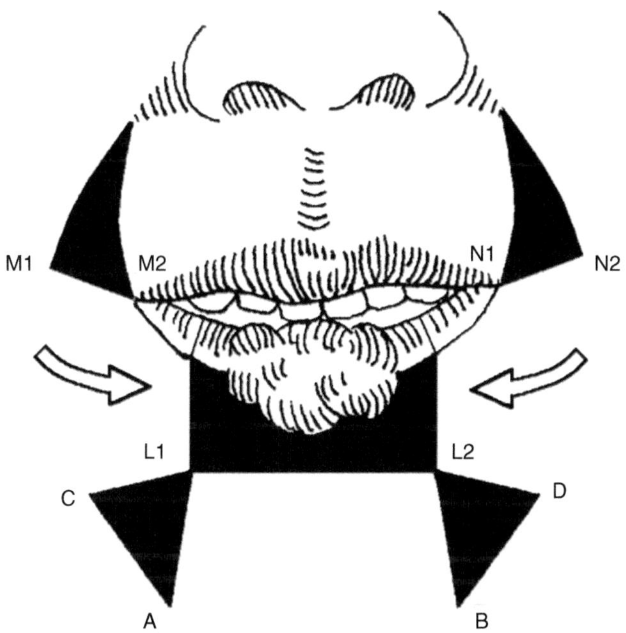

Fig. 15.15 Illustration of the surgical design

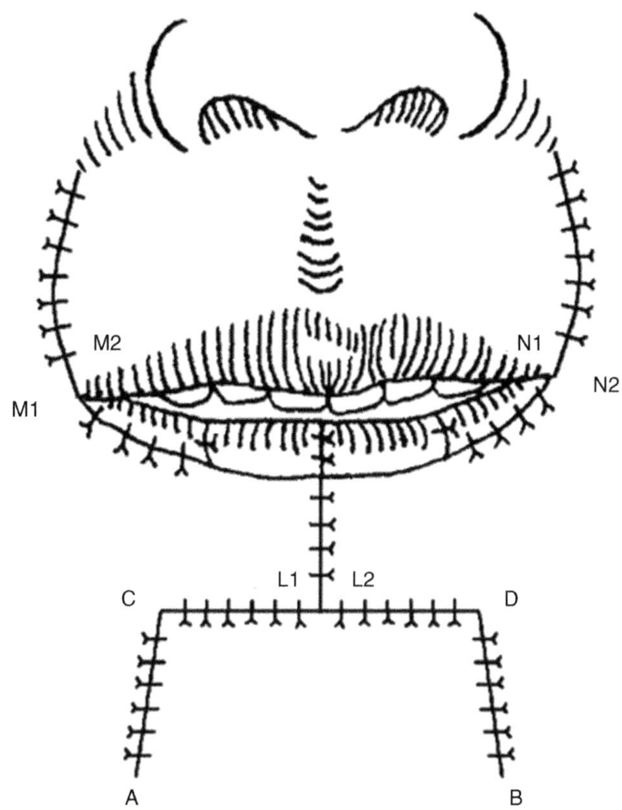

Fig. 15.16 Illustration of the surgical design

The appearance after completion of the suture.

Note: The left and right edges of the vermillion of the lower lip are formed using the mucosa retained and inverted from the two triangles at the upper lip, respectively. Therefore, the mucosa layer of the triangles of the upper lip should only be cut at the two triangular lengths. The base of the triangles should not be incised.

Clinical Example of the Surgical Procedure:

The patient suffers from a lower lip squamous cell carcinoma. Pre-operatively, after the addition of more than 0.5 cm safety surgical margin all-round the tumor, the width of the surgical excision required is two-third to four-fifth of the total width of the lower lip. During the design of the triangular excision at the upper lip, do note that the inner line should coincide with the corner of the mouth, and the outer line should be placed along the nasolabial fold as much as possible. The sum of the base of the two triangles at the lower lip should be approximately two-third the width of the lower lip defect (Fig. 15.17).

After excising the skin and muscle layers, the mucosa layer should be incised at the sides of the triangles. The base of the triangle should not be cut. The loose connective tissue beneath the mucosa should also be preserved (Fig. 15.18).

After removal of the skin and muscle layers of the upper lip, the wound is approximated and sutured. The base of the mucosa layer of the upper lip is not excised fully, and instead,

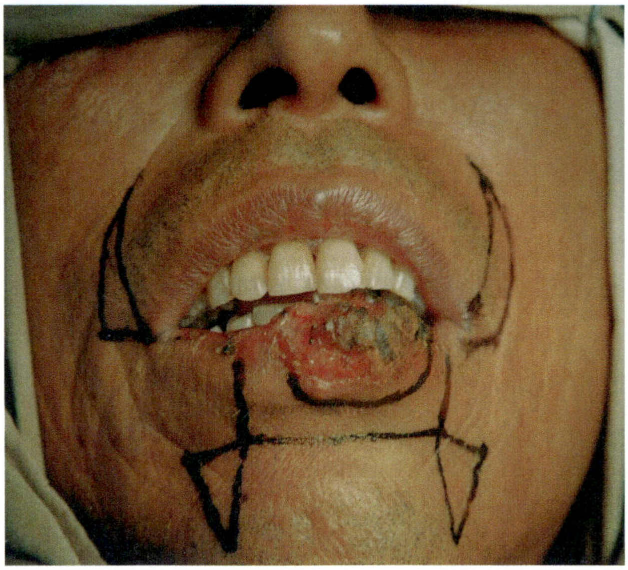

Fig. 15.17 Surgical step

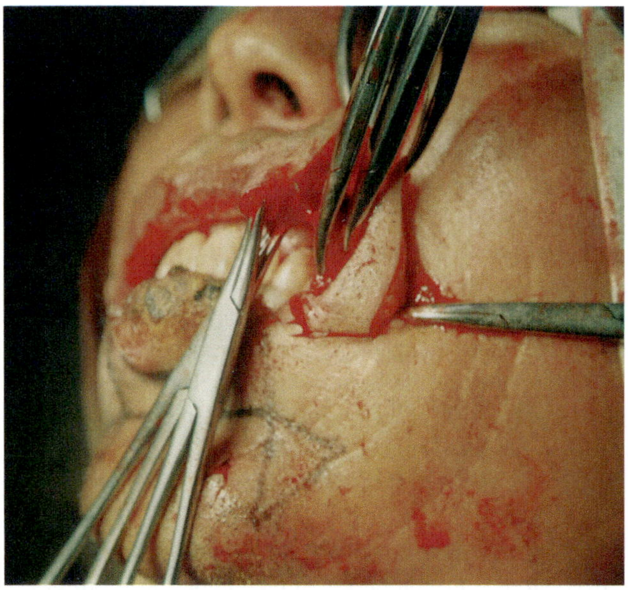

Fig. 15.18 Surgical step

it is inverted, trimmed, and sutured to the corner of the lip, forming the new vermillion of the lower lip (Fig. 15.19).

After suture closure, the sutures are removed in about 7 days, and sutures with more tension are removed in 10–12 days (Fig. 15.20).

Classical Example 1

Pre-operatively, the lower lip squamous cell carcinoma tumor, together with the surgical safety margin, extends to approximately four-fifth of the total lower lip width (Fig. 15.21).

One month post-operatively, the lower lip width does not appear to be significantly reduced compared to that pre-operatively (Fig. 15.22).

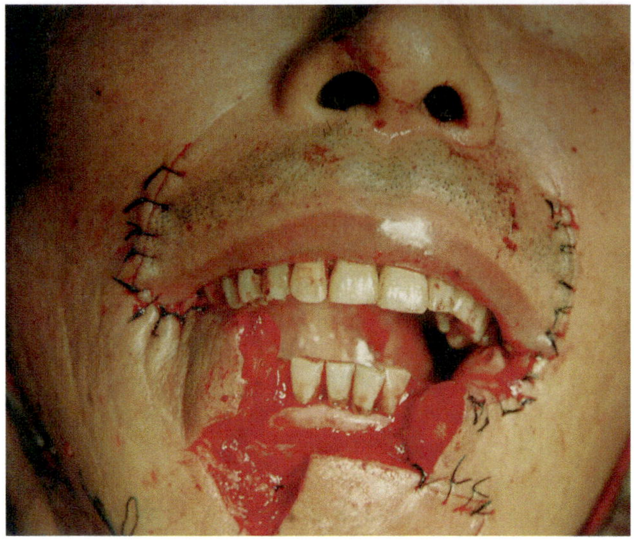

Fig. 15.19 Surgical step

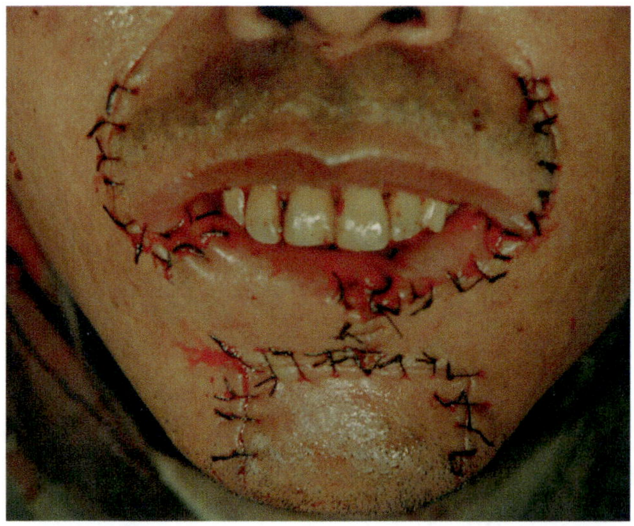

Fig. 15.20 Surgical step

Post-operative function is good (Fig. 15.23).

Classical Example 2

An example of a lower lip tumor relapse. The patient had undergone a V-shaped excision 2 years ago, and the wound was closed primarily. This time, a 1 cm surgical safety margin is chosen, and the width of the lower lip defect is four-fifth that of the total width of the lower lip (Fig. 15.24).

One week post-operatively, after removal of partial sutures (Fig. 15.25).

The left photo (a) depicts the patient pre-operatively, and the right photo (b) depicts the patient post-operatively. Even though four-fifth of the lower lip has been excised, the width of the lower lip is still larger than that pre-operatively, achieving ideal results (Fig. 15.26).

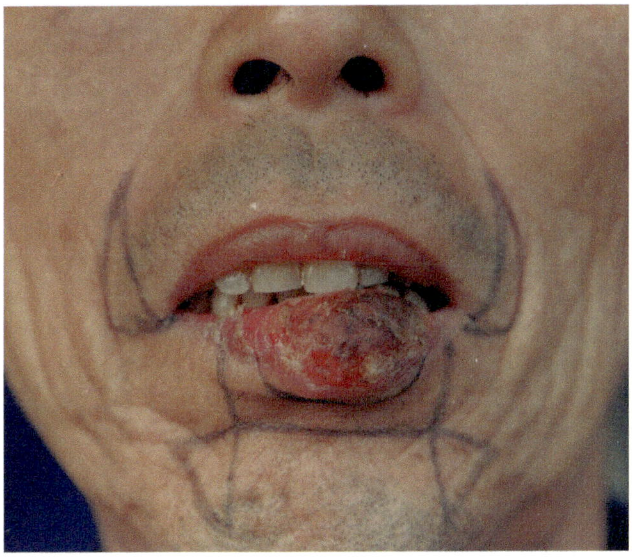

Fig. 15.21 Classical example 1

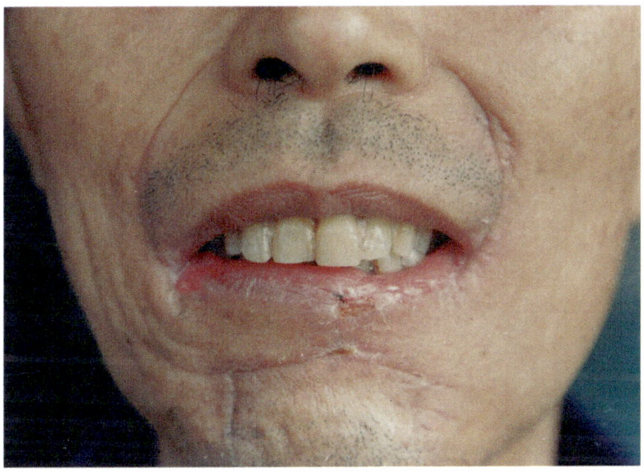

Fig. 15.22 Classical example 1

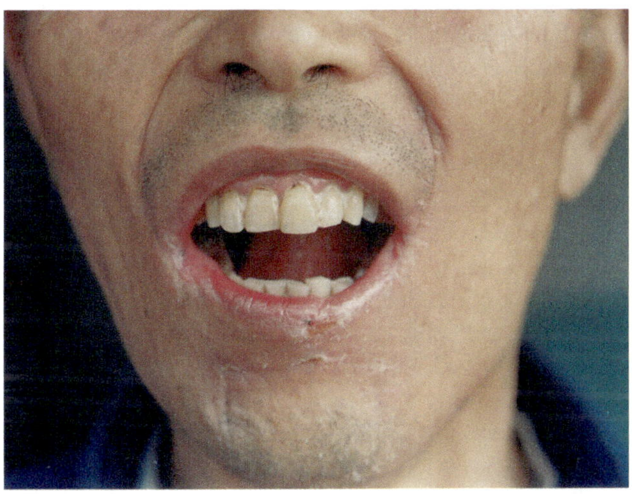

Fig. 15.23 Classical example 1

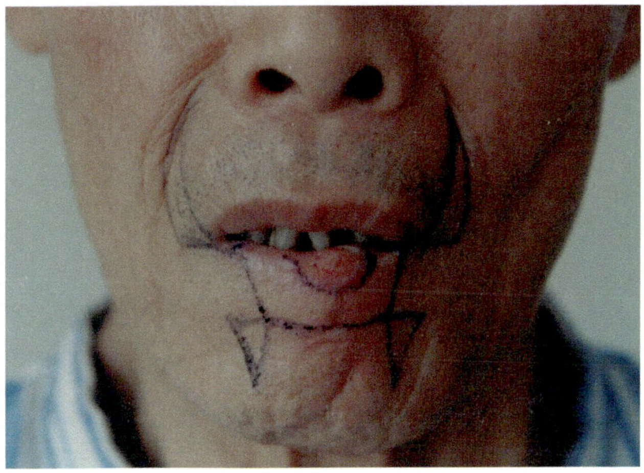

Fig. 15.24 Classical example 2

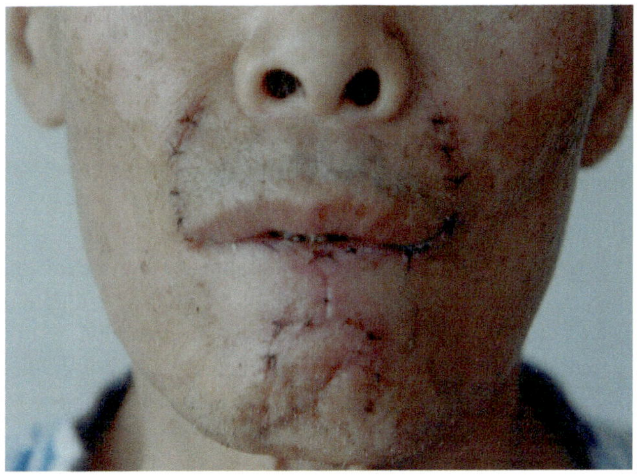

Fig. 15.25 Classical example 2

3. Precautions
   (i) Most of the literature reported a safety surgical margin of 5–7 mm, with the smallest margin reported as 3 mm. If the tumor margin is clear and well-demarcated, we suggest a safety surgical margin of 5 mm. In addition, the safety surgical margin is also dependent on the type of lip tumor and its level of differentiation, as well as, whether or not the intraoperative frozen section of the surgical margin returns as positive or negative.
   (ii) The surgical excision margin should not extend below the deepest point of the lower lip sulcus. If the lip tumor is larger and requires the extension of the surgical margin below the deepest point of the lower lip sulcus, the surgical blade can be directed upwards in order to ensure that the adjacent sliding flaps can move towards the center.
   (iii) After surgical excision of the lip tumor, if there is too much tension following the primary closure of the

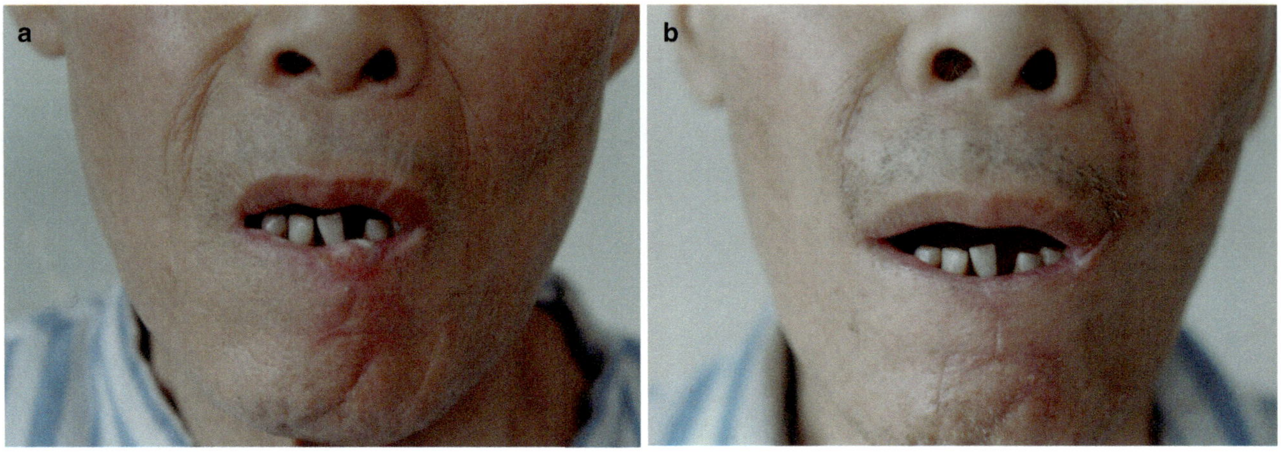

Fig. 15.26 (**a**, **b**) Classical example 2

sliding flaps, there is a need to enlarge the width of the two additional triangles.

15.3 Immediate Reconstruction of Larger Lateral Lower Lip Defect

1. Indications
   (i) The lip defect secondary to trauma or tumor excision is approximately two-third of the total lip width and involves the corner of the mouth unilaterally.
   (ii) The inferior margin of the defect does not extend beyond the deepest point of the lower lip sulcus.
   (iii) The lip defect involves full thickness of skin, muscle, and labial mucosa.
   (iv) The simultaneous repair for the malignant lip tumor shows clear frozen margins after surgical excision.
2. Surgical Method and Procedure

   This surgical repair is suitable for a lower lip defect that involves two-third of the lower lip and is located unilaterally towards the side of the lip. This is a modification of Bernard's sliding flap reconstruction (see Sect. 15.1), together with an additional triangular excision at the unilateral nasolabial fold of the upper lip to improve the sliding ability of the flap.

At the surgical safety margin of the rectangular excision, the combined width of the two triangles (L1-C-A and L2-D-B) is equivalent to two-third of the length of the rectangle. The width of the additional triangular excision at the nasolabial fold is smaller or equal to two-third of the length of the rectangle. The shaded areas indicate the areas that require excision (Fig. 15.27).

The illustration shows that after excision of the shaded areas, the left and right flaps are approximated and sutured. A thing to note is that the shaded triangular excision at the nasolabial fold should only excise the skin and muscle layers. The mucosa layer should be preserved and inverted to form the new vermillion of the lower lip.

Clinical Example of the Surgical Procedure:

The patient suffers from a lower lip squamous cell carcinoma. Pre-operatively, after the addition of more than 0.5 cm safety surgical margin all-round the tumor, the width of the surgical excision required is two-third of the total width of the lower lip. During the design of the triangular excision at the upper lip, do note that the inner line should coincide with the corner of the mouth, and the outer line should be placed along the nasolabial fold as much as possible. The sum of the base of the two triangles at the lower lip should be approximately two-third the width of the lower lip defect (Fig. 15.28).

After the rectangular excision of the lower lip, the specimen should be sent for a frozen section to verify the surgical margins of the mucosa. Sutures are placed to orientate the specimen (Fig. 15.29).

Neck dissection can be performed while waiting for the results of the frozen section (Fig. 15.30).

Excision of the skin and muscle layers of the triangle at the left nasolabial fold. The mucosa at the sides of the triangle is excised, while the mucosa at the base of the triangle is preserved (Fig. 15.31).

The mucosa from the triangular excision at the nasolabial fold is inverted and converted into the vermillion of the lower lip (Fig. 15.32).

After excision of the skin and muscle layers of the triangle at the lower left lip, the mucosa is transected, and the lower lip flap is slide towards the center and sutured. Submental and submandibular neck dissection have been completed (Fig. 15.33).

After excision of the triangle at the lower right lip, the flap is advanced towards the left and sutured to the flap from the left (Fig. 15.34).

Classical Example 1

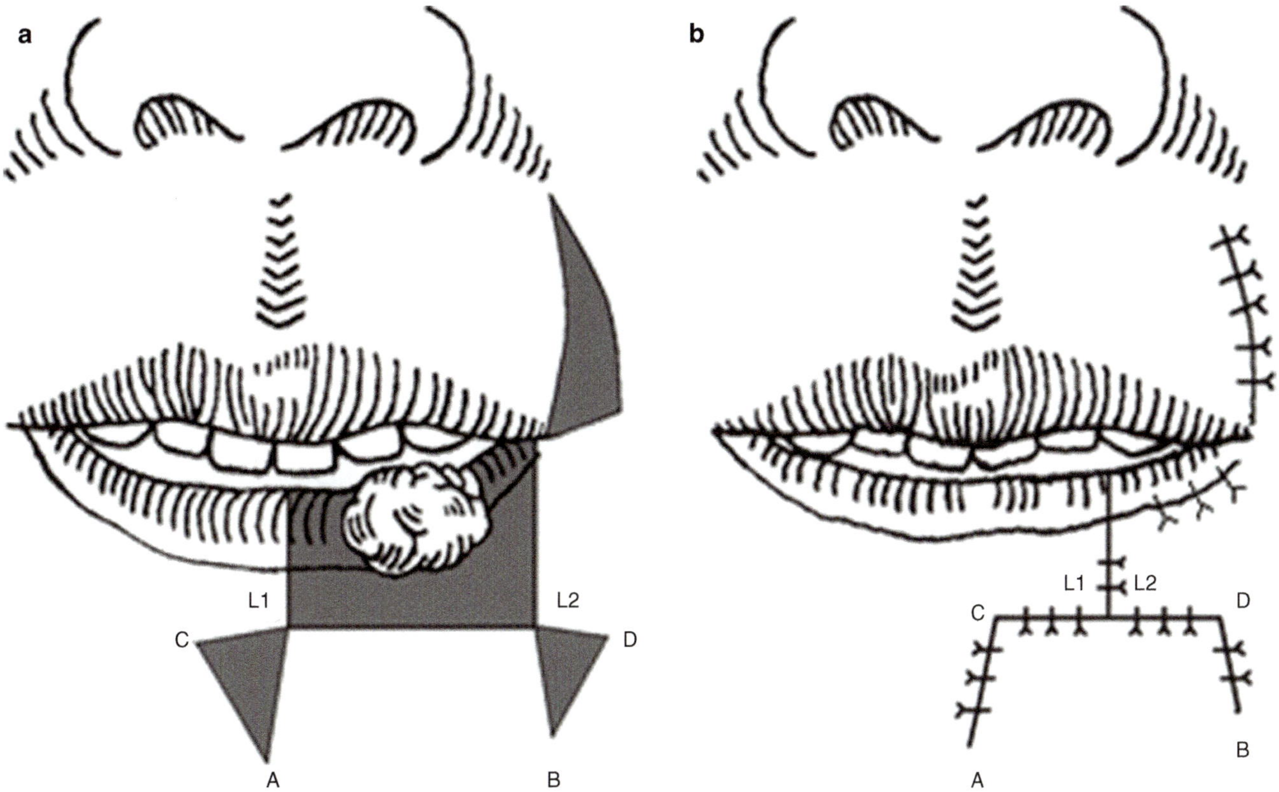

Fig. 15.27 (**a**) Illustration of the surgical excision design. (**b**) Illustration of surgical design

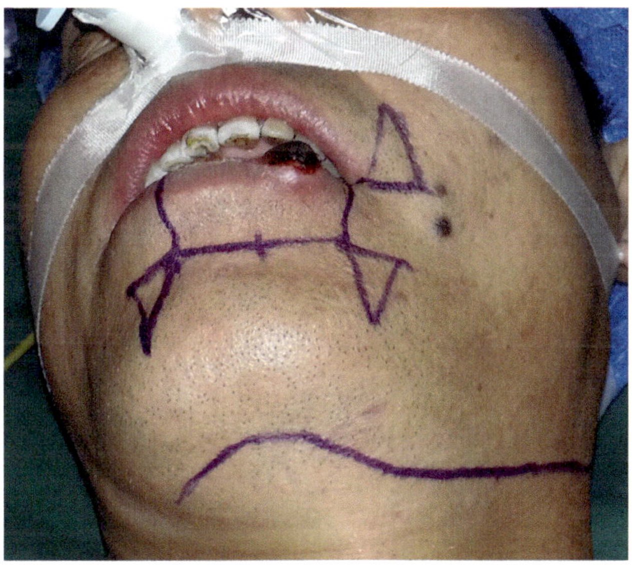

Fig. 15.28 Surgical step

The tumor is located at the lower left lip. The surgical excision design involves two-third the width of the lower lip (Fig. 15.35).

Intra-operatively (Fig. 15.36).

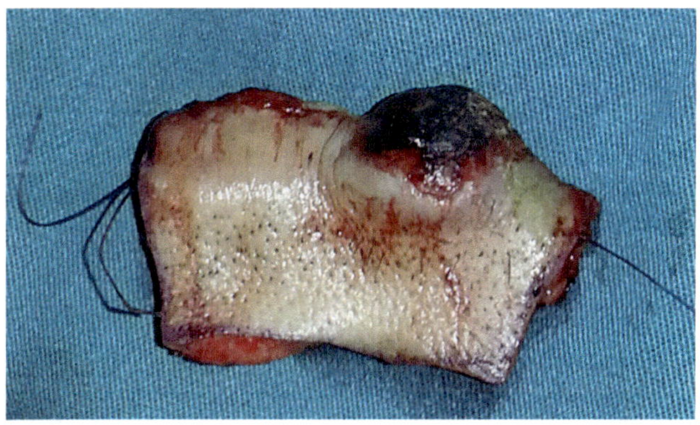

Fig. 15.29 Surgical step

Post-operatively, the width of the lower lip is slightly smaller, but the corner of the mouth has no obvious deviation (Fig. 15.37).

Classical Example 2

The tumor is located at the lower left lip. The surgical excision design involves one and half of the lower lip width (Fig. 15.38).

Intra-operatively (Fig. 15.39).

1-month post-operative review. Both the function and esthetics are ideal (Fig. 15.40).

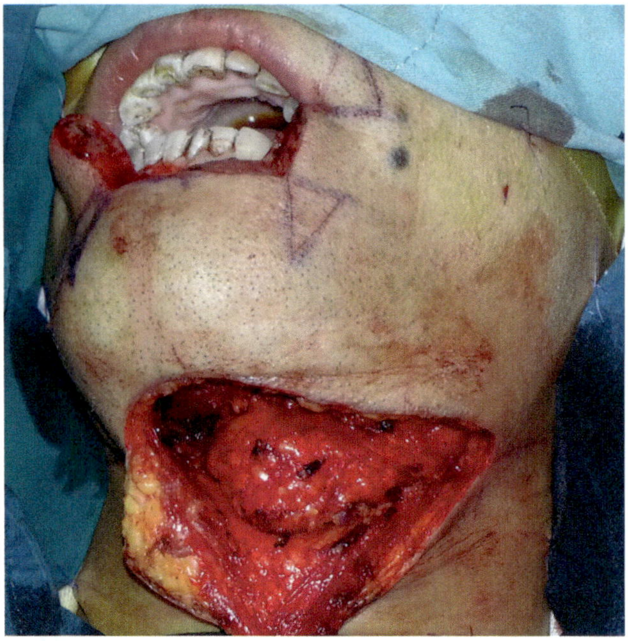

Fig. 15.30 Surgical step

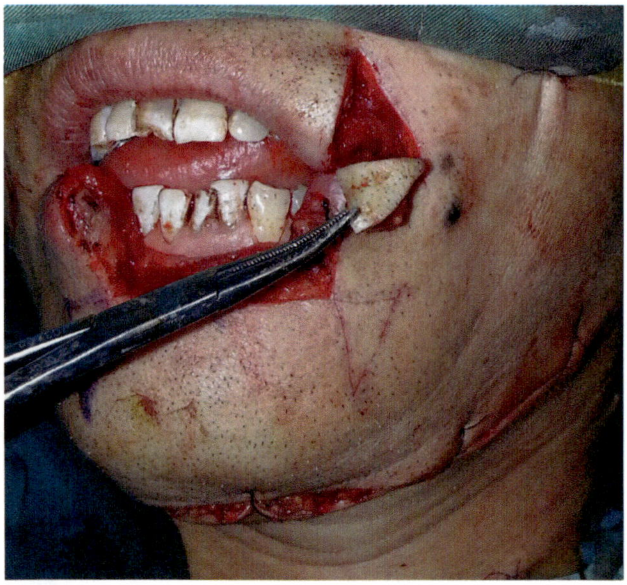

Fig. 15.31 Surgical step

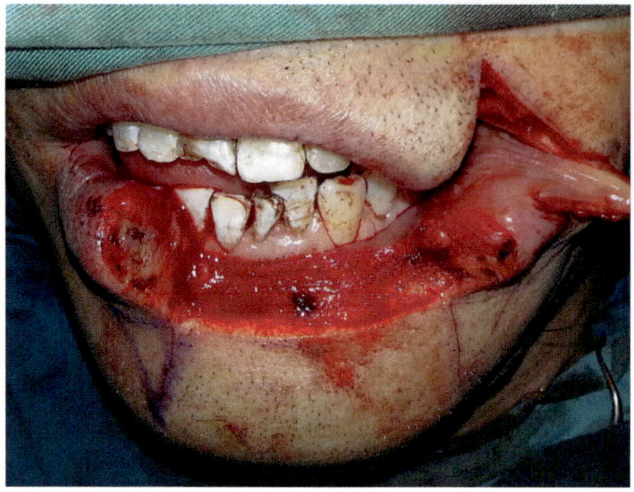

Fig. 15.32 Surgical step

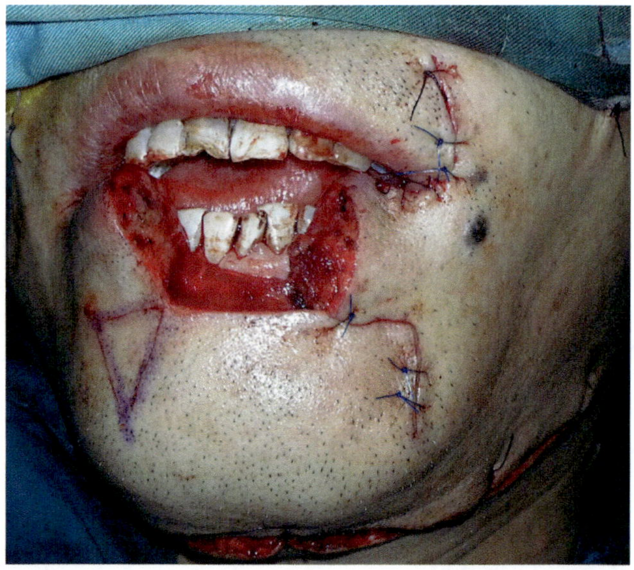

Fig. 15.33 Surgical step

3. Precautions
   (i) Most of the literature reported a safety surgical margin of 5–7 mm, with the smallest margin reported as 3 mm. If the tumor margin is clear and well-demarcated, we suggest a safety surgical margin of 5 mm. In addition, the safety surgical margin is also dependent on the type of lip tumor and its level of differentiation, as well as, whether or not the intra-operative frozen section of the surgical margin returns as positive or negative.
   (ii) The surgical excision margin should be above the lower lip sulcus. If the lip tumor is larger and requires the extension of the surgical margin below the deepest point of the lower lip sulcus, the surgical blade can be directed upwards, in order to ensure that the adjacent sliding flaps can move towards the center.
   (iii) After surgical excision of the lip tumor, if there is too much tension following the primary closure of the sliding flaps, there is a need to enlarge the width of the two additional triangles. Alternatively, the immediate reconstruction of large (two-third) lower lip defect can be considered.
   (iv) With regards to the need for neck dissection: If there are suspicious enlarged submental or submandibular

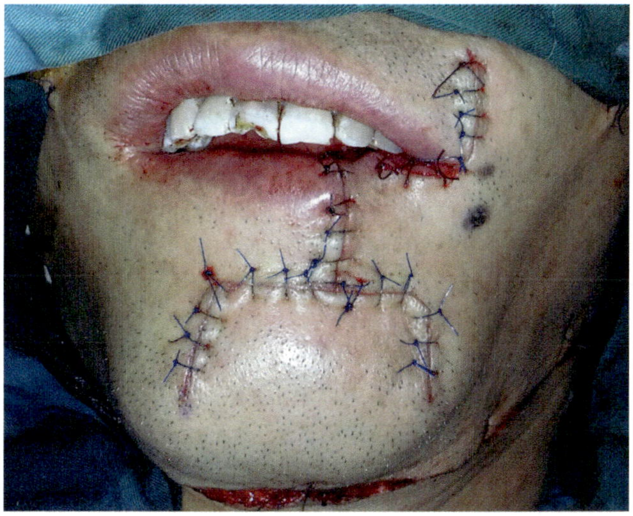

Fig. 15.34 Surgical step

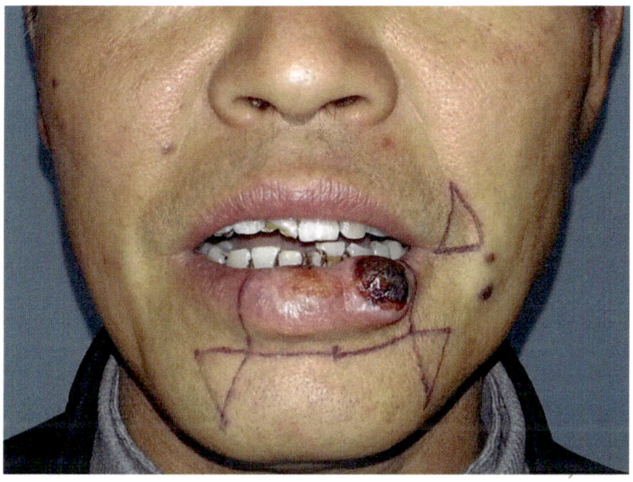

Fig. 15.35 Classical Example 1

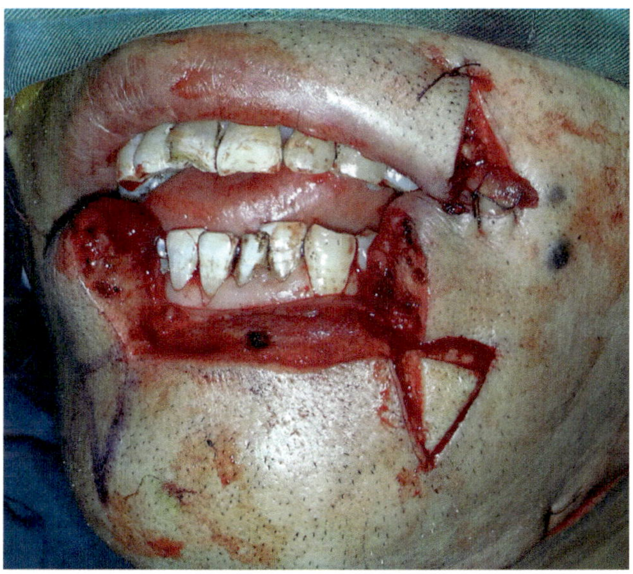

Fig. 15.36 Classical Example 1

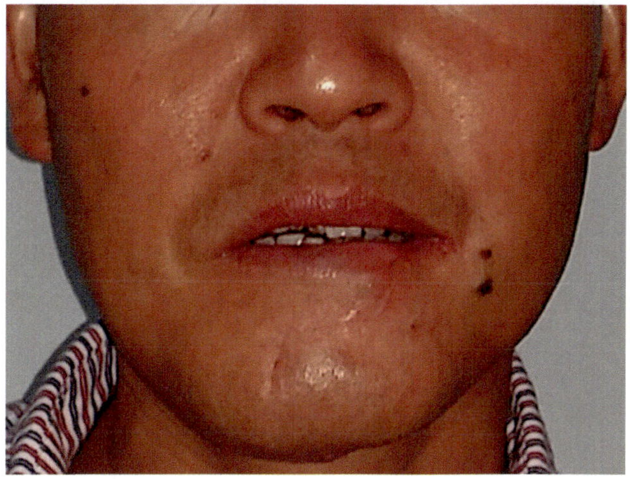

Fig. 15.37 Classical Example 1

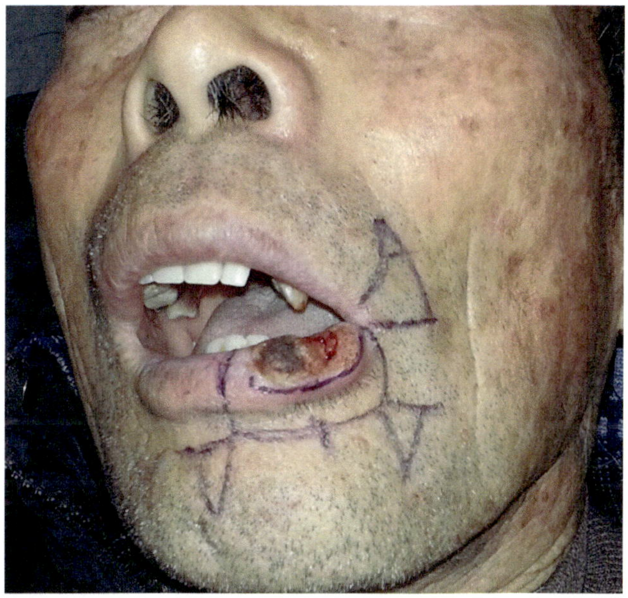

Fig. 15.38 Classical Example 2

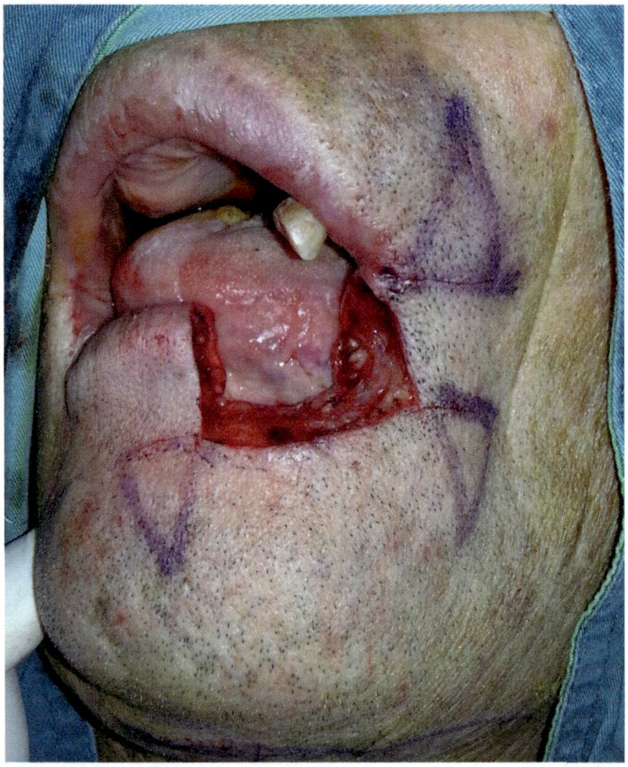

Fig. 15.39 Classical Example 2

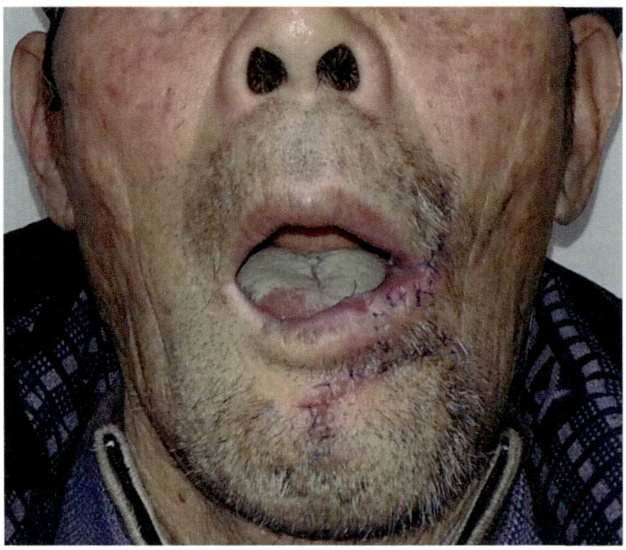

Fig. 15.40 Classical Example 2

lymph nodes, it would require submental and unilateral submandibular neck dissection. In addition, endophytic tumors have a higher risk of metastasis as compared to exophytic tumors, and hence simultaneous neck dissection should be performed. Endophytic upper lip tumors should include neck dissection of submental, submandibular, and superior deep cervical lymph nodes.

References

1. Ru-Yao S, Zhang-Lin F. Cosmetic and plastic surgery (in Chinese). 2nd ed. Beijing: Beijing Publish House; 1992. p. 132–9.
2. Campbell JP. Surgical management of lip carcinoma. J Oral Maxillofac Surg. 1998;56:955–61.
3. Yi L, Ting-Man J, Jian-Hua L, Zhi-Qiang C. Modified bernard sliding flap on defect after lip carcinoma resection (in Chinese). Acad J Hangzhou Teachers College. 2003;24(5):25–6.

Reconstructive Surgery After Total Lower Lip Resection

16

Huiyong Zhu and Jianhua Liu

There are many causes for the loss of lower lip soft tissue, the most common one being the consequence of therapeutic resection of the tumor. The resultant tissue defects require meticulously planned reconstruction with local or free flaps [1, 2].

16.1 Adjacent Soft Tissue Sliding Flaps for Total Lower Lip Defect

This design is suitable for the reconstruction of the total lower lip defect, based on the Bernard-Webster flap with modifications.

1. Indications
   (i) Traumatic or post-resection lower lip defect greater than two-third of and up to almost the entire width of the lower lip.
   (ii) Tissue defect not beyond the labial-buccal sulcus.
   (iii) Full thickness tissue defect involving skin, muscle, and mucosae.
   (iv) Primary repair after resection of lower lip malignancy; all frozen section margins must be negative.
   (v) Older patients with facial tissue laxity. This flap is less suitable for patients below 60 years of age.
2. Surgical Steps

Shaded areas on the left picture indicate areas to be resected, followed by inward sliding of flaps L1 and L2. As illustrated by the picture of the right, M1 is then sutured to M2 and L1 to L2. The combined length of C-L1 and L2-D equals or is slightly less than L1–L2 (Fig. 16.1).

16.1.1 Case Report and Surgical Process

Two reverse triangles are planned below the lower lip, with bases parallel to the stoma. Similarly, two upright triangles are drawn at the sides of the upper lip where each hypotenuse lies within the nasolabial fold. The base of each triangle should equal to or slightly short of half of the anticipated lower lip defect (Fig. 16.2).

Note: the two lower lip triangles shown here were drawn slightly smaller than the actual incision (Fig. 16.3).

Operative steps:

(a) Excise the lower lip tumor with safety margin and send for frozen section. If margins are positive for cancer, to include further resective margins.
(b) Carry out skin incisions as designed pre-surgically and remove the skin and part of the muscle of the triangles. Incise the mucosal surfaces of the bases of the lower lip triangles at the level just above the buccal sulcus. Ensure the mucosal base of the upper lip triangles is kept intact. Incise through all remaining mucosal surfaces. Mobilize the lower lip skin flaps towards the midline.
(c) If any submental lymph nodes are palpable, neck dissection and removal of the lymphatic structures of the submental region are mandatory.
(d) Perform alternative skin suture removal at post-operative days 7 to 10, and complete skin suture removal at post-operative day 14.

Photos of surgical procedures are representative of the reconstruction of a defect comprising two-third of the lower lip width (Figs. 15.17, 15.18, 15.19, 15.20).

H. Zhu · J. Liu (✉)
Department of Oral and Maxillo-facial Surgery, First Affiliated Hospital, Zhejiang University School of Medicine, Hangzhou, China

J. Liu, B. Shi (eds.), *Atlas of Lip and Nose Plastic and Cosmetic Surgery*, https://doi.org/10.1007/978-981-16-1911-3_16

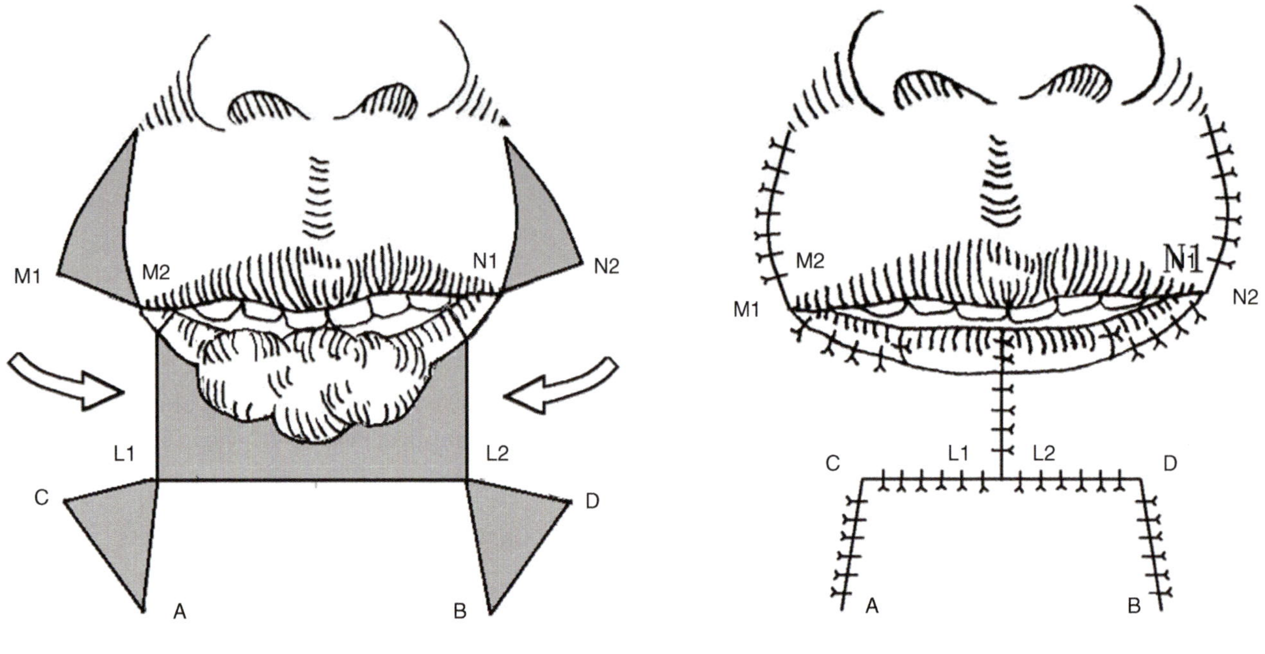

Fig. 16.1 Modified Bernard-Webster sliding flap to reconstruct lower lip defect

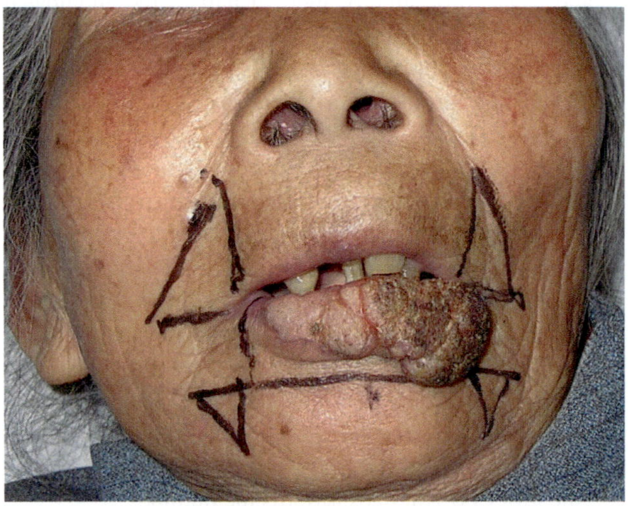

Fig. 16.2 Pre-operative incision design

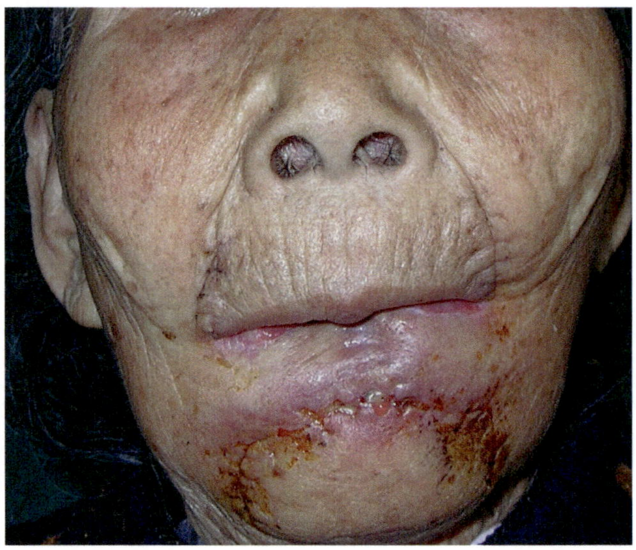

Fig. 16.3 Immediately after skin suture removal

3. Special Considerations
   - (i) The post-resection tissue defect should be anticipated pre-operatively, and the lower lip triangles be designed accordingly. The additional incision at the nasolabial fold allows the utilization of a new sliding flap with both lips with greater flexibility and tissue mobilization.
   - (ii) The triangles should be designed as isosceles with their sides longer than the bases. The base of each triangle should equal or be slightly shorter than one and half the length of the tissue defect.
   - (iii) The base of each lower lip triangle is slightly shorter than one and half the length of the tissue defect. However, if significant tissue tension is encountered during mobilization, the outer incision can be extended.
   - (iv) Particular attention should be paid intra-operatively to ensure the mucosal surfaces of the nasolabial fold incisions are kept intact. This mucosal surface is later flipped and sutured to the remaining lower lip skin surface to form the new vermilion. Brunches of

the facial artery near the nasolabial folds should be preserved.

(v) Given the local tissue tension after sliding flap, suture removal can be delayed slightly and be removed at post-operative day 10–14.

16.2 Vascularized Soft Tissue Free Flaps for Total Lower Lip Defect

1. Indications
   (i) Total lower lip defect after trauma or tumor resection.
   (ii) Defect involving vermilion and considerable surrounding skin.
   (iii) Full thickness tissue defect involving skin, muscle, and mucosae.
   (iv) Limited skin laxity rendering local sliding or rotating flaps unsuitable.
   (v) Primary repair after resection of lower lip malignancy; all frozen section margins must be negative.
2. Surgical Steps

Case study and operative procedures.

Tumor involving the entire lower lip and surrounding skin (Fig. 16.4).

The large tissue defect after resection of the entire lower lip, mental soft tissue, and corresponding mandibular alveolus (Fig. 16.5).

Antero-lateral thigh free flap with the pedicled vessel, muscle, skin, and subcutaneous tissue is harvested from the patient (Figs. 16.6, 16.7, 16.8, 16.9).

3. Special Considerations
   (i) Ensure the tumor is resected as wide as necessary to obtain clear margins.

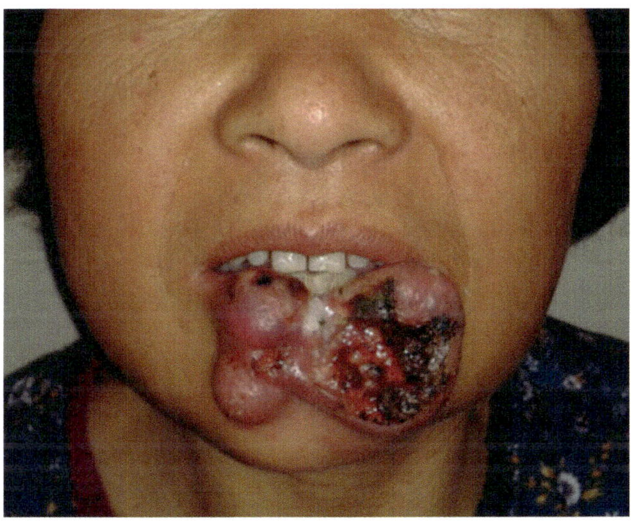

Fig. 16.4 Lower lip malignancy, pre-operative

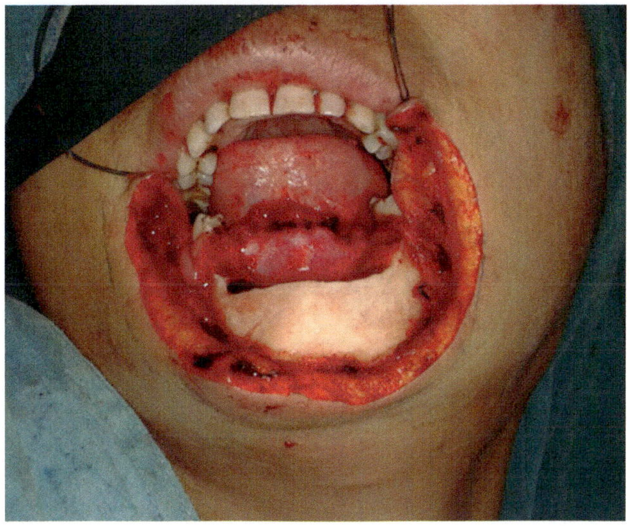

Fig. 16.5 After wide excision of the tumor

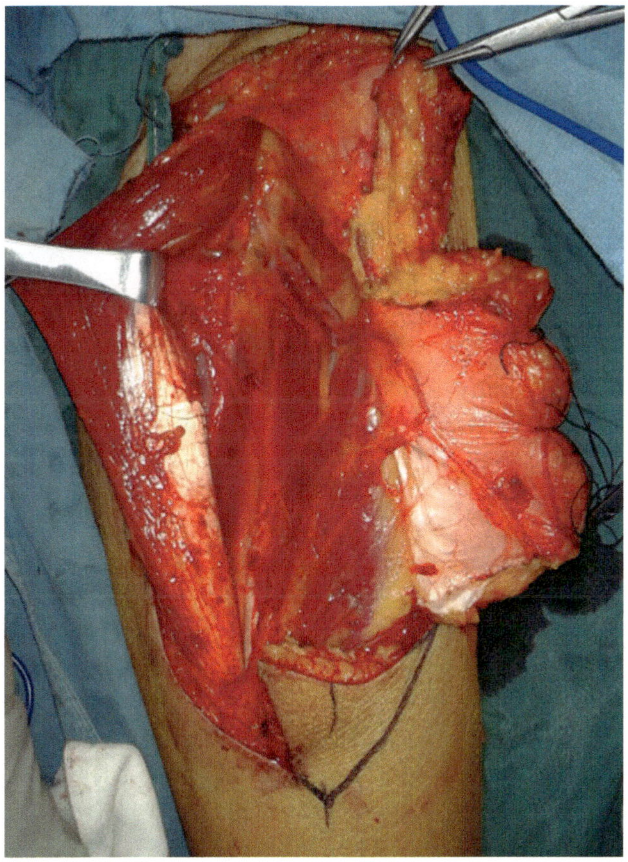

Fig. 16.6 Antero-lateral thigh (ALT) flap is prepared

   (ii) Select the appropriate free flap pre-operatively depending on the size and thickness of the anticipated tissue defect. The commonly used free flaps are the forearm skin flap and ALT flap. However, after the reconstruction, the lower lip vermilion will

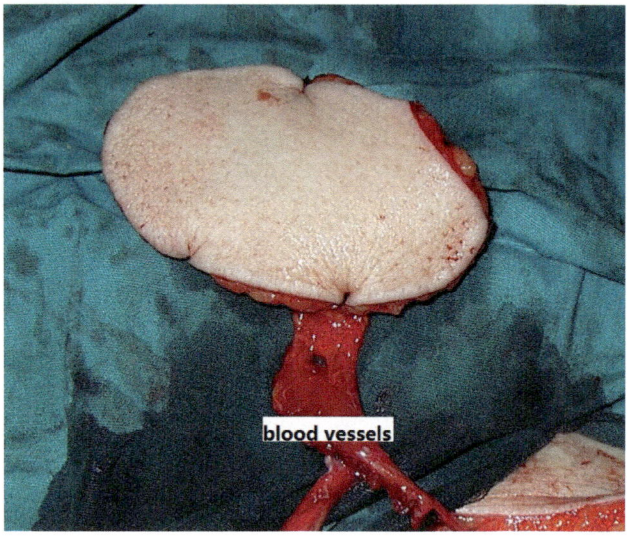

Fig. 16.7 The harvested ALT flap

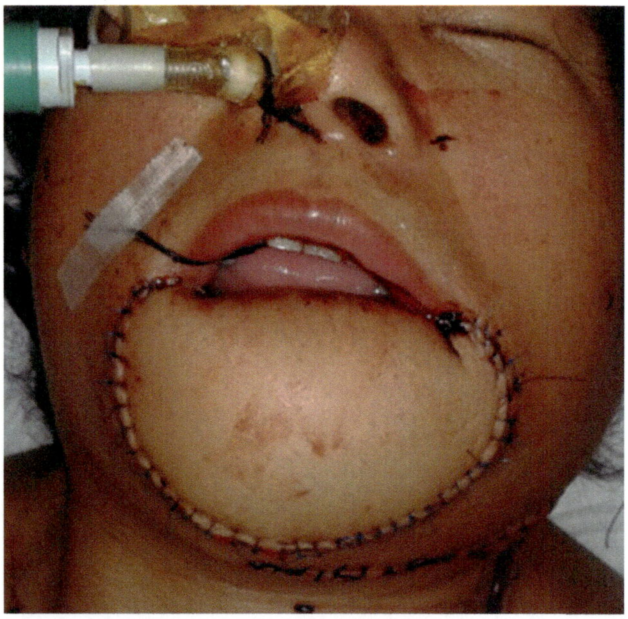

Fig. 16.8 Defect reconstruction and closure with ALT flap

need to be recreated with a skin tattoo. It is also possible with a second reconstruction procedure; however, a certain level of surgical difficulty could be anticipated.

(iii) The pedicles of the ALT flap are tunneled through the skin bridge of the neck and micro-anastomosed with suitable arteries and veins from the recipient bed. Within 72 hours immediately after reconstruction, close monitoring of the color, texture, turgor, temperature, pulse, and capillary refill of the flap is crucial. Immediate interventions are required in case of any abnormalities.

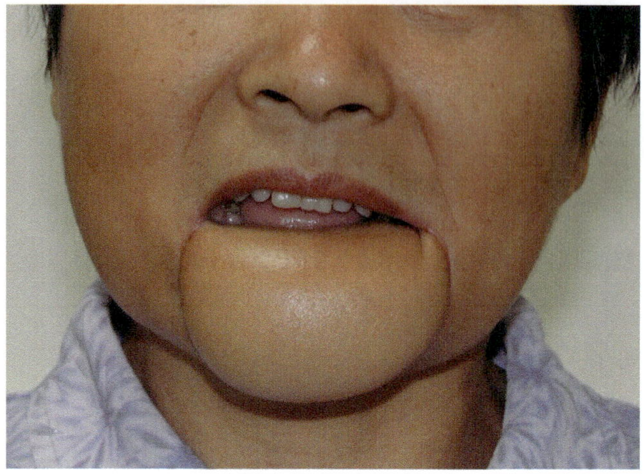

Fig. 16.9 Three-month post-surgery

(iv) For cases of free flap reconstruction with excessive flap thickness, a second surgery to thin down the flap can be performed 3 to 6 months later. However, care to be taken to avoid excessive trimming of tissue leading to flap necrosis.

16.3 Fan-Shaped Tissue Flaps for Total Lower Lip Defect

1. Indications
   (i) Traumatic or post-resection lower lip defect greater than two-third of and up to almost the entire width of the lower lip.
   (ii) Tissue defect not beyond the buccal sulcus.
   (iii) Full thickness tissue defect involving skin, muscle, and mucosae.
   (iv) Adequate peri-oral skin laxity.
   (v) Primary repair after resection of lower lip malignancy; all frozen section margins must be negative.
2. Surgical Steps

A fan-shaped skin flap is formed by linking points 1–2–3–4. Point 4 is located at the upper lip vermilion border. Part of the orbicularis oris muscle is preserved as the flap pedicle. The flap is rotated towards the midline of the lower lip in a clockwise direction and sutured with the opposing flap. Note that the reconstructed lower lip length is depended on the distance between point 1 and 4. The right side flap is as same as the left flap.

Case Study and Operative Procedures:

For lower lip SCC, complete resection is required. The local fan-flap is used for this case. Note the slight difference in flap design compared to Fig. 16.10 with the preservation of soft tissue beyond resection margin (Fig. 16.11).

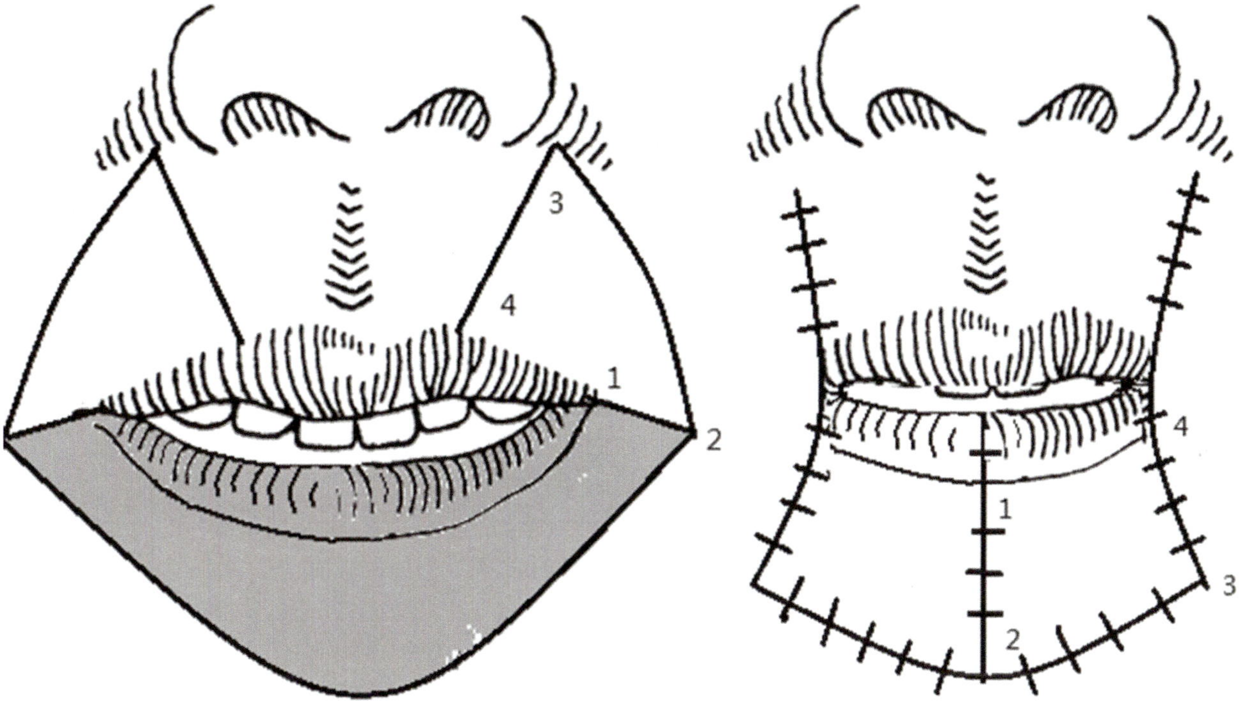

Fig. 16.10 Fan-shaped buccal tissue flap for total lower lip reconstruction

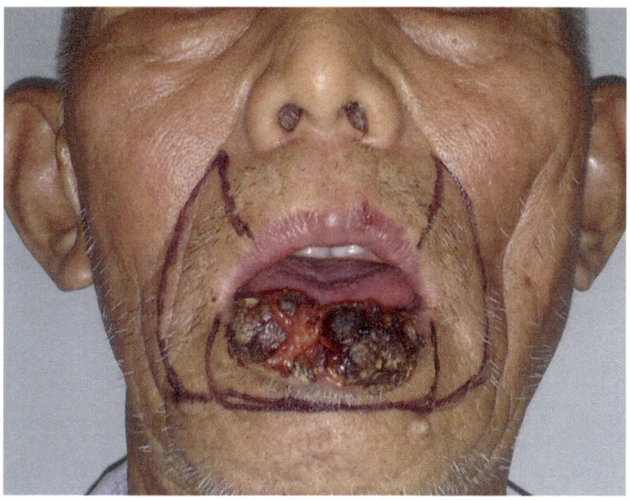

Fig. 16.11 Pre-surgical incision design for lower lip SCC resection

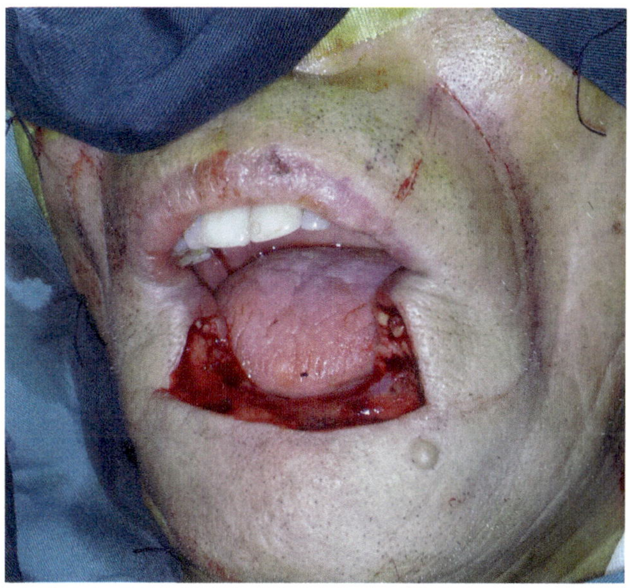

Fig. 16.12 Wide resection of lower lip tumor

Total lower lip defect after wide excision of tumor with safety margin (Fig. 16.12).

The right fan-flap is prepared, care is taken to preserve the distal end of the facial artery (Fig. 16.13).

The left fan-flap is prepared, care is taken to preserve the distal end of the facial artery (Fig. 16.14).

Bilateral skin flaps are secured at the midline. Skin, muscle, and mucosa are sutured in layers (Fig. 16.15).

Reduced oral stoma as wound contracts (Figs. 16.16 and 16.17).

Three months after reconstruction, the oral stoma is still restricted, precluding fabrication of dentures. The patient is planned for oral commissurotomy (Fig. 16.18).

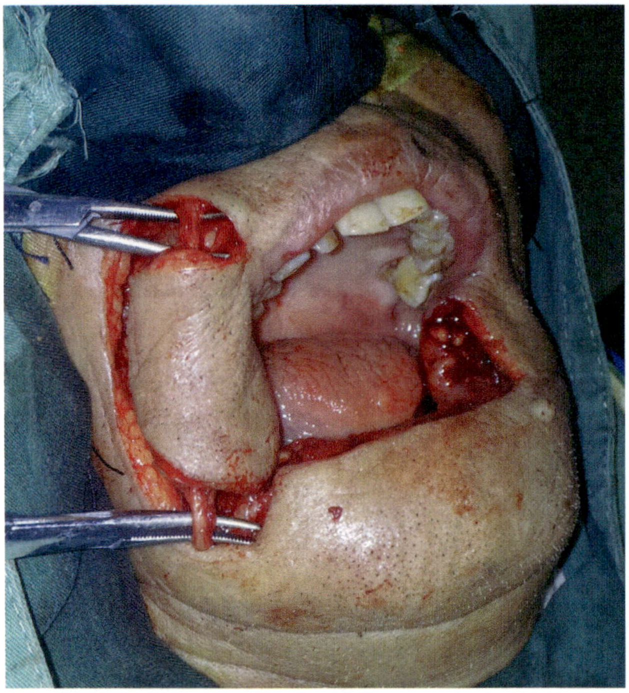

Fig. 16.13 Preparation of the right fan-flap

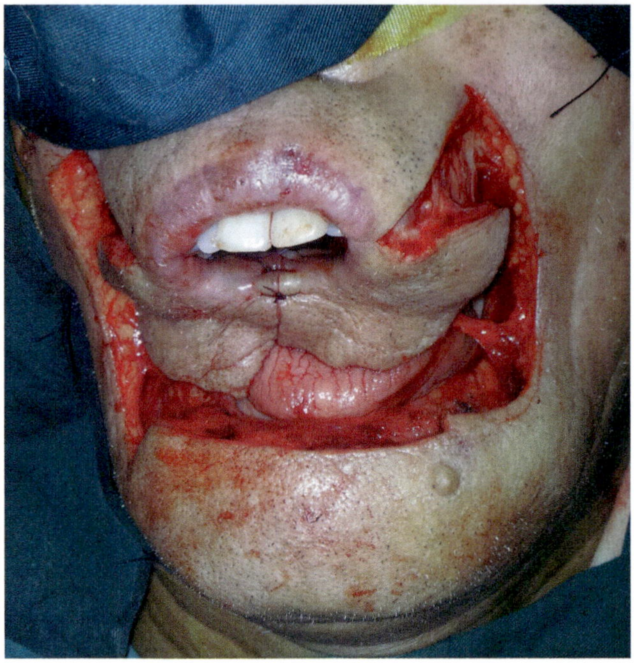

Fig. 16.15 Bilateral skin flaps are rotated and secured

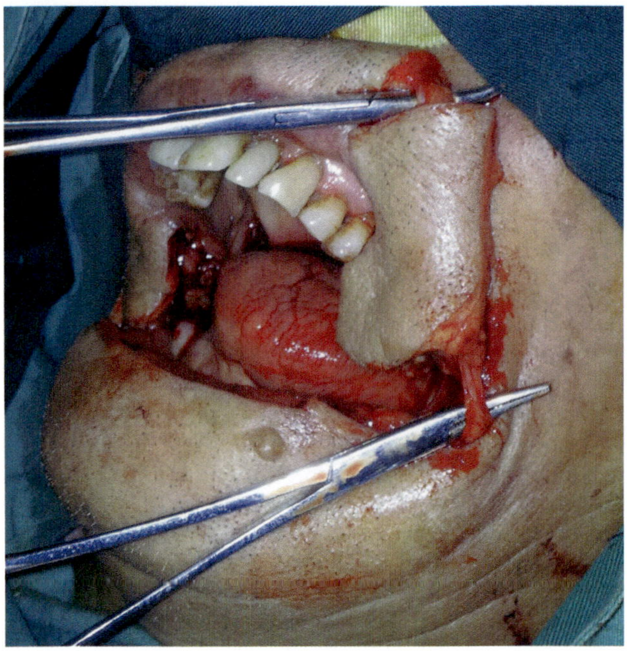

Fig. 16.14 Preparation of the left fan-shaped flap

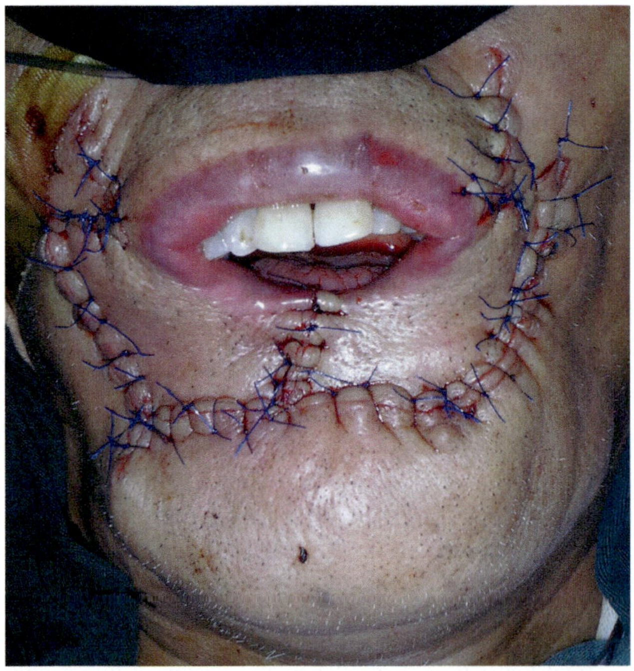

Fig. 16.16 Flaps rotated and secured with sutures

Second stage oral commissurotomy can be performed 4–6 months after primary reconstruction. The new oral commissures are usually placed at the intersection of a vertical line dropped from the pupil, and the existing oral stoma extended. The procedure can be performed under local anesthesia (Fig. 16.19).

3. Special Considerations
   (i) When designing the fan-flap, ensure the reconstructed lower lip vermilion is half the width of the original upper lip.
   (ii) The upper lip incision should stop near the vermilion, avoiding injuries to its arterial supply.

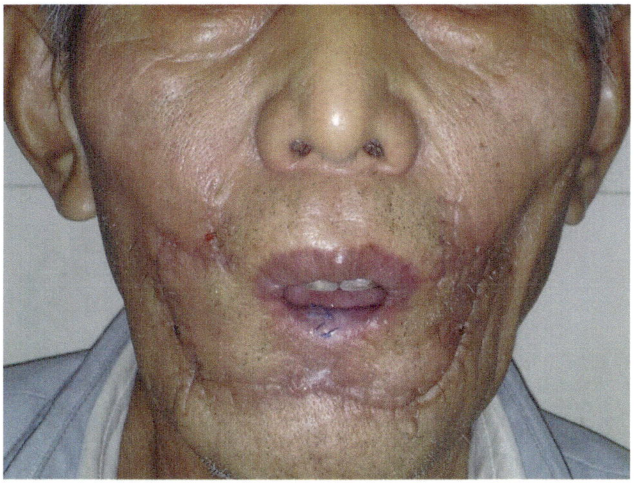

Fig. 16.17 Two weeks after fan-flap reconstruction

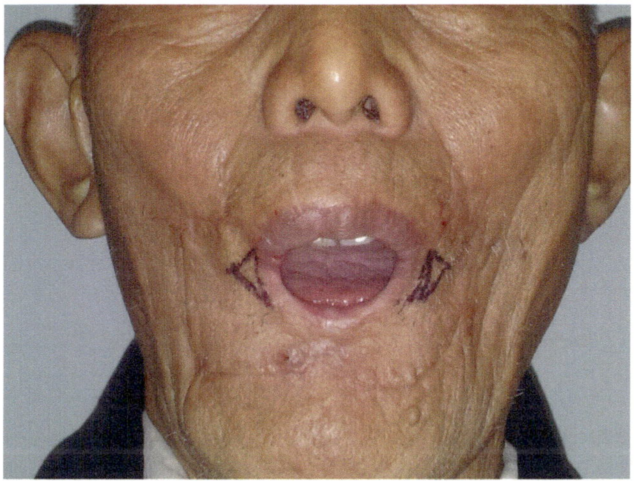

Fig. 16.18 Three-month post-op

(iii) Efforts should be made to preserve some of the buccal sulcular mucosa intra-operatively to facilitate complete closure of oral mucosa. When sulcular tissues are inadequate, the periosteum of the preserved gingivae could be elevated and then sutured to the mucosal surfaces of the fan-flap [3].

(iv) Muscular layers should be matched carefully to avoid undesired rotation and compression of the flap pedicle. Excessive tissue tension and formation of dead space should be minimized during closure. If excessive tension is observed after flap rotation, a 0.5 cm incision could be made buccal to the labial sulcus bilaterally, and periosteum elevated to release tension.

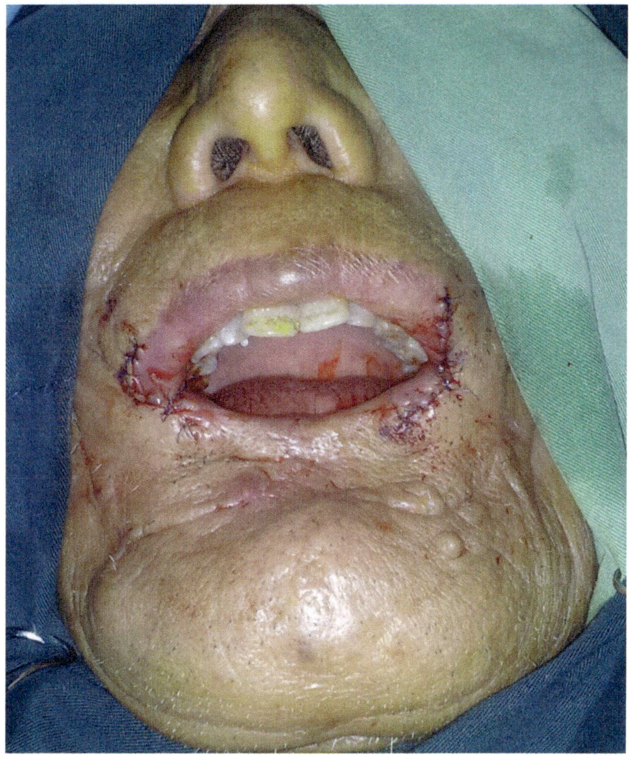

Fig. 16.19 Second stage oral commissurotomy

(v) Minimize risk of infection with thorough scaling pre-operatively, antibiotic coverage post-operatively, and oral hygiene care.

(vi) Commonly 3–4 weeks after fan-flap reconstruction, bilateral oral commissurotomy is performed in cases of restricted stoma or rounded commissures.

References

1. Zilinsky I, Winkler E, Weiss G, et al. Total lower lip reconstruction with innervated muscle bearing flaps. A modification of the webster flap. Dermatol Surg. 2001;27(7):687–91.
2. Bradley C, Leake JE. Compensatory reconstruction of the lips and mouth after major tissue loss. Clin Plast Surg. 1984;11(5):637–42.
3. Long X. Fan shaped flap on lower lip defect (in Chinese). Gansu Med J. 2012;31(5):353–5.

17 Reconstruction of Upper Lip Defect After Tumor Resection

Jianhua Liu

17.1 Labial and Buccal Sliding Flaps for One and Half Upper Lip Defect

1. Indications
   - (i) Rectangular defect of the upper lip due to trauma or tumor resection, with the width approaching half of entire upper lip.
   - (ii) Defects not involving nasal base.
   - (iii) Full thickness defects involving skin, muscle, and mucosa.
   - (iv) For first stage reconstruction after resection of malignant upper lip tumor, all frozen section margins must be negative.
2. Surgical Steps

This method is suitable for defects involving ½ of the upper lip. It utilizes a sliding flap of lip and cheek tissues on both sides of the defect to reconstruct the missing upper lip. When the defect is smaller, a unilateral sliding flap would suffice, whereas bilateral flaps could be considered for larger defects [1, 2].

Additional triangles are removed adjacent to the rectangular defect along the nasolabial fold, with its width approximately two-third that of the actual defect. If the flap is expected to slide across a greater distance, an additional triangle can be excised at the ipsilateral lower lip, which width is slightly smaller than that of the upper lip triangle. After excision of the triangles as planned, the resultant flaps are advanced and sutured accordingly [3].

J. Liu (✉)
Department of Oral and Maxillo-facial Surgery, First Affiliated Hospital, Zhejiang University School of Medicine, Hangzhou, China

17.1.1 Case Report and Surgical Process

Picture showing a trauma patient approximately 1 week after the initial injury. The upper lip defect has been debrided of scabs and fresh wound surfaces exposed (Fig. 17.1).

Surgical design of unilateral labial and buccal sliding flap (Fig. 17.2).

The existing lip defect is trimmed, and the additional triangles excised as planned. Hemostasis is achieved (Fig. 17.3).

Skin and muscle of the nasolabial triangle are removed. The mucosa at the base of the triangle is incised to facilitate mobilization of the flap (Fig. 17.4).

The mucosal and muscular layers are closed first, followed by matching of the vermillion border. Skin closure is completed last (Fig. 17.5).

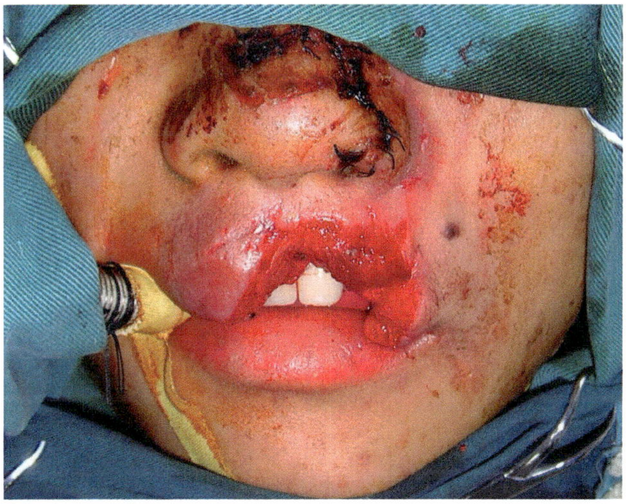

Fig. 17.1 One and half width upper lip defect

J. Liu, B. Shi (eds.), *Atlas of Lip and Nose Plastic and Cosmetic Surgery*, https://doi.org/10.1007/978-981-16-1911-3_17

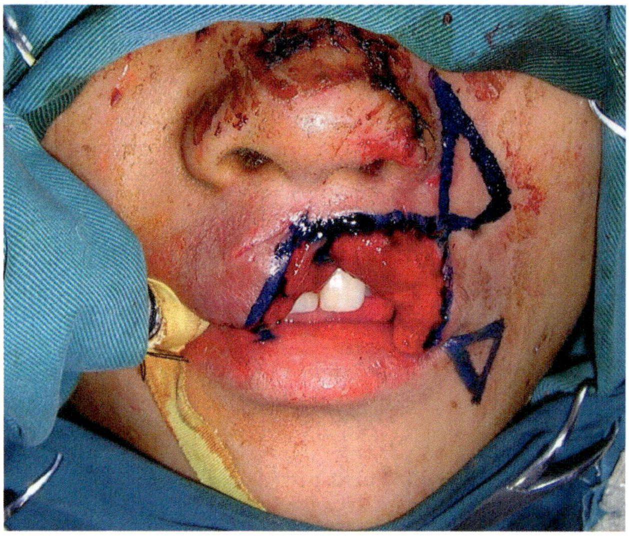

Fig. 17.2 Surgical flap design

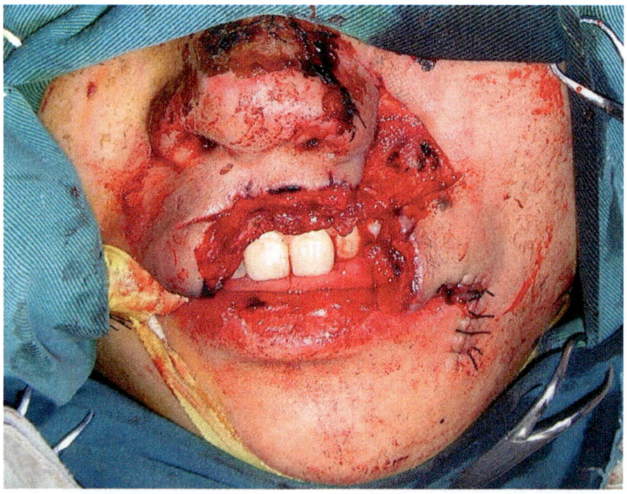

Fig. 17.3 Resection of the additional triangles

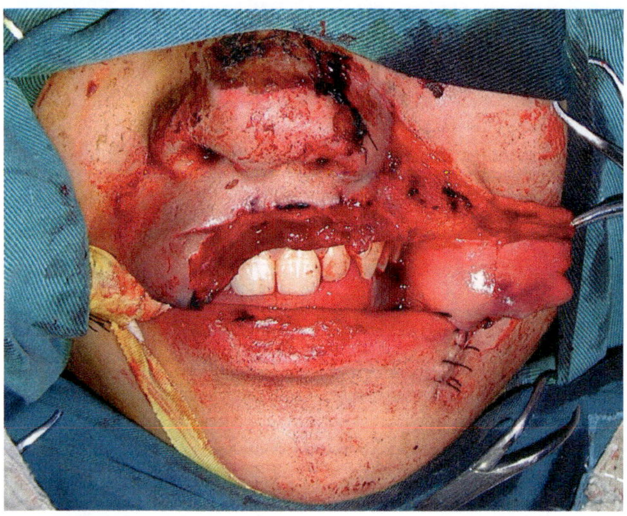

Fig. 17.4 Prior to mobilization of flap

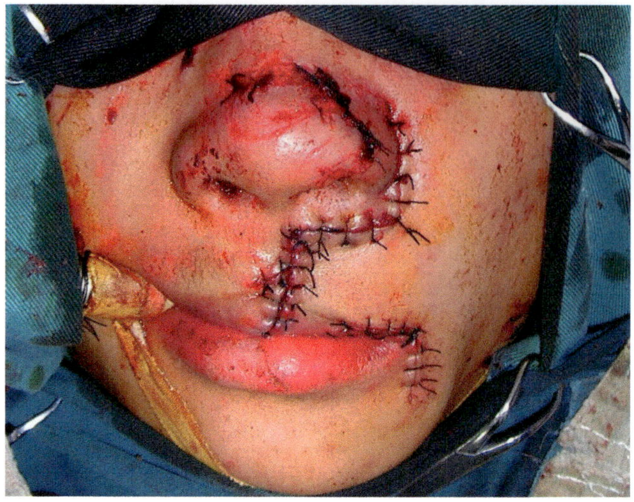

Fig. 17.5 After flap mobilization and closure

17.1.2 Classic Case Study (Fig. 17.6)

3. Special Considerations
   (i) In cases of wound contamination due to trauma, thorough wound debridement prior to reconstruction is crucial to prevent infection and poor healing. For infected cases, a second stage reconstruction is recommended.
   (ii) Irregularly shaped defects should be trimmed into rectangular shapes to facilitate flap-design and reconstruction while preserving as much lip tissues as possible.
   (iii) Additional isosceles triangles are drawn at the ipsilateral nasolabial fold and lower lip. The width of the nasolabial triangle should be slightly shorter than the width of the upper lip defect, whereas the base of the lower lip triangle is slightly smaller than that of the nasolabial triangle.
   (iv) When reconstructing the upper lip defect with local sliding defect, the vermillion is often deficient. Therefore, during flap preparation, the mucosal tissue of the lower lip triangle can be preserved and flipped later to form the new upper lip vermillion.

17.2 Lower Lip Rectangle-Like Flap for One and Half Upper Lip Defect

1. Indications.
   (i) Unilateral defect of the upper lip due to trauma or tumor resection, with the width approaching half of entire upper lip.
   (ii) Defects not involving nasal base.
   (iii) Full thickness defects involving skin, muscle, and mucosa.

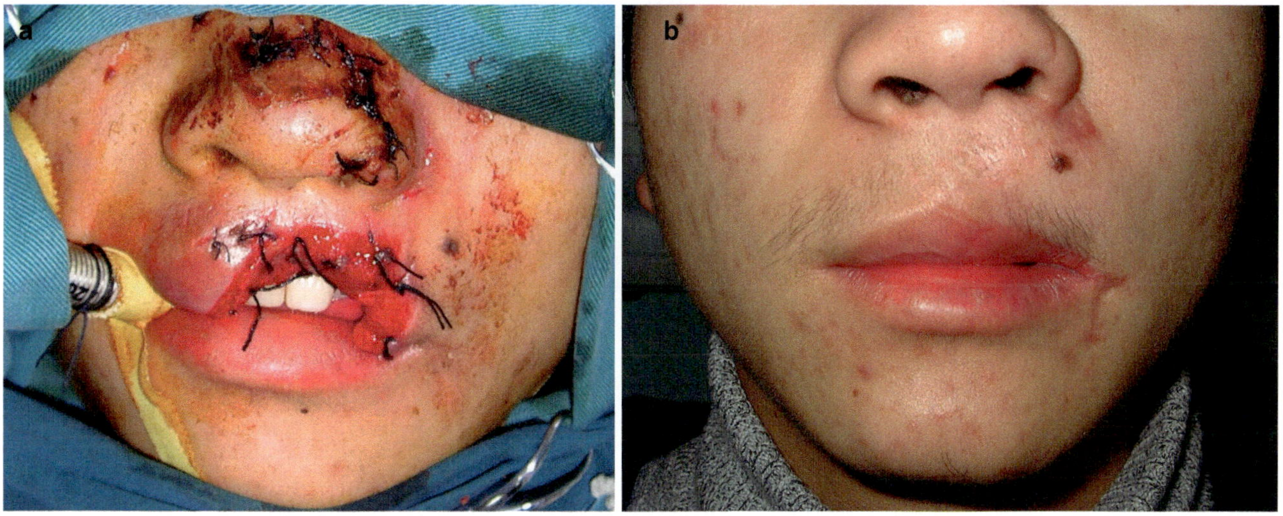

Fig. 17.6 (**a**, **b**) Pre- and post-reconstruction. (**a**) On the left: Pre-reconstruction of left upper lip defect. (**b**) Taken at 6 months review after upper lip reconstruction with labial and buccal sliding flap demonstrating adequate function and aesthetic

(iv) For first stage reconstruction after resection of malignant upper lip tumor, all frozen section margins must be negative.

2. Surgical Steps

This method is a modification of the Abbe-Estlander flap. The flap is designed as a rectangle to reconstruct a defect approximately one and half of the width of the upper lip.

Design a rectangular flap on lower lip same side as the defect. The width of the flap should approximate ½ of the defect. The vermilion muscles, vessels, and part of mucosa adjacent to the flap should be preserved to ensure healthy vascularity and prevent flap necrosis. The lower lip rectangular flap is prepared accordingly and rotated towards the upper lip. The defect is reconstructed and closed in layers.

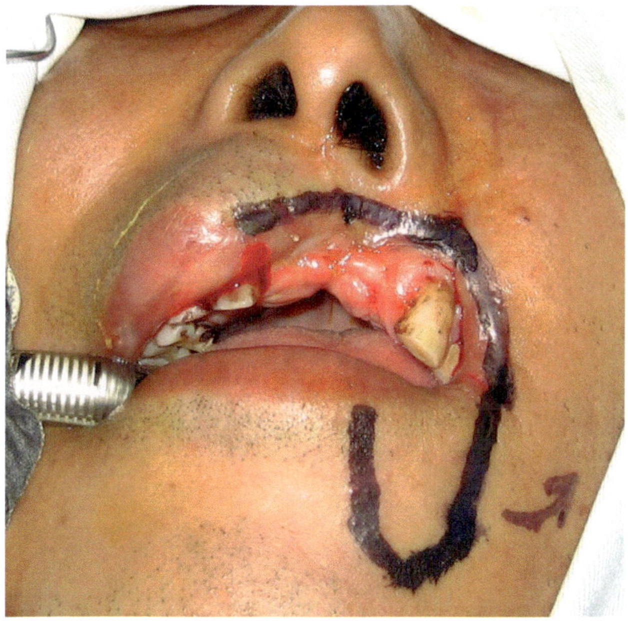

Fig. 17.7 Planned surgical incisions

17.2.1 Case Presentation

Incisions are planned for the lower lip rectangular flap (Fig. 17.7).

Prepare the lower lip rectangular flap according to the size of the defect and planned incision. Care must be taken to preserve the inferior labial artery at the base of the flap (Fig. 17.8).

Rotate the prepared flap 180 degrees to repair the upper lip defect (Fig. 17.9).

Position and suture the corresponding mucosal, muscular, and skin layers and ensure the vermillion border is well-matched (Fig. 17.10).

17.2.2 Classic Case 1 (Fig. 17.11)

The patient was a male elderly with cancer of the upper lip. He received wide excision of the lesion, with a resultant lip defect approaching one and half of the entire width. A lower lip rectangular-shaped flap was planned for stage-1 reconstruction; width of the flap approximate one and half of the defect (Fig. 17.12).

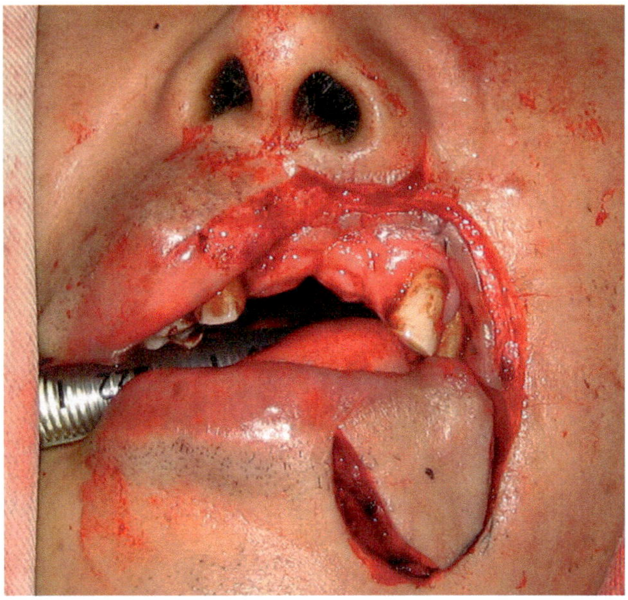

Fig. 17.8 Preparation of the lower lip rectangular flap

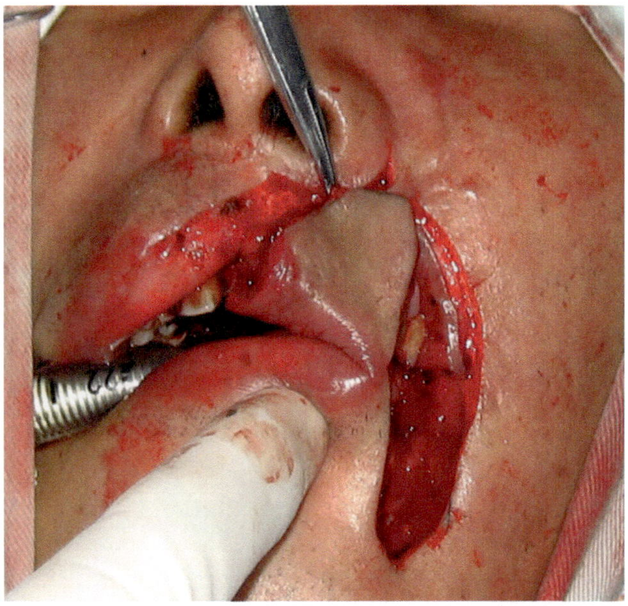

Fig. 17.9 After rotation of the lower lip rectangular flap

The upper lip defect was successfully reconstructed. However, the patient required a second-stage commissurotomy due to constricted oral stoma.

17.2.3 Classic Case 2

Left upper lip defect with adjacent tissue scarring. Reconstruction is relatively difficult (Fig. 17.13).

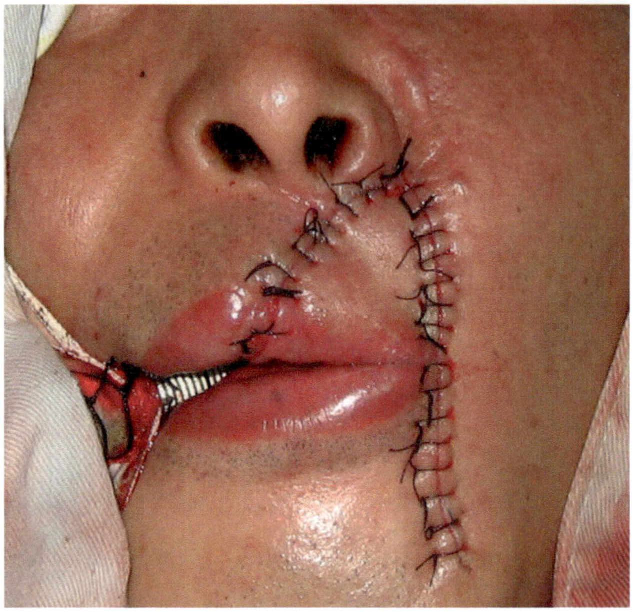

Fig. 17.10 After layered closure

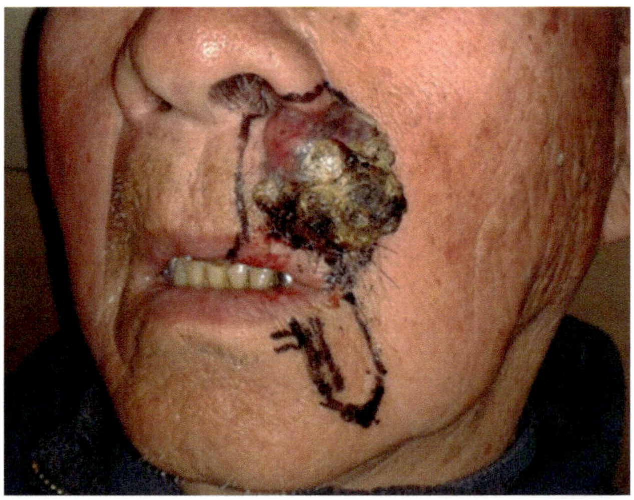

Fig. 17.11 Cancer on the left side of the upper lip, surgical incision design

Intra-operative marking of left-sided lower lip rectangular-like flap for the reconstruction of ipsilateral upper lip defect (Fig. 17.14).

Successful reconstruction of upper lip defect using rectangular-like lower lip flap with satisfactory outcome (Fig. 17.15).

3. Special Considerations
   (i) Plan the lower lip rectangular flap based on the width of the upper lip defect. It is advisable to obtain a flap one and half the width of the defect for a harmonious width ratio of the upper and lower lips after reconstruction.

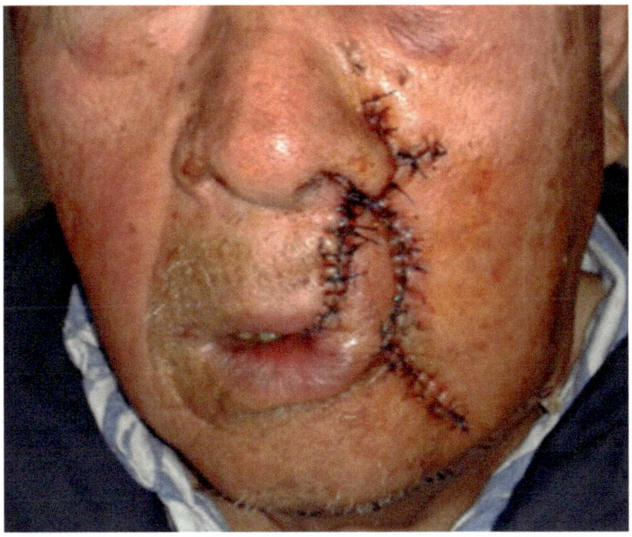

Fig. 17.12 Prior to suture removal

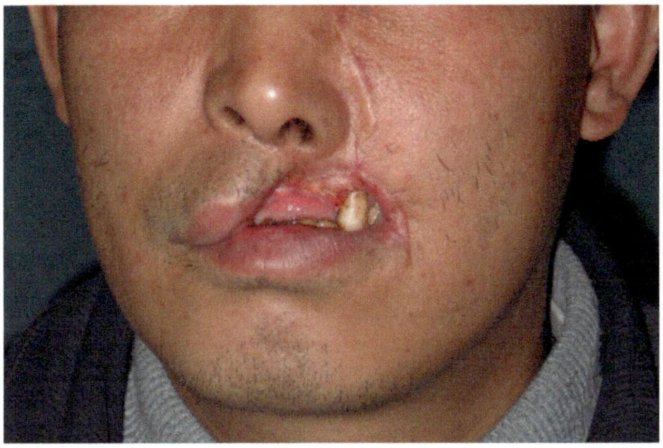

Fig. 17.13 Post-traumatic left upper lip defect

(ii) When preparing the rectangular flap, the vertical incision close to the midline should stop short of the vermilion. Care must be taken to preserve the inferior labial artery at the pedicle of the flap.

(iii) Patients commonly present with asymmetrical commissures after reconstruction, which would require second-stage surgical corrections.

17.3 Lower Lip Flap for Median Upper Lip Defect

1. Indications
   (i) Triangular upper lip defect due to trauma or tumor resection, with the width approaching half of entire upper lip.
   (ii) Full thickness defects involving skin, muscle, and mucosa.

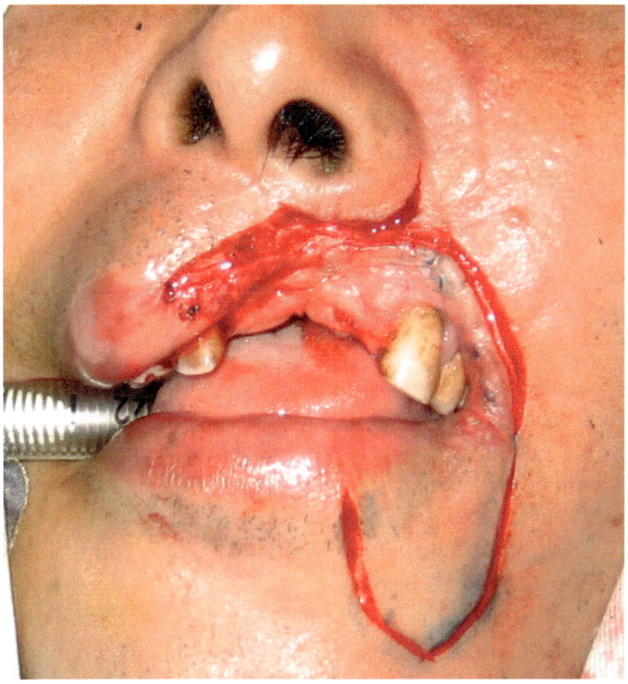

Fig. 17.14 Planned incision of lower lip rectangular-like flap for upper lip defect reconstruction

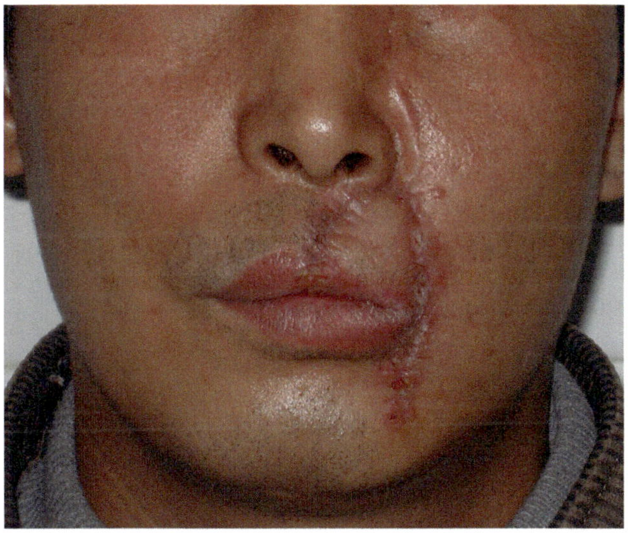

Fig. 17.15 Two weeks after surgery

   (iii) For first stage reconstruction after resection of malignant upper lip tumor, all frozen section margins must be negative.
2. Surgical Steps

This is known as the Abbe flap, which is suitable for reconstructions of both upper and lower lip midline defects of about one and half of the lip length. Applications for upper lip reconstructions: prepare a midline flap at the lower lip of similar shape to and one and half the width of the upper lip defect. Preserve the inferior labial artery at the lower lip and close the lower lip incision first. Rotate the lower lip flap 180°to reconstruct the upper lip defect and close in layers. A second surgery to separate the rotated flap from its pedicle is performed 21 days after the first surgery.

17.3.1 Case Presentation

Design the resection margin of upper lip tumor (carcinoma). In this case, the tumor is well-demarcated, therefore a 5 mm safety margin is adequate, and otherwise, a larger margin should be considered. The lower lip flap is designed accordingly (Fig. 17.16).

Excise the lesion with desired safety margin and send for frozen sections and histology (Fig. 17.17).

Prepare the median lower lip flap according to the extent of upper lip defect and pre-operative design. Preserve a part of the vermilion mucosa and blood vessels. Note: there are anatomical variations of the inferior labial arteries. After incising through the skin, locate the vessels carefully within the muscles without transecting vessels traveling into the flap. In this case, anatomical variation of the blood vessel was encountered (Fig. 17.18).

Rotate the lower lip flap towards the upper lip defect. Position and suture the corresponding mucosal, muscular, and skin layers. Ensure the vermillion border is well-matched. A second surgery to separate the rotated flap from its pedicle is performed 21 days after the first surgery (Fig. 17.19).

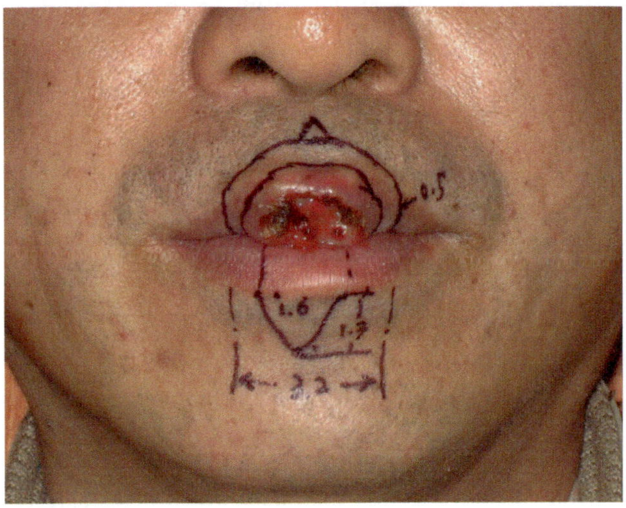

Fig. 17.16 Planned incision

17.3.2 Classic Case

The lower lip flap design shown here was slightly smaller than desired. A wider flap was used during surgery (Fig. 17.20).

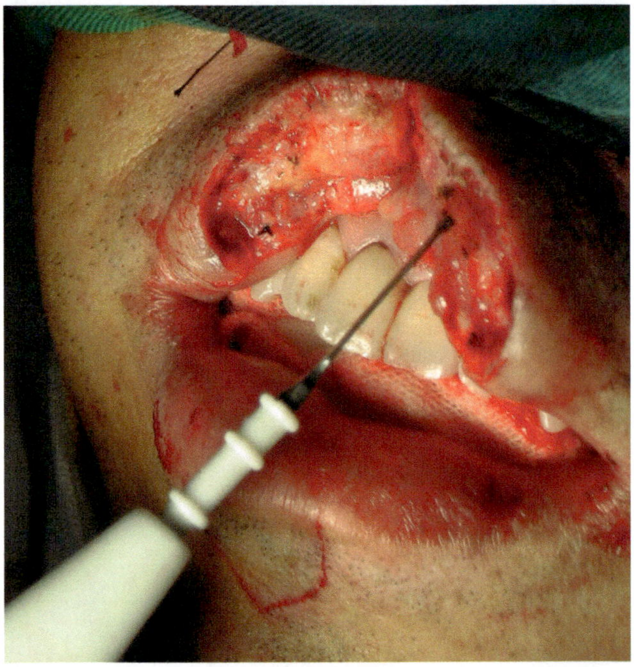

Fig. 17.17 Wide excision of upper lip cancer

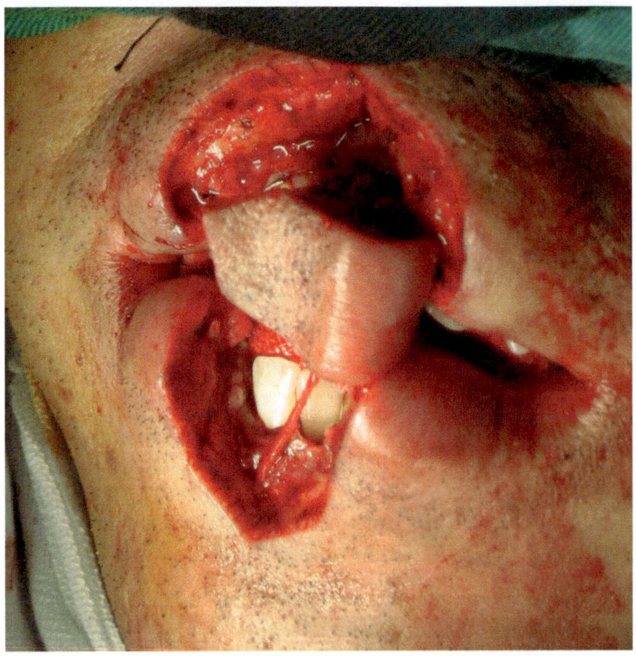

Fig. 17.18 Preparation of median lower lip flap

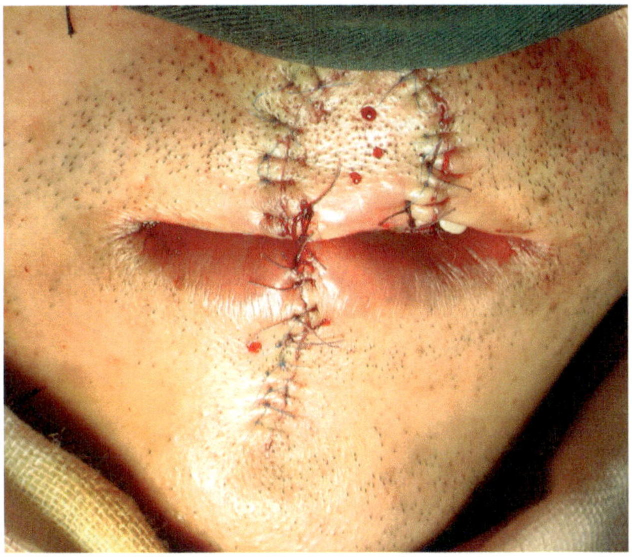

Fig. 17.19 Reconstruction of upper lip defect with rotation of median lower lip flap

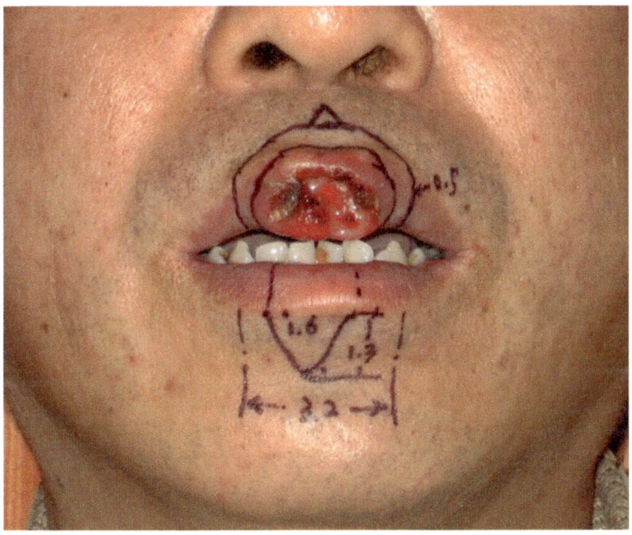

Fig. 17.20 Pre-operative design for upper lip malignancy

21 months after reconstruction demonstrating superb aesthetic and function of both lips (Fig. 17.21).

3. Special Considerations
   (i) Plan the lower lip flap based on the width of the expected upper lip defect. It is advisable to obtain a flap one and half the width of the defect for a harmonious ratio of the upper and lower lips after reconstruction.
   (ii) Care must be taken while dissecting around the vermilion region to preserve the inferior labial artery at the pedicle of the flap.
   (iii) A second surgery is commonly performed 3 weeks later to divide the flap from its pedicle. Special attention must be given in the meanwhile to prevent tearing of the vascular pedicle due to excessive mouth-opening or jaw movement.

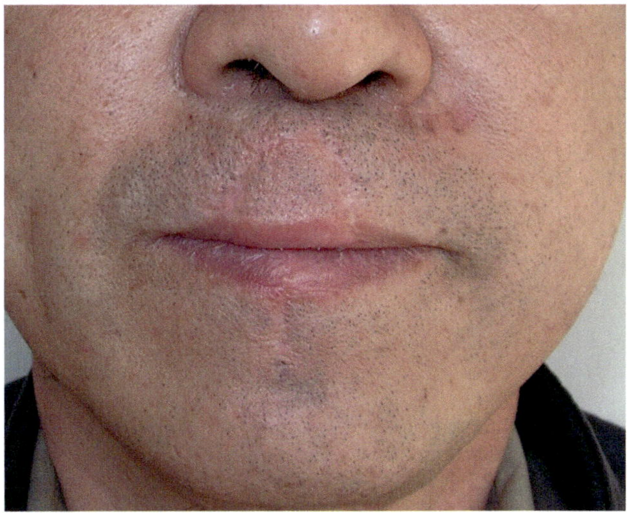

Fig. 17.21 Twenty-one months after reconstruction

17.4 Pedicled Naso-Labial Groove Flap for Unilateral Upper Lip Defect

1. Indications
   (i) Round or oval-shaped unilateral upper lip defect due to trauma or after tumor resection, the width of which approximates one-third–one and half of the entire upper lip.
   (ii) Defects involving skin, muscle but preferably sparing the mucosa. When the labial mucosa is involved, a combination rotational mucosal flap is necessary.
   (iii) For first stage reconstruction after resection of malignant upper lip tumor, all frozen section margins must be negative.
2. Surgical Steps (Fig. 17.22)

First design a flap of appropriate size at the ipsilateral nasolabial groove. The brunches of the inner canthal artery and superior labial artery of the facial artery superior and inferior to the flap should be preserved and dissected free for about 0.5 to 1 cm away from the flap to form a double-pedicled nasolabial groove flap. If the distance between the defect and the flap is considerable, the superior arterial pedicle can be divided. The blood supply from the inferior arterial pedicle is adequate to ensure flap vitality. Muscles of facial expressions inferior to the flap can be divided and rotated to repair ipsilateral lip defects. The missing vermilion can be reconstructed with rotational labial mucosal flaps [4].

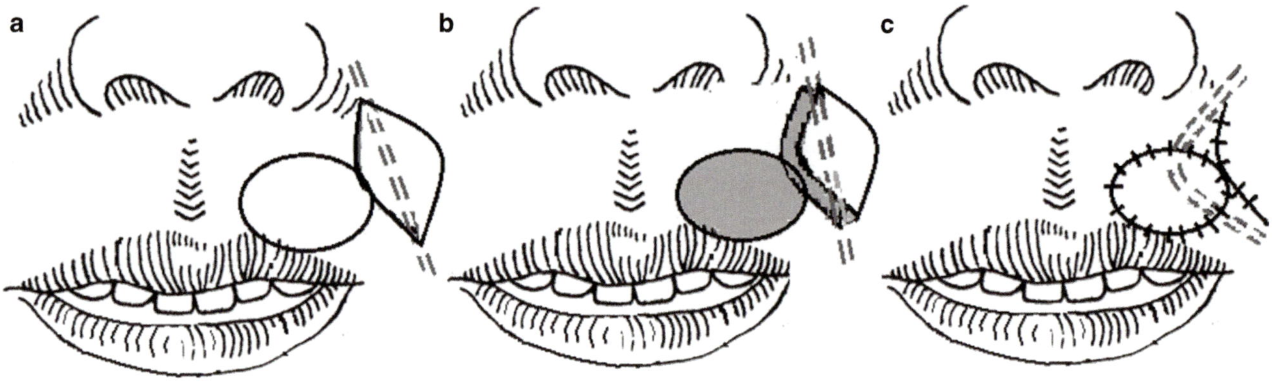

Fig. 17.22 Illustration of the surgical steps. (**a**) Design a double-pedicled nasolabial groove flap of appropriate size according to the shape and extent of the defect. (**b**) Dissect and separate superior and inferior arterial pedicles to allow smooth rotation of the flap towards lip defect. (**c**) Post-operative appearance of upper lip reconstruction

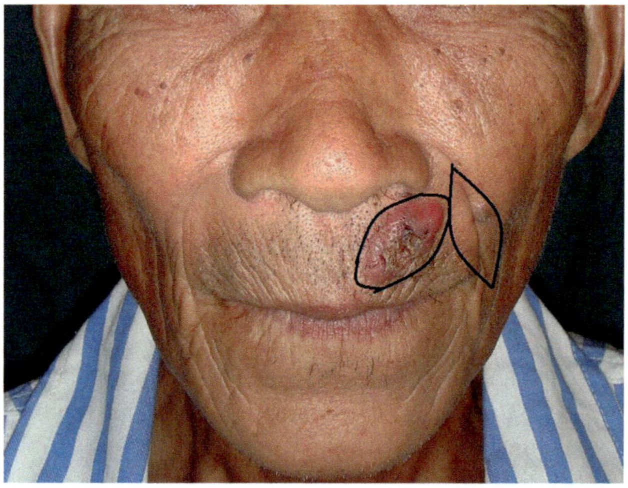

Fig. 17.23 Design of surgical incisions

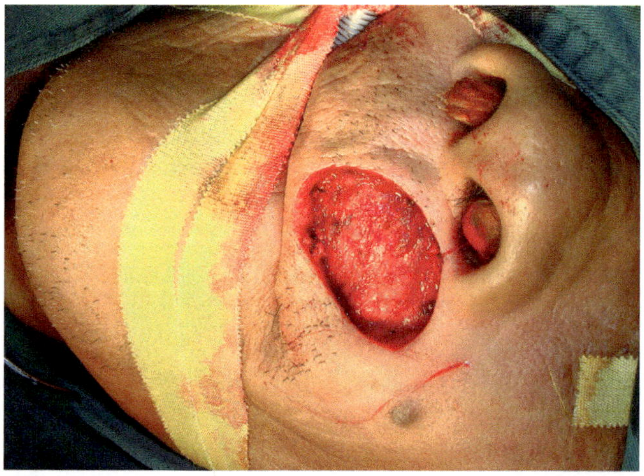

Fig. 17.24 After wide excision of tumor

17.4.1 Case Presentation

Plan for the extent of tumor excision, and design the double-pedicled nasolabial groove flap accordingly (Fig. 17.23).

Excise the tumor with the appropriate margin to form an oval-shaped defect (Fig. 17.24).

Locate the inferior arterial pedicle after skin incision, and dissect it free as shown (Fig. 17.25).

When the pedicles on both ends have been dissected free, the flap incisions are carried deeper into the muscles. Once the muscular layers have been dissected, the flap is readily mobile (Fig. 17.26).

The prepared flap is then mobilized and rotated towards the defect (Fig. 17.27).

The nasolabial groove flap is brought to the intended position and secured with sutures (Fig. 17.28).

17.4.2 Classic Case 1

This patient presented with a right-sided upper lip malignancy. The expected defect after resection involves vermilion and adjacent skin tissues. A double-pedicled nasolabial groove flap is designed for first-stage reconstruction (Fig. 17.29).

At 6 months review, the healed flap appears satisfactory (Fig. 17.30).

17.4.3 Classic Case 2 (Fig. 17.31)

3. Special Considerations
   (i) The nasolabial groove flap is preferably designed elliptical with the nasolabial groove as its long axis to minimize tissue distortion after flap rotation and closure.

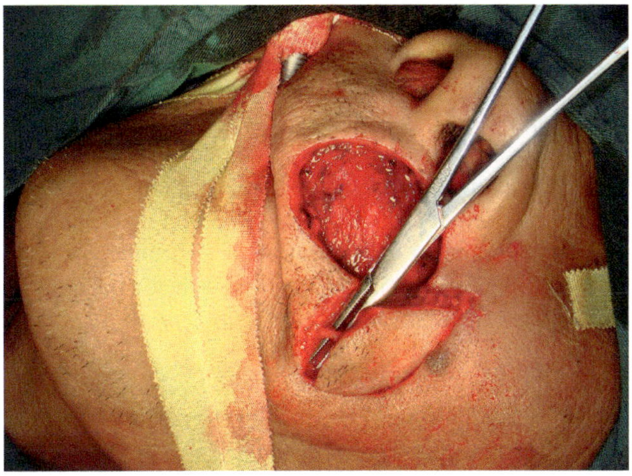

Fig. 17.25 Inferior arterial pedicle is dissected free

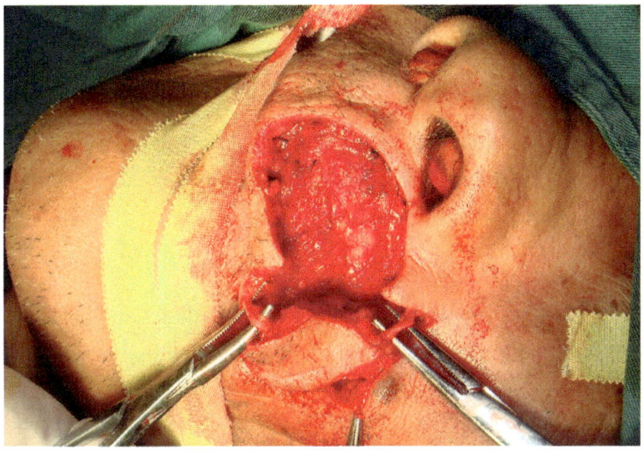

Fig. 17.26 The skeletonized double pedicles

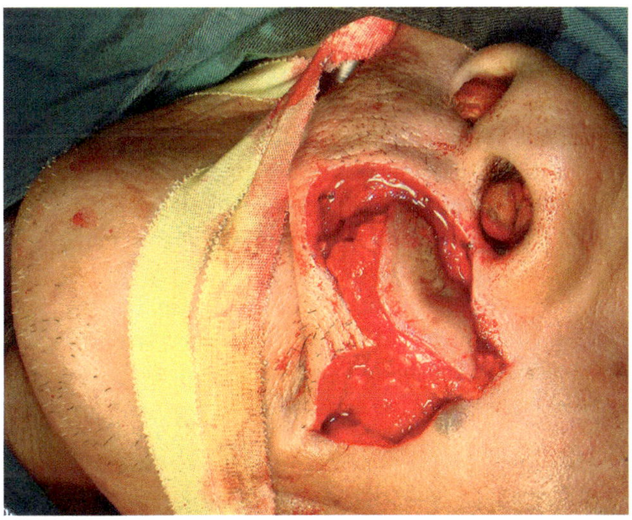

Fig. 17.27 Flap is rotated and mobilized

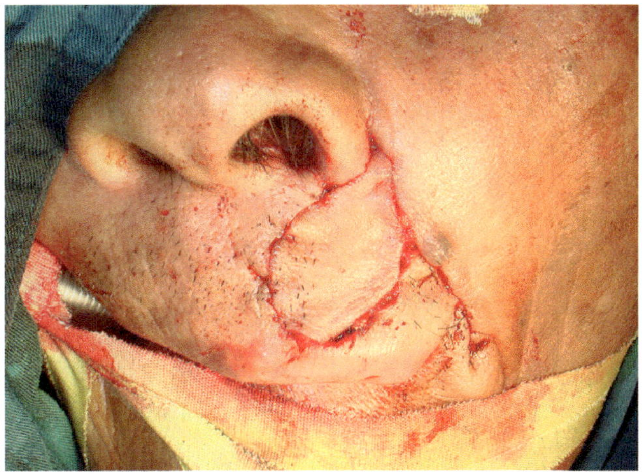

Fig. 17.28 The double-pedicled nasolabial groove flap secured at the intended position

(ii) It is imperative to preserve blood supplies during flap preparation and to avoid over compression of vessels during flap rotation. As much as possible, both proximal and distal extensions of the arterial supply should be preserved to form a double-pedicled flap for better vascularity and flap survival.

(iii) In cases where the corresponding labial mucosae are not harvested during flap preparation, the reconstruction of vermillion defects can be achieved with local mucosal rotational flaps.

17.5 Bilateral Sliding Flaps for Upper Lip Defect

1. Indications
   (i) Upper lip defects due to trauma or tumor resection, the width of which approximates half of the entire upper lip.
   (ii) Full thickness defects involving skin, muscle, and mucosa.
   (iii) For first stage reconstruction after resection of malignant upper lip tumor, all frozen section margins must be negative.
2. Surgical Steps

This method is similar to the modified Bernard-Webster flap for lower lip reconstruction described earlier in Sect. 17.3. The upper lip lesion is first excised with a safe margin to form a rectangular defect. Additional triangular tissues at bilateral nasolabial grooves are then removed to form sliding flaps which are mobilized towards the defect and secured with sutures.

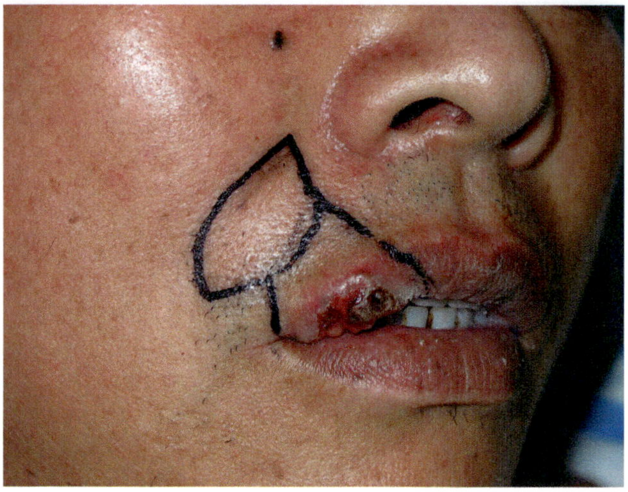

Fig. 17.29 Planned incision for right upper lip malignancy

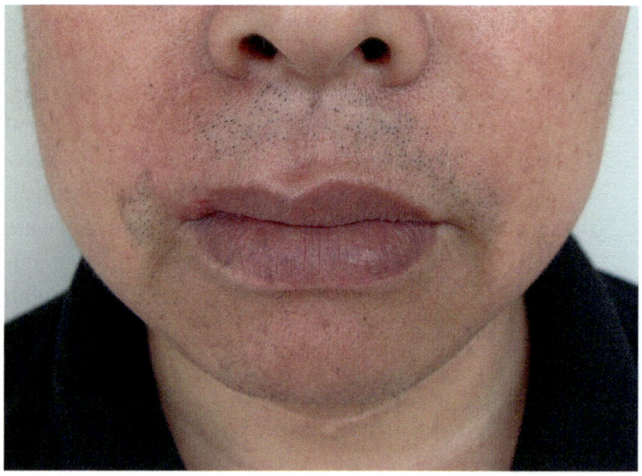

Fig. 17.30 Six months after reconstruction

17.5.1 Case Presentation

Right-sided upper lip intra-muscular malignant tumor. Picture showing pre-operative design of the rectangular resective section and bilateral sliding flaps (Fig. 17.32).

Part of the upper lip is resected to form the rectangular defect. Additional triangular tissues at bilateral nasolabial grooves are removed to form the sliding flaps (Fig. 17.33).

The bilateral sliding flaps are repositioned and secured to close the upper lip defect (Fig. 17.34).

3. Special Considerations
   (i) The lateral edges of the nasolabial triangles can be designed with curves similar to the existing natural nasolabial grooves for less conspicuous post-operative scarring. The bases of the triangles should parallel the base of the nose; after closure, the sutures can be hidden well underneath the nose.
   (ii) Irregularly shaped defects should be trimmed into rectangular shapes to facilitate flap-design and reconstruction while preserving as much healthy lip tissues as possible.
   (iii) Given the natural facial soft tissue laxity, generally a base of each nasolabial groove flap slightly short of one and half of the upper lip defect is adequate. If considerable tissue tension is encountered during flap mobilization, the bases of each additional triangle can be extended.

17.6 Fan-Shaped Tissue Flap for Unilateral Upper Lip Defect

1. Indications
   (i) Upper lip defects due to trauma or tumor resection, the width of which exceeds two-third of the entire upper lip.
   (ii) Full thickness defects involving skin, muscle, and mucosa.
   (iii) For first stage reconstruction after resection of malignant upper lip tumor, all frozen section margins must be negative.
2. Surgical Steps

The upper lip lesion is first excised with a safe margin to form a relatively large defect. A fan-shaped labial and buccal flap is designed to reconstruct the upper lip defect. The vascular supply of this flap comes from branches of the facial artery from the contralateral lower lip. Common post-operative complications are reduced oral stoma and lip asymmetry.

Tissue defect approaching two-third of the upper lip after wide excision of malignancy. Reconstruction is planned with fan-shaped tissue flap (Fig. 17.35).

Upper lip tumor is excised with a safety margin (Fig. 17.36).

Fan-shaped tissue flap is rotated towards the defect; the mucosal layer has been closed surgically (Fig. 17.37).

Fan-shaped flap is brought to its desired position and the muscular layer sutured (Fig. 17.38).

Immediate before suture removal, the flap demonstrating healthy blood supply. However, the reduced oral stoma and asymmetry are apparent. A second stage surgical correction is necessary (Fig. 17.39).

3. Special Considerations
   (i) During flap preparation, the vertical incision must stop short of the lower lip vermilion. It is essential to preserve blood vessels at the tissue pedicle to ensure flap survival. Intra-operatively and during the closure, care must be taken to prevent over-compression

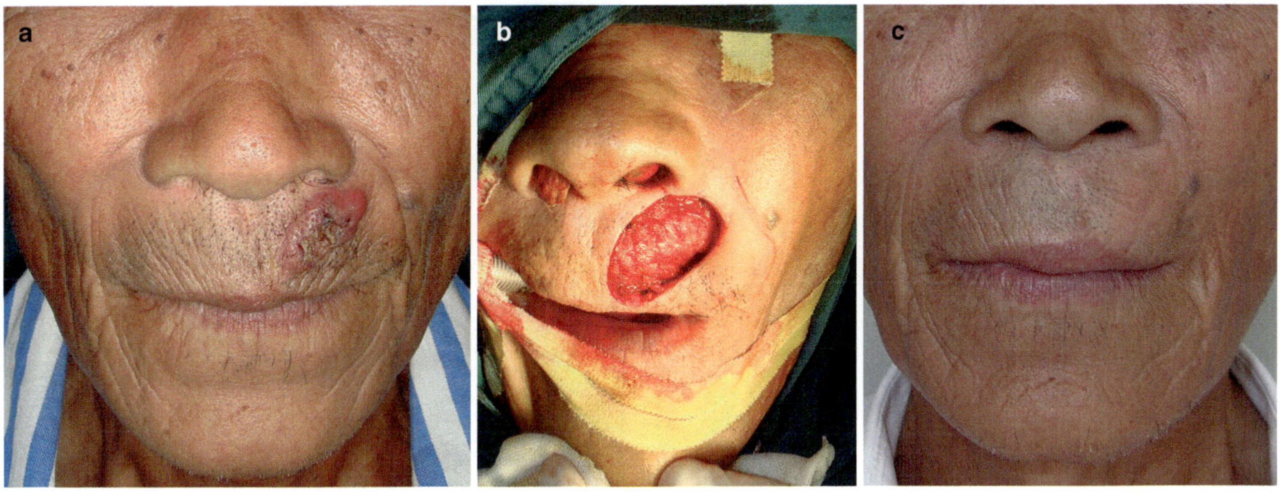

Fig. 17.31 (**a**, **b**, **c**) Left-sided upper lip defect reconstructed with double-pedicled nasolabial groove flap. (**a**) Left-sided upper lip cancer; (**b**) After wide excision; (**c**) 2 years after initial surgery

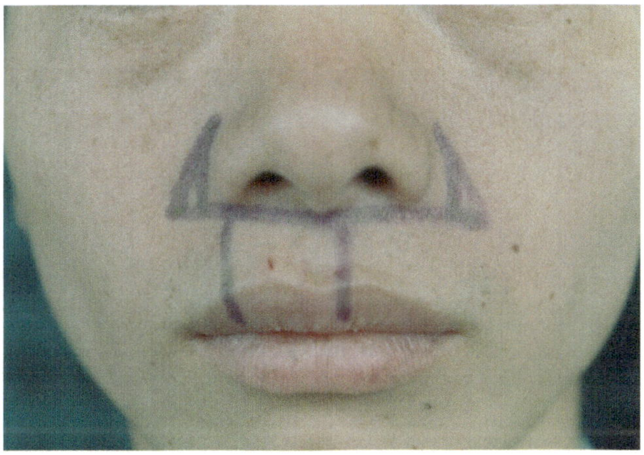

Fig. 17.32 Planned surgical incision

of the pedicle tissue from excessive rotations or surgical manipulations.

(ii) Considering the relatively large resective defect; considerable tissue tension and full thickness incision from the skin through the oral mucosa, stringent layered closure is imperative. Oral mucosa is usually closed first. Muscles should be matched and closed separately.

(iii) Avoid excessive pressure and distortion of flap pedicles. Surgical wounds should be closed with minimal tissue tension as well as to avoid the creation of dead space. If excessive tension is encountered after flap rotation, additional releasing incisions should be considered to reduce the stress on soft tissue. Alternate suture removal should be delayed until post-operative day 10.

(iv) Microstome and rounded commissures are commonly observed after reconstruction. A second stage commissurotomy is usually performed 3–4 weeks after the initial fan-shaped flap reconstruction.

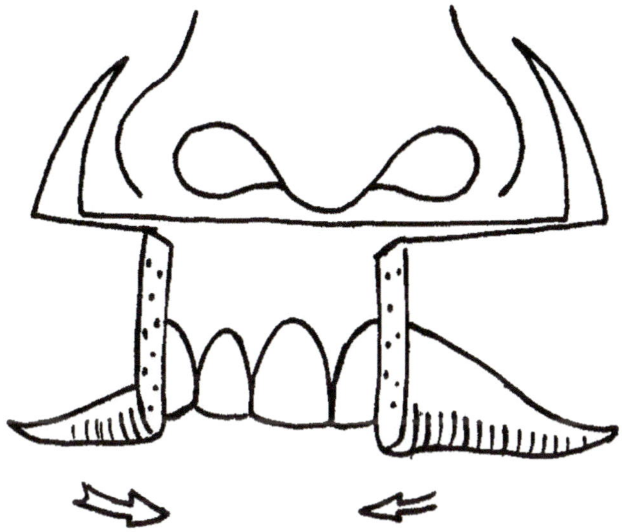

Fig. 17.33 Preparation of bilateral sliding flaps

17.7 Second Stage Repairing of Microstome

1. Indications
   (i) Patients with microstome or asymmetrical oral commissures after fan-shaped tissue reconstruction of upper lip defects.
   (ii) Second stage repair with bilateral commissurotomy should ideally be performed 6 months after initial flap reconstruction and no earlier than 3 weeks post-op.

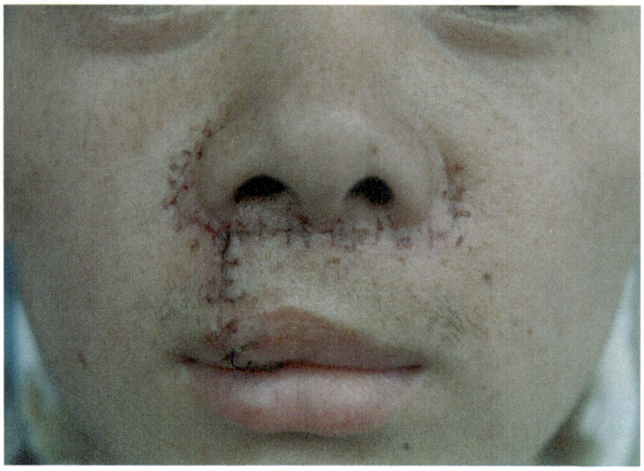

Fig. 17.34 The reconstructed upper lip

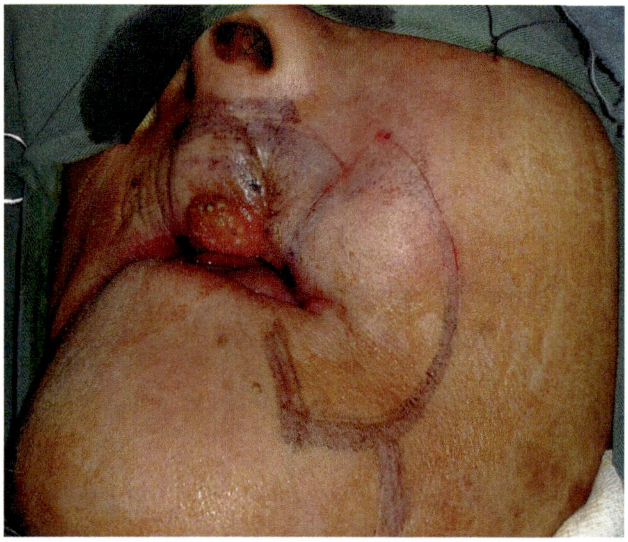

Fig. 17.35 Unilateral fan-shaped sliding flap

2. Surgical Steps

Plan the desired new position of the deformed commissure with reference to the contralateral normal commissure and vermilion, commonly along the vertical line dropped from the ipsilateral pupil. Draw out a triangular area accordingly, of which the skin and part of the subcutaneous tissues are to be removed. The remaining soft tissue through oral mucosa are then incised at the level of the desired oral commissure. The oral mucosa superior and inferior to the incision is rotated outwards and sutured to the respective skin surface to form the new extended commissures. Submucosal dissection might be necessary to reduce tissue tension.

Picture showing patient with microstome and asymmetrical oral commissures after wide excision of left-sided upper lip tumor excision and fan-shaped flap reconstruction (Fig. 17.40).

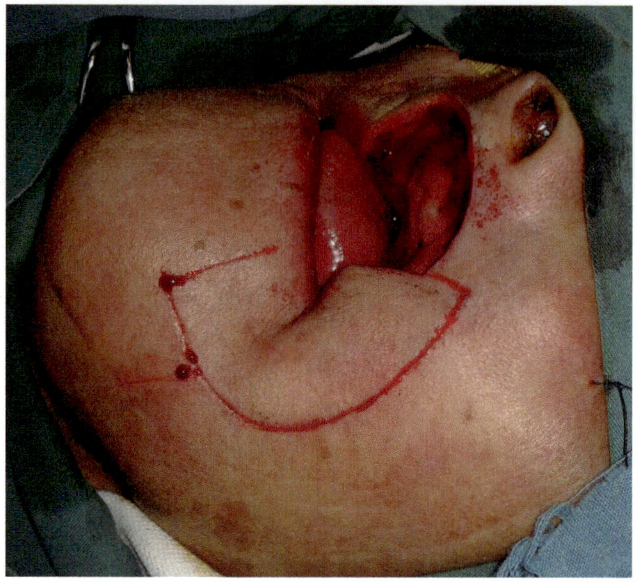

Fig. 17.36 Upper lip tumor excised

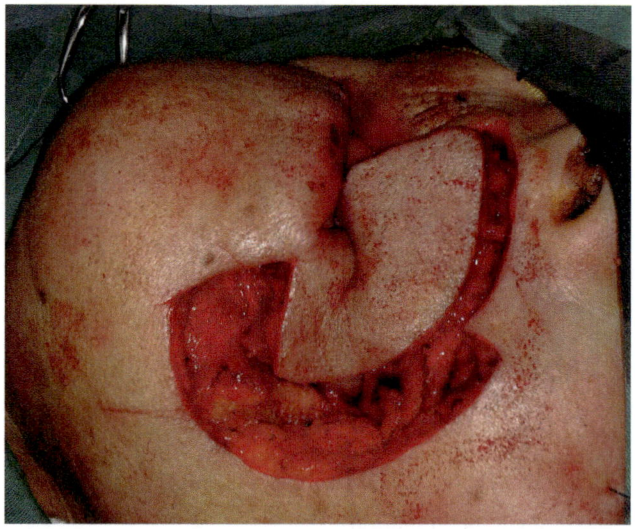

Fig. 17.37 Fan-shaped tissue flap is rotated

Plan the surgical incision with reference to the positions of contralateral commissure and vermilion (Fig. 17.41).

The skin, subcutaneous tissue, and part of the muscles within the triangular area are resected. The mucosal layer is then dissected, trimmed and sutured to the opposing skin surface (Fig. 17.42).

Labial mucosa of the upper lip is trimmed and secured in place with sutures (Fig. 17.43).

Labial mucosa of upper and lower lips are trimmed and secured in place with sutures (Fig. 17.44).

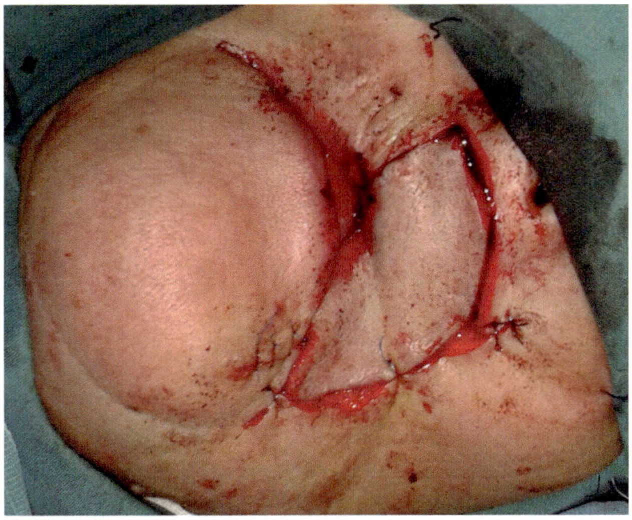

Fig. 17.38 Fan-shaped flap in the desired position

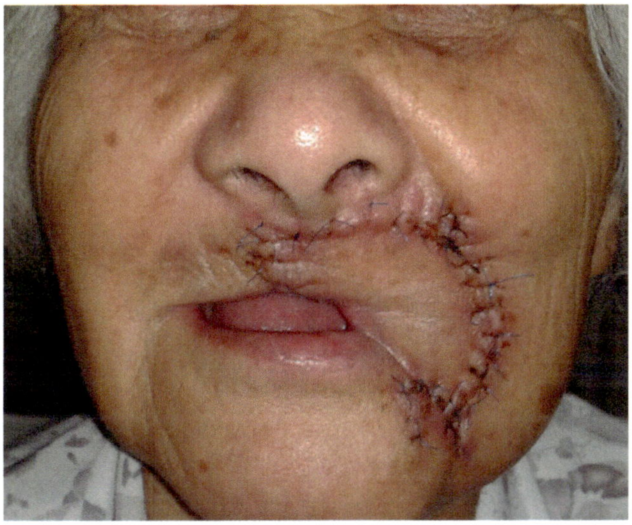

Fig. 17.39 After first stage reconstruction

17.7.1 Classic Case

After left-sided upper lip cancer resection and fan-shaped labial and buccal flap reconstruction, consequent microstome and restricted mouth opening are apparent (Fig. 17.45).

Pre-operative incision design according to the contralateral commissure (Fig. 17.46).

Patient presented at 3 month review since commissurotomy showing satisfactory lip symmetry and function (Fig. 17.47).

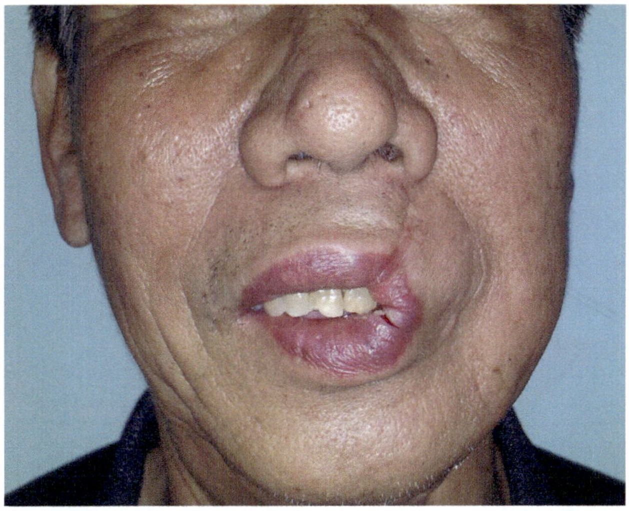

Fig. 17.40 Ten months after fan-shaped flap reconstruction

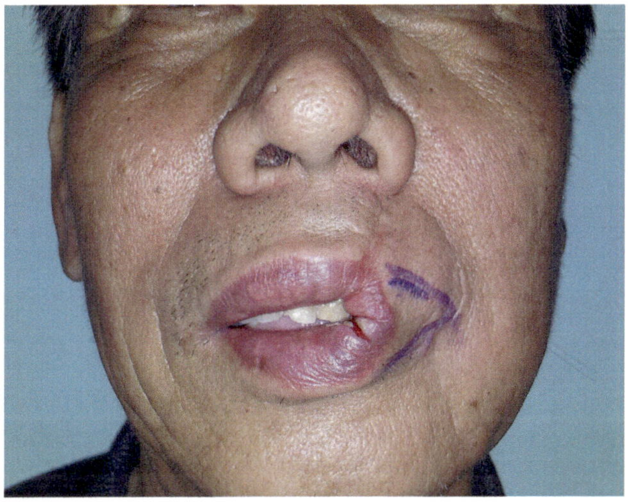

Fig. 17.41 Planned surgical incision

3. Special Considerations
   - (i) Prior to surgery, the desired position of the new commissure and vermilion should be designed accurately to be symmetrical to the normal contralateral side.
   - (ii) Only the skin and part of the subcutaneous tissue within the triangular area are removed, the remaining muscular and mucosal layers are incised horizontally at the level of the oral commissure.
   - (iii) The superior and inferior ends of the cut oral mucosa should be preserved and rotated outwards to form the new vermilion. Ensure natural continu-

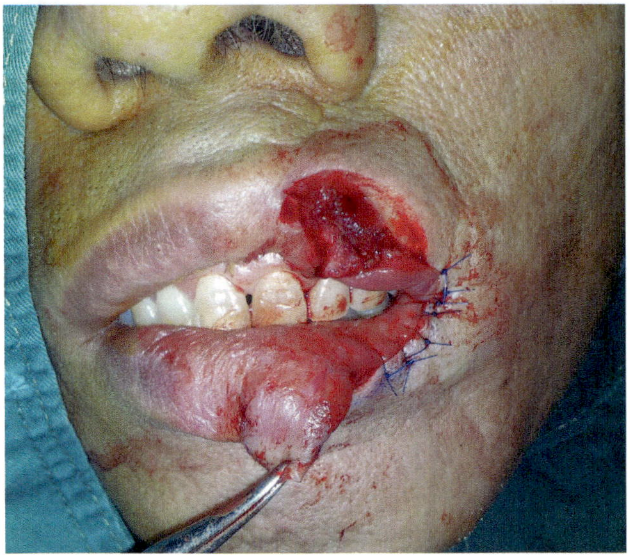

Fig. 17.42 Lower lip vermilion reconstruction

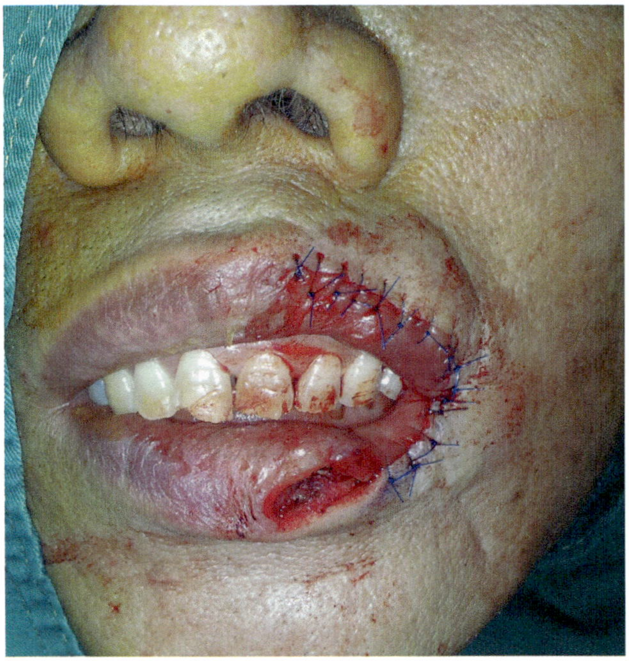

Fig. 17.43 Reconstructed upper lip vermilion

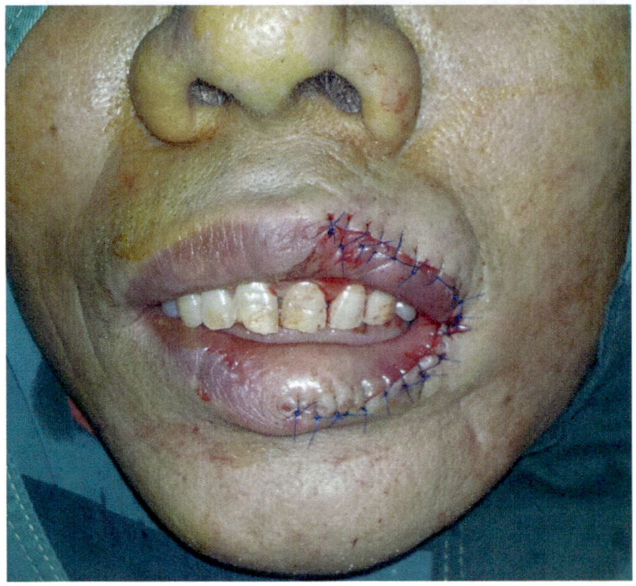

Fig. 17.44 Labial mucosa of both lips are secured in place

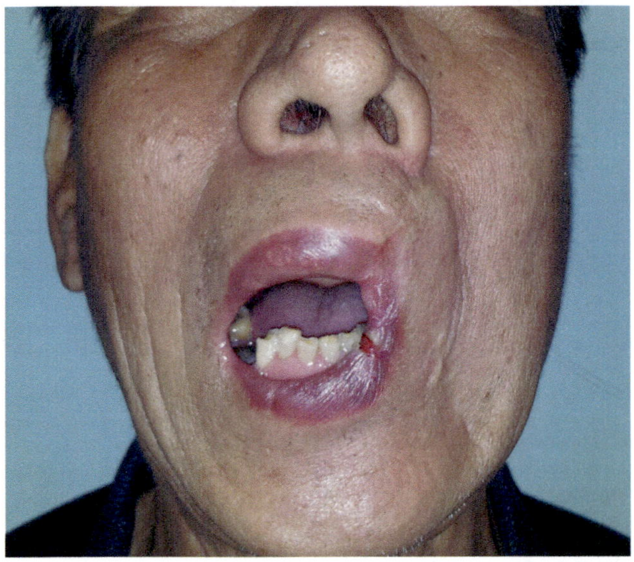

Fig. 17.45 After fan-shaped flap reconstruction

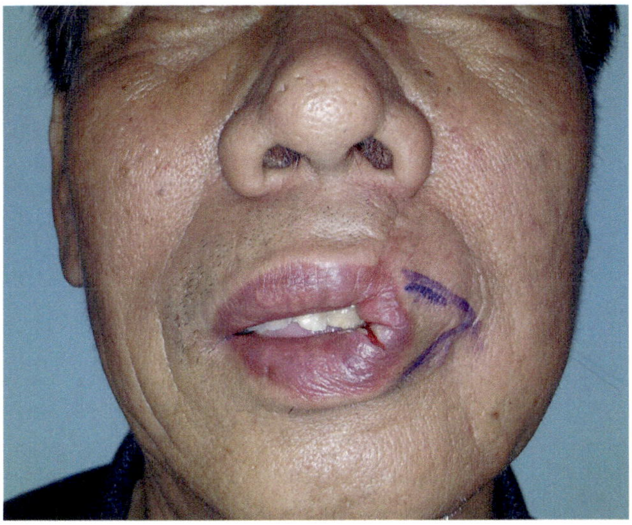

Fig. 17.46 Planned surgical incisions

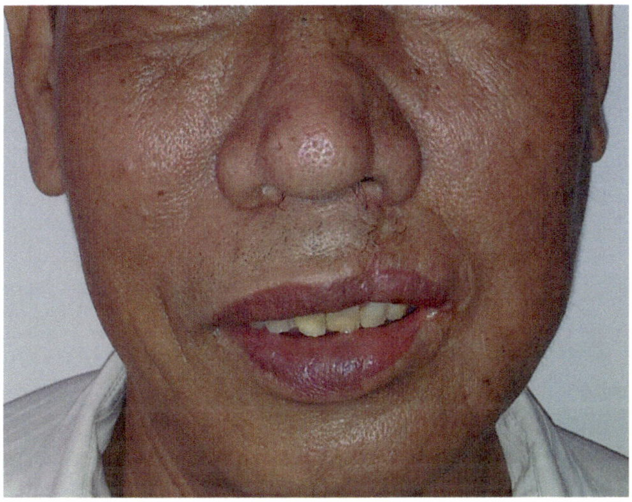

Fig. 17.47 After commissurotomy

ation and symmetry with the native labial vermilion border.

References

1. Yu-Zhe Q, Wen-Guang Z, Shu-Jie S. 120 Cases of reconstructing of lip defects (in Chinese). Beijing Oral Med J. 2001;9(2):88–9.
2. Campbell JP. Surgical management of lip carcinoma. J Oral Maxillofac Surg. 1998;56:955–61.
3. Lu M, Jian-Hua L. Four cases of labial and buccal sliding flap repairing lager upper lip defects (in Chinese). J Clin Oral Med. 2007;23(11):682–3.
4. Bao T-W, Wang R, Xu H, Jian-Hua L. Double pedicled naso-labial groove myocutaneous flap for upper lip defect: with 2 cases report (in Chinese). Chin J Reparat Reconst Surg. 2009;23(6):746–7.

Reconstruction of Irregular Lip Defects

18

Xu Huang and Jianhua Liu

18.1 Repairing After Broad Nasolabial Tumor Resection

1. Indications

   Benign tumors of lip or nasolabial region, such as neurofibromatosis; patients who responded poorly to laser, medication and steroid therapies.
2. Surgical Steps

For irregular lip defects, the pre-surgical flap design is relatively flexible, usually customized to each individual patient. During resection, normal skin, muscle and mucosa should be preserved as much as possible. Tissues at bilateral nasolabial grooves are frequently used during the design of sliding or rotational flaps. When the lesion is relatively extensive, the contralateral nasolabial tissues may need to be used as well to maintain soft tissue midline and facial asymmetry after reconstruction [1].

We present a case of generalized neurofibromatosis of the nasolabial region, which was severely disfiguring. The patient required tumor reduction and cosmetic reconstruction improve facial aesthetics. Simple resection with local advancement flaps would result in severe facial asymmetry and deformity.

Method:

(i) Plan for the bilateral nasolabial groove tissues to be removed surgically and ensure symmetrical upper lip height post-operatively.

(ii) Additional incisions are planned at the nasal base to facility smooth advancement of the upper lip tissue flap. Columella and bilateral nares should be largely symmetrical post-operatively.

(iii) During tumor resection, preserve normal tissues including skin, muscle, and mucosa as much as possible.

(iv) Close the mucosa, muscle, and skin in layers tension-freely.

18.1.1 Case Presentation

Frontal view of the planned incisions for broad nasolabial neurofibromatosis (Fig. 18.1).

Right profile view of the planned incisions for broad nasolabial neurofibromatosis (Fig. 18.2).

Left profile view of the planned incisions for broad nasolabial neurofibromatosis (Fig. 18.3).

The arrows demonstrating the moving direction of bilateral advancement flaps (Fig. 18.4).

Frontal view—the mucosal layer is closed first, followed by muscles and then skin (Fig. 18.5).

Right profile view—the mucosal layer is closed first, followed by muscles and then skin (Fig. 18.6).

Left profile view—the mucosal layer is closed first, followed by muscles and then skin (Fig. 18.7).

18.1.2 Classic Case (Fig. 18.8)

3. Special Considerations

   (i) During pre-surgical planning, the size and extent of post-resective tissue defect should be estimated, and the advancement of remaining nasolabial tissues planned accordingly.

X. Huang
Department of Stomatology, Fourth Affiliated Hospital, Zhejiang University School of Medicine, Yiwu, China

J. Liu (✉)
Department of Oral and Maxillo-facial Surgery, First Affiliated Hospital, Zhejiang University School of Medicine, Hangzhou, China

J. Liu, B. Shi (eds.), *Atlas of Lip and Nose Plastic and Cosmetic Surgery*, https://doi.org/10.1007/978-981-16-1911-3_18

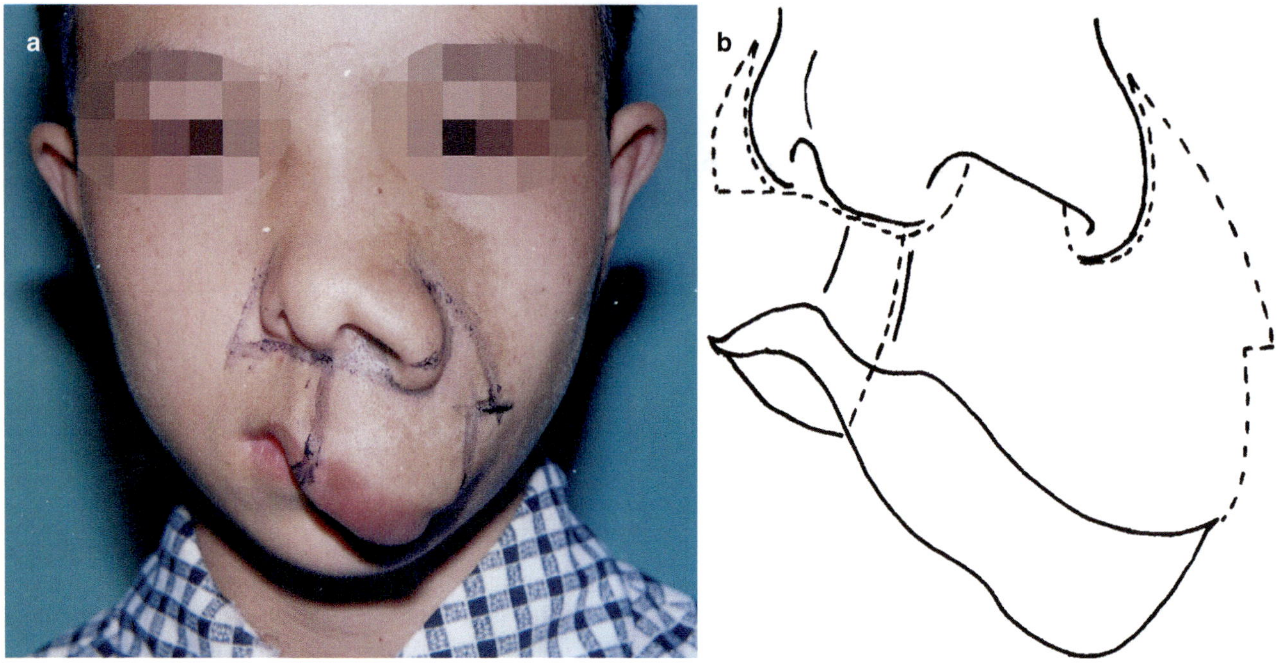

Fig. 18.1 (**a**, **b**) Planned incisions—frontal view

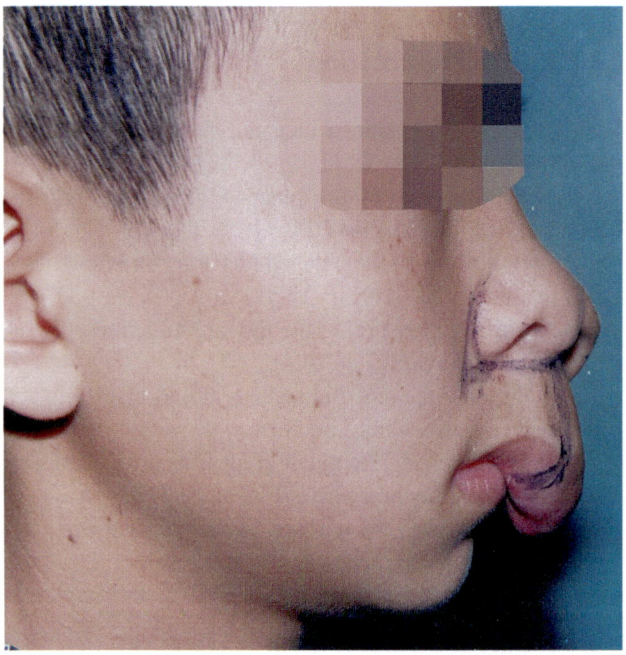

Fig. 18.2 Planned incisions—right profile view

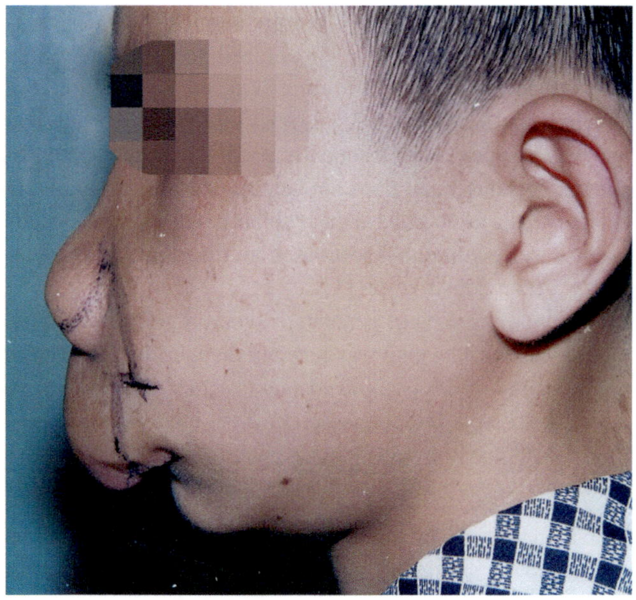

Fig. 18.3 Planned incisions—left profile view

(ii) The bases of additional triangular resective areas at bilateral nasolabial grooves should parallel the alar base.

(iii) Design linear incisions on both sides of the lesion to be removed; ensure the incisions are of similar lengths and approximates the height of the healthy contralateral upper lip.

(iv) Ensure symmetry of bilateral nares post-op.

(v) Anticipate considerable intra-operative bleeding could be encountered during partial tumor resections; standby for blood transfusion if necessary.

18.2 Reconstruction of Irregular Upper Lip Defects After Tumor Resection

1. Indications
   (i) Irregular upper lip defects after tumor resection.
   (ii) Full thickness defects involving skin, muscle, and mucosa.
   (iii) For first stage reconstruction after resection of malignant upper lip tumor, all frozen section margins must be negative.
2. Surgical Steps

   This method is suited for irregular upper lip defects close to oral commissures. For tumors occurring in this area, resections commonly leave a rectangular-shaped defect. A triangular flap is prepared beneath the defect about one and half its size. Care must be taken to preserve the inferior labial artery.
   (i) Surgical plan: excise the tumor with a safety margin leaving a rectangular defect; prepare a triangular tissue flap beneath the defect.
   (ii) Depending on the extent of the tumor, the superior resective margin can be carried to the nasal base, and the inferior margin parallel the commissures.
   (iii) Design the flap as a reversed triangle with the inferior border of the rectangular defect as its base, extending to the ipsilateral commissure or slightly into the labial mucosa.
   (iv) Rotat0e the tissue flap about 180 degrees towards the defect.
   (v) Secure the flap accordingly. The new lower lip defect formed by the triangular flap can be easily closed primarily [2].

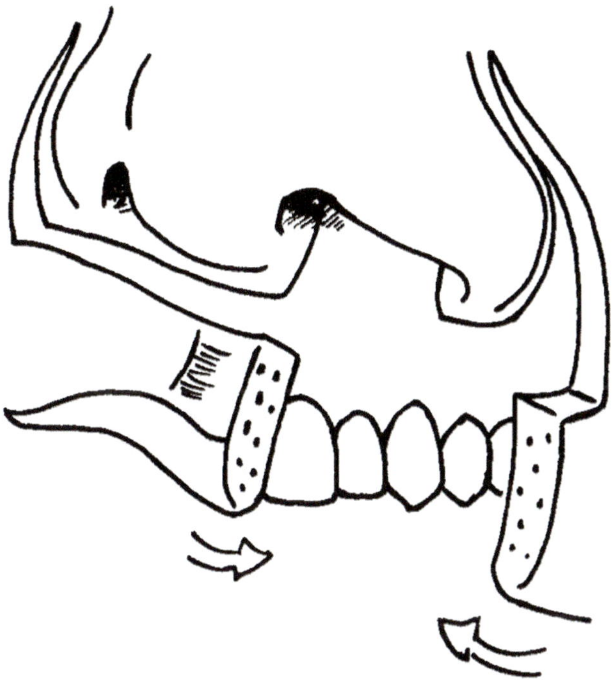

Fig. 18.4 Tumor resection and additional incisions made

18.2.1 Case Presentation

Picture illustrating the size and position of the upper lip carcinoma (Fig. 18.9).

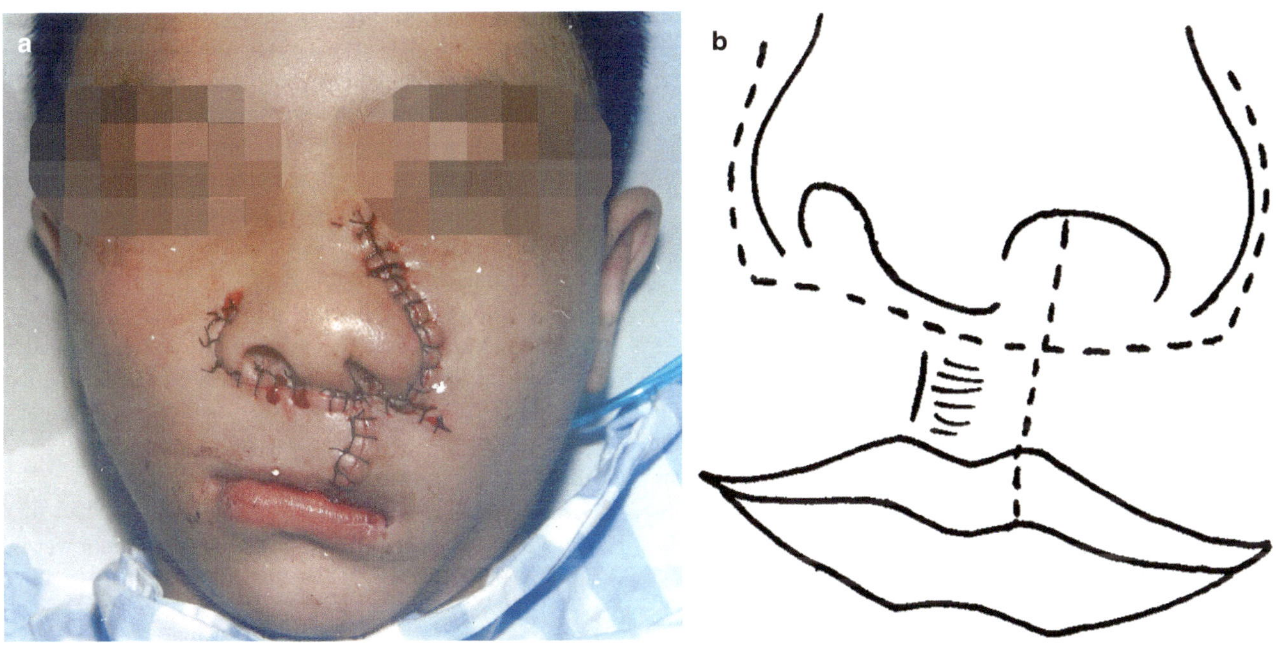

Fig. 18.5 (**a**, **b**) Completed tumor resection and reconstruction with local advancement flap—frontal view

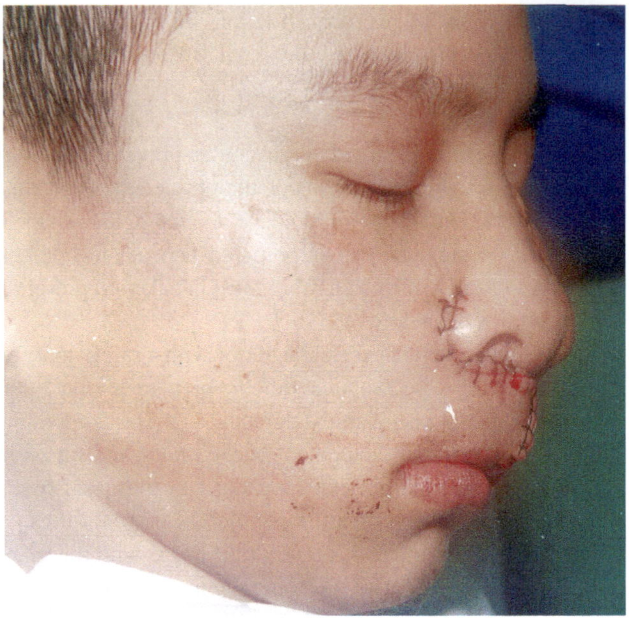

Fig. 18.6 Completed tumor resection and reconstruction with local advancement flap—right profile view

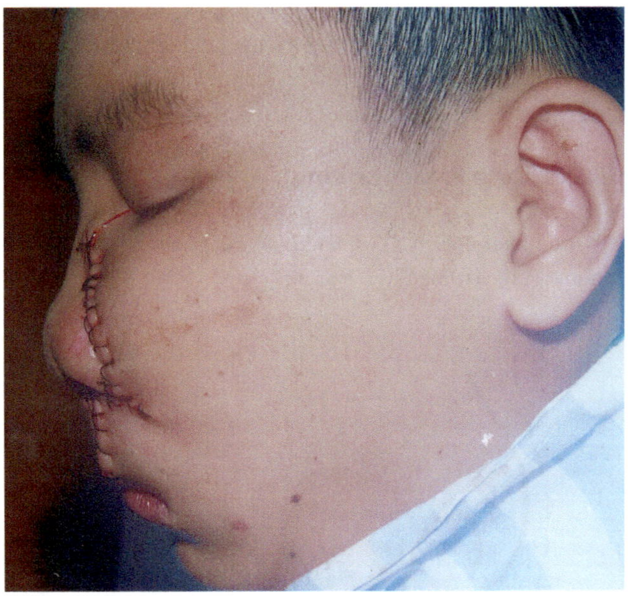

Fig. 18.7 Completed tumor resection and reconstruction with local advancement flap—left profile view

Planned incisions for tumor resection and rotational flap (straight arrow indicates the position of the vascular pedicle; the curved arrow indicates direction of flap rotation) (Figs. 18.10 and 18.11).

All incisions were closed primarily and healing well. Resultant upper lip aesthetics were satisfactory (Fig. 18.12).

18.2.2 Classic Case (Fig. 18.13)

3. Special Considerations
   (i) Ensure complete resection of tumor with adequate margins. Plan the lower lip rotational flap based on the width of the expected upper lip defect. It is advisable to obtain a flap one and half the width of the defect for a harmonious width ratio of the upper and lower lips after reconstruction.
   (ii) When preparing the lower lip flap, the mesial vertical incision should stop short of the vermilion. Blunt dissection should be carried out at the vermillion border to locate and preserve the inferior labial artery; a cuff of muscle should be attached preferably for better protection. Good vascular supply at the pedicle is crucial for flap survival.
   (iii) Patients with resultant asymmetrical commissures after reconstruction would require second-stage surgical corrections.

18.3 Reconstruction of Total Lower Lip Vermilion Defect with Tongue Flap

1. Indications
   (i) Extensive pathology involving lower lip mucosa but sparing the muscle and skin.
   (ii) Defects involving mucosal layer sparing muscle and skin.
   (iii) Normal tongue and lingual mucosa.
2. Surgical Steps

   For defects after resection of extensive pathology involving lower lip mucosa, reconstruction using tissue flap from the dorsal surface of the tongue can achieve satisfactory functional and aesthetic results [3].
   (i) Resect the lower lip mucosal lesion.
   (ii) Based on the extent of the defect, a curvilinear incision of similar length is made on the dorsal surface of the anterior one-third of the tongue. The mucosal layer is incised and dissected free from the underlying muscle to form the flap.
   (iii) The tongue flap is sutured to the lower lip defect.
   (iv) Three weeks later, the pedicle is divided and sutured to the lip. The resultant tongue defect is closed primarily.

18.3.1 Case Presentation 1:

Extensive lesion involving but limited to the entire lower lip vermilion (Fig. 18.14).

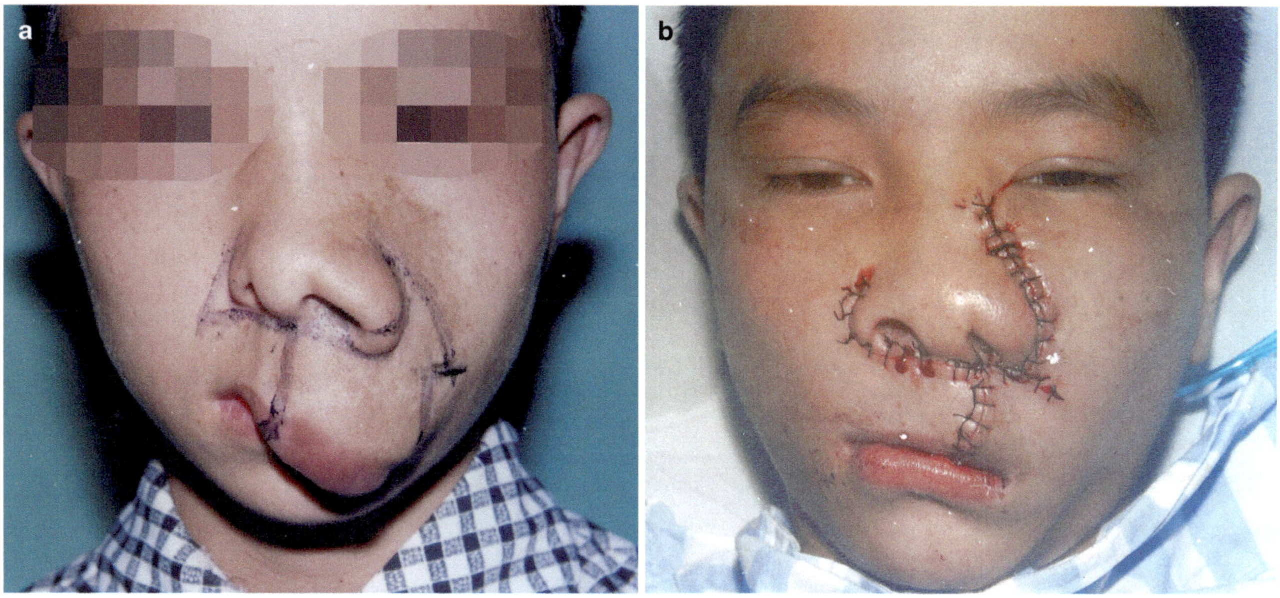

Fig. 18.8 (**a**, **b**) Pre- and post-op appearances. (**a**) Pre-surgical planned incisions for broad nasolabial neurofibromatosis resection. Part of the left nasal base should be resected to correct the enlarged alar. (**b**) After tumor resection and flap reconstruction, the upper lip form was significantly improved, and the left alar reduced

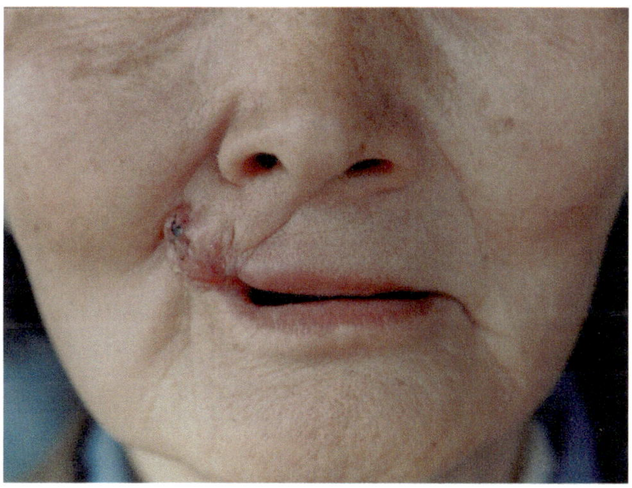

Fig. 18.9 Pre-operative photo of a right-sided upper lip acinic cell carcinoma

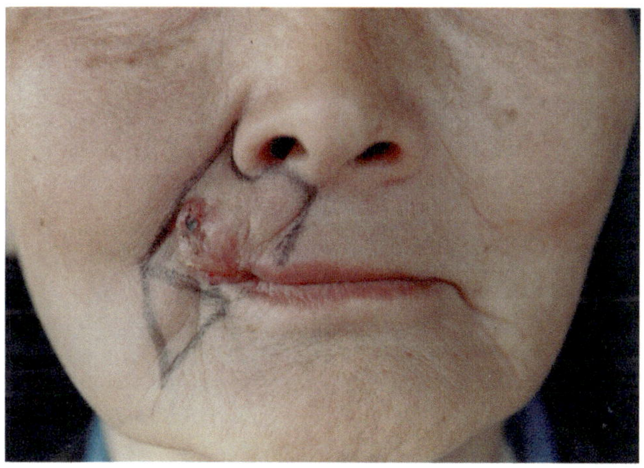

Fig. 18.10 Planned surgical incisions

Tumor resection leaving a total vermilion defect; note that the shallow tumor infiltration (Fig. 18.15).

Based on the extent of the defect, plan for a tongue flap with a curvilinear incision of similar length on the dorsal surface of the tongue (Fig. 18.16).

The desired tongue flap is raised, exposing the underlying muscular layer (Fig. 18.17).

Suture the dorsal mucosa of the tongue flap to the labial mucosa of the lip defect first, then proceed to secure the flap to the skin of the lower lip (Fig. 18.18).

Three weeks post-op, the pedicled tongue flap is healing well with good form (Fig. 18.19).

The flap is divided from its pedicle 3 weeks after the initial surgery. Tongue mobility is satisfactory (Fig. 18.20).

Post-op the tongue mobility remained satisfactory, and the lower lip vermillion well healed (Fig. 18.21).

18.3.2 Case Presentation 2:

Malignant transformation of the lower lip of a patient with systemic lupus erythematosus (SLE) (Fig. 18.22).

Resection is planned, including a 3 mm margin involving part of the skin (Fig. 18.23).

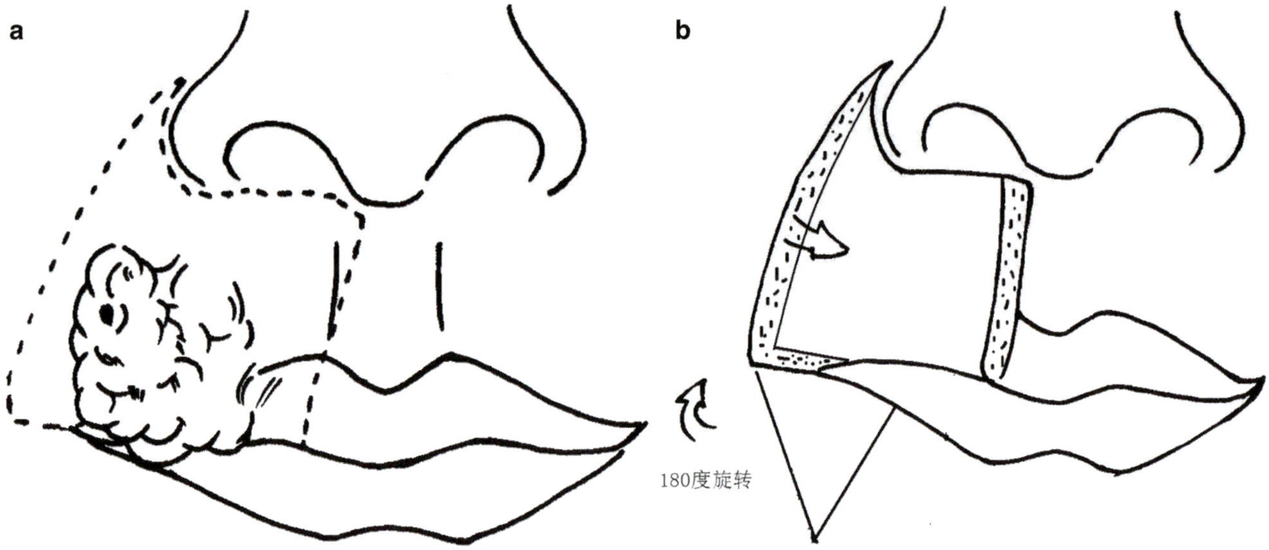

Fig. 18.11 (**a**, **b**) Illustration showing tumor resection and flap rotation. (**a**) Illustration of planned tumor resection. (**b**) Illustration of post-resection defect and planned rotational flap.

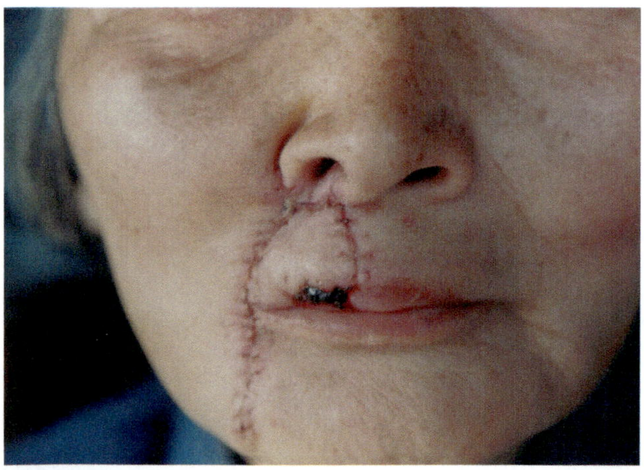

Fig. 18.12 Two-week post-op

A total vermilion defect was formed after tumor resection, and the tongue flap was designed accordingly (Fig. 18.24).

The tongue flap was matched and secured to the lower lip to form the new vermilion (Fig. 18.25).

Threeweeks post-op, the pedicled tongue flap is healing well with good form and color (Fig. 18.26).

The flap is divided from its pedicle 3 weeks after the initial surgery (Fig. 18.27).

After the division of the pedicle, the tongue defect and vermilion are closed primarily (Fig. 18.28).

At 1-month post-op the tongue mobility remained satisfactory and lower lip vermillion well healed (Fig. 18.29).

18.3.3 Classic Case 1

Extensive disease involving the lower lip mucosa with local malignant transformation (Figs. 18.30 and 18.31).

At post-op review the tongue mobility remained satisfactory, and lower lip vermillion well healed.

18.3.4 Classic Case 2

Malignant transformation of the lower lip of a patient with systemic lupus erythematosus (SLE) (Figs. 18.32 and 18.33).

Patient received total vermilionectomy and reconstruction with tongue flap. 1 month after flap division, tongue mobility remained satisfactory, and lower lip vermillion well healed.

3. Special Considerations
   (i) This method is indicated for simple but extensive vermillion lesion of the lower lip, preferably benign. Application to malignant cases should be considered with caution. The dorsal mucosa of the tongue must be histologically proven to be healthy and free from tumor involvement.
   (ii) During the 3 weeks prior to flap division, the tongue is pulled forward and secured to the lower lip. Patient must be informed of and mentally prepared for the expected difficulty during feeding and speech.
   (iii) The inherent difference in color between dorsal mucosa of tongue and native lower lip vermilion must be recognized.

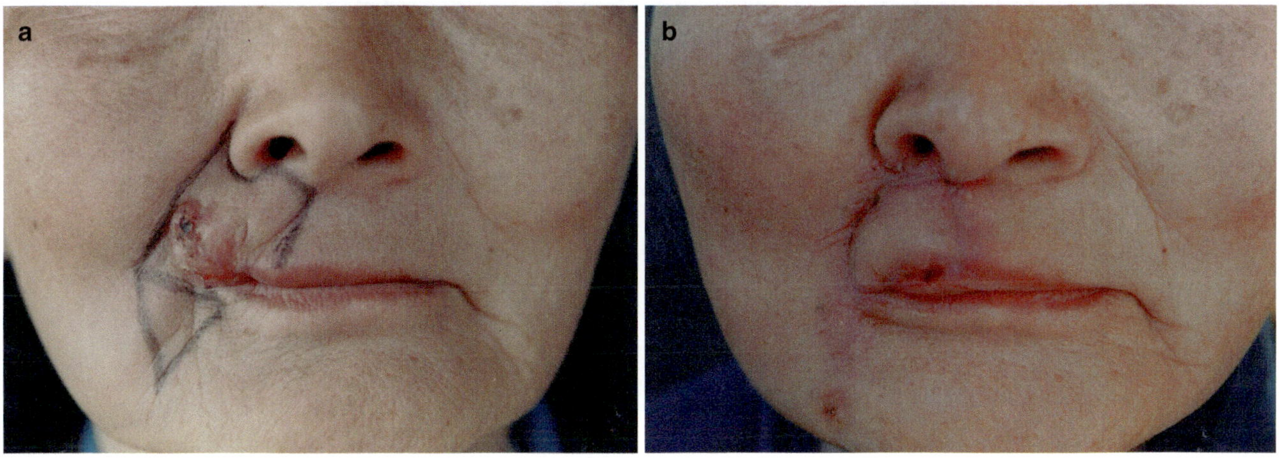

Fig. 18.13 (**a**, **b**) Pre- and post-op photos of resection and reconstruction of a right-sided acinic cell carcinoma of upper lip. (a) Pre-surgical plan of resection and rotational flap. The lower lip flap is rotated clockwise into the upper lip defect. (b) 1-month review.

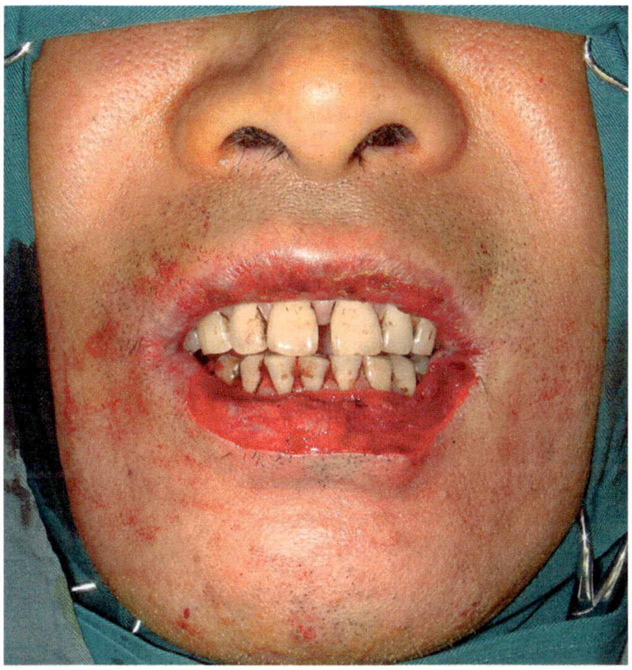

Fig. 18.15 After tumor resection

(iv) After flap preparation, match the base of the tongue flap to the inferior border of the lower lip defect first and secure with sutures. The external edges should be closed last to form the future vermilion border of the lower lip.

18.4 Reconstruction of Unilateral Upper and Lower Lip Vermilion Defect with Tongue Flap

Jianhua Liu and Hui-yong Zhu

1. Indications

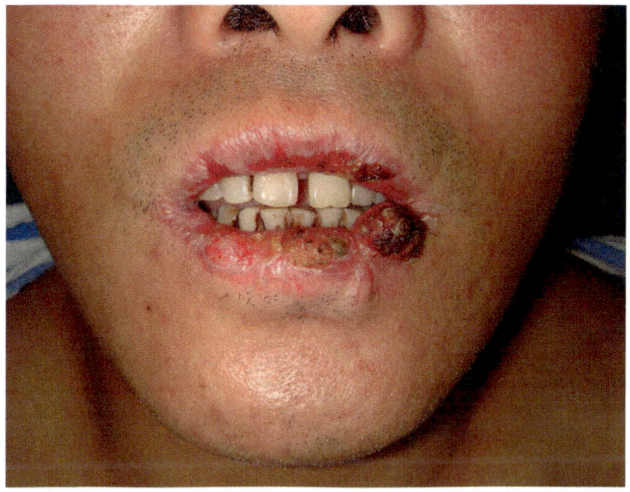

Fig. 18.14 Well-differentiated SCC of the lower lip

Lesions involving unilateral oral commissure and both upper and lower lip vermilions where part of the skin and muscles are spared.

2. Surgical Steps

For lesions involving unilateral oral commissure and both upper and lower lip vermilions, the post-resective defects can be repaired with tongue flaps similarly to vermilions with satisfying results.

(i) Resect the lower lip mucosal lesion.
(ii) Based on the extent of the defect, a curvilinear incision of similar length is made on the dorsal surface of the anterior one-third of tongue. The mucosal layer is incised and dissected free from the underlying muscle to form the flap.
(iii) The tongue flap is sutured to the upper and lower lip defect.
(iv) Three weeks later, the pedicle is divided and sutured to the lip. The resultant tongue defect is closed primarily.

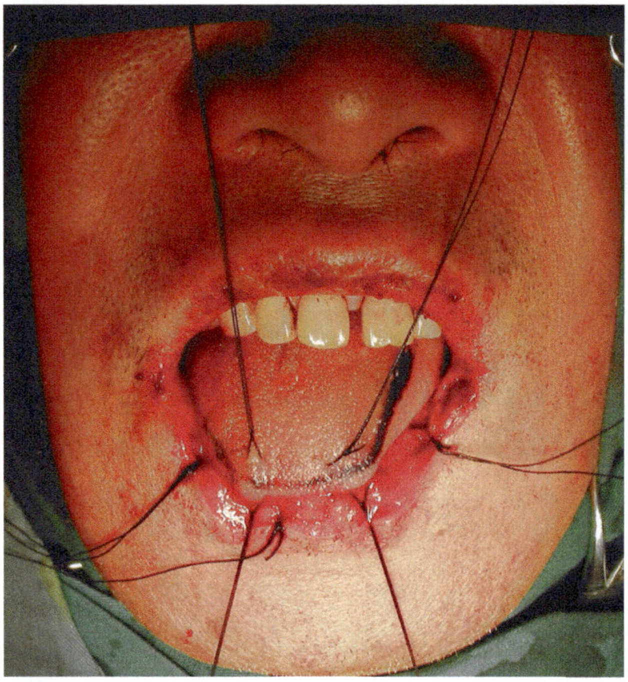

Fig. 18.16 Tongue flap design

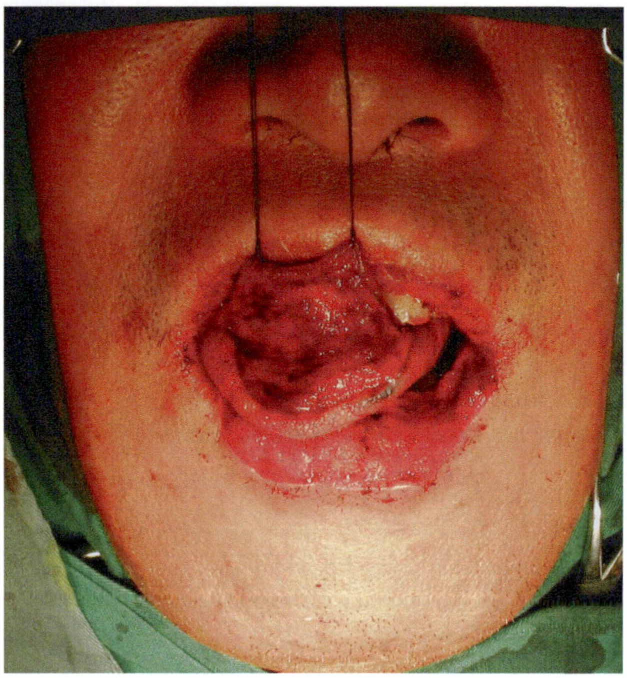

Fig. 18.17 The desired tongue flap is raised

18.4.1 Case Presentation

Lower lip SCC involving left oral commissure and part of upper lip vermilion tissue. A frontal view of the surgical incisions (Fig. 18.34).

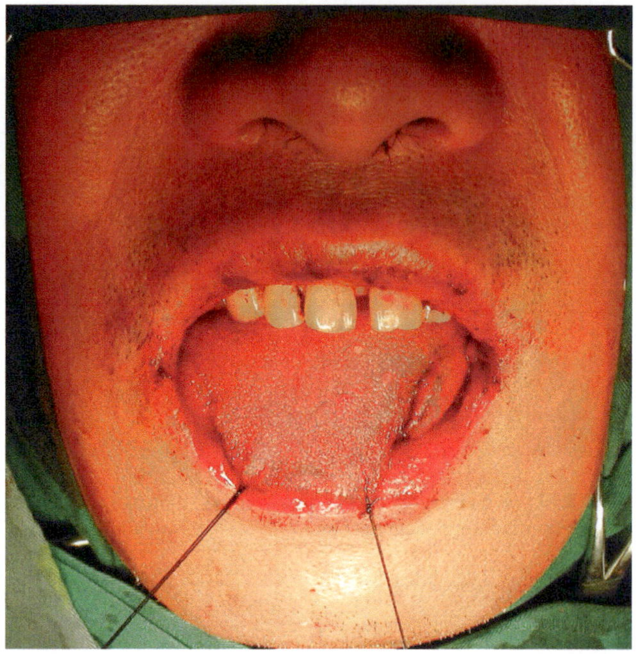

Fig. 18.18 The tongue flap is sutured to the lower lip defect

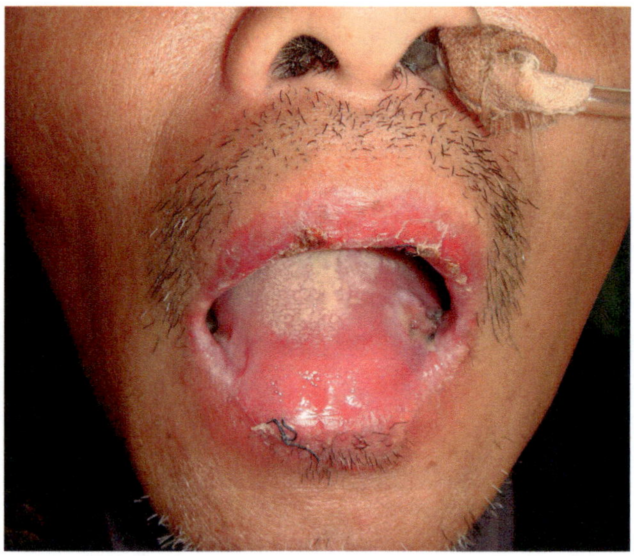

Fig. 18.19 The healing tongue flap before the division of the pedicle

Lower lip SCC involving left oral commissure and part of upper lip vermilion tissue. A side view of the surgical incisions (Fig. 18.35).

The resultant tissue defect after tumor resection (Fig. 18.36).

The tongue flap is designed and prepared according to the length and configuration of the tissue defect (Fig. 18.37).

The incisions on ventral surfaces of the tongue are sutured to the corresponding labial mucosa margin of defect. The

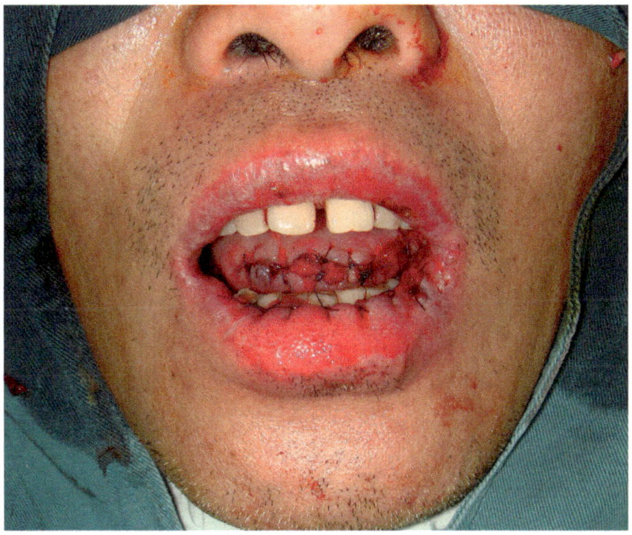

Fig. 18.20 The flap is divided from its pedicle

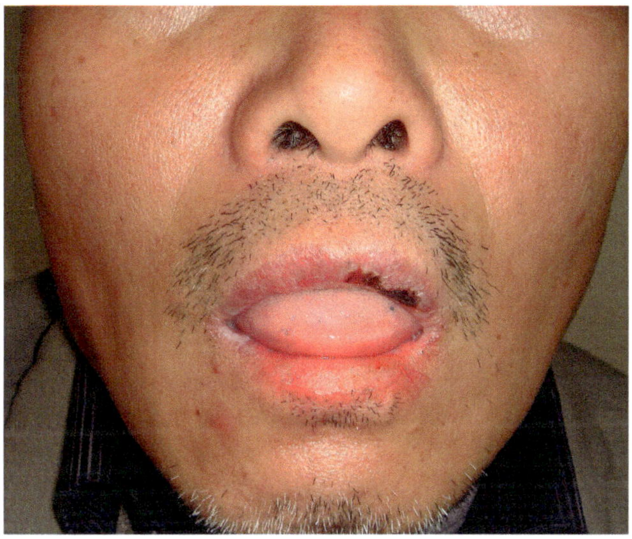

Fig. 18.21 At post-op review

dorsal margin of the tongue flap is fitted to form the new vermilion margin (Fig. 18.38).

The tongue flap is sutured to the skin (Fig. 18.39).

The pedicled flap is healing well at 3 weeks after initial reconstruction (Fig. 18.40).

The pedicle is divided after 3 weeks. Wound edges are approximated and sutured accordingly (Fig. 18.41).

18.4.2 Classic Case

Lower lip SCC involving left oral commissure and part of upper lip vermilion tissue. A frontal view of the surgical incisions (Figs. 18.42 and 18.43).

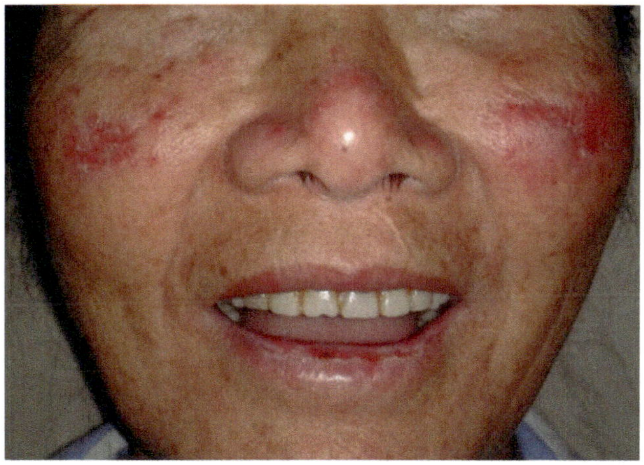

Fig. 18.22 Pre-operative picture of lower lip lesion

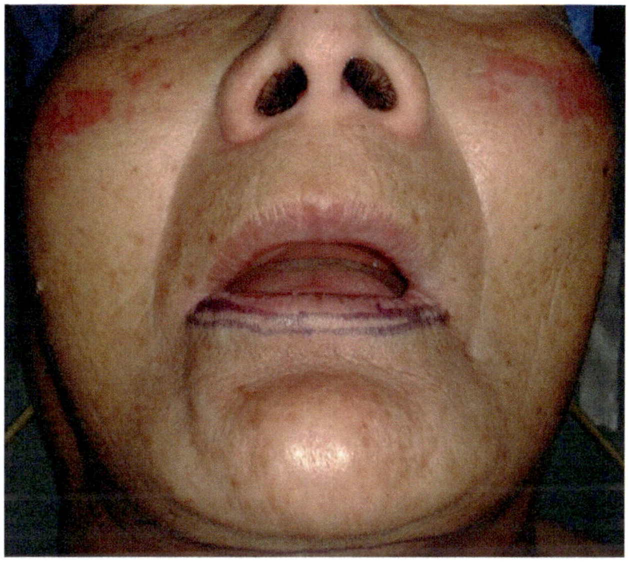

Fig. 18.23 Planned resection

At 2-month after flap division, the flap is well healed. Tongue mobility and lower lip aesthetics remained satisfactory. The excess vermilion tissue can be removed during a second surgery.

3. Special Considerations
   (i) This method is indicated for simple lower lip lesions, preferably benign. Application to malignant cases should be considered with caution. The dorsal mucosa of the tongue must be histologically proven to be healthy and free from tumor involvement.
   (ii) During the 3 weeks prior to flap division, the tongue is pulled forward and secured to the lower lip. Patient must be informed of and mentally prepared for the expected difficulty during feeding and speech.

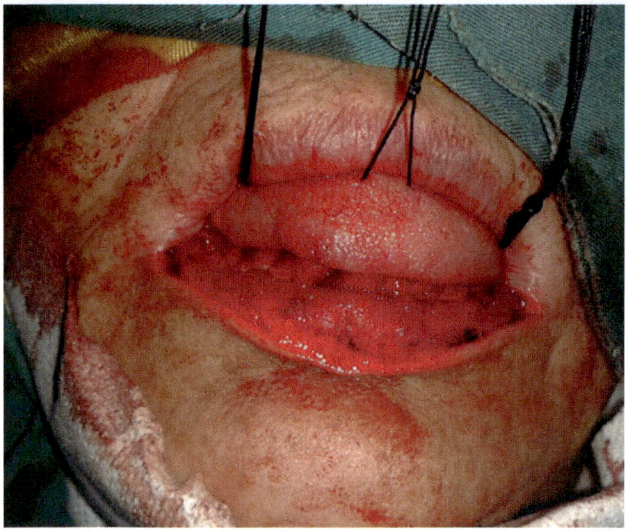

Fig. 18.24 Complete resection of the tumor with lower lip vermilion and preparation of the tongue flap

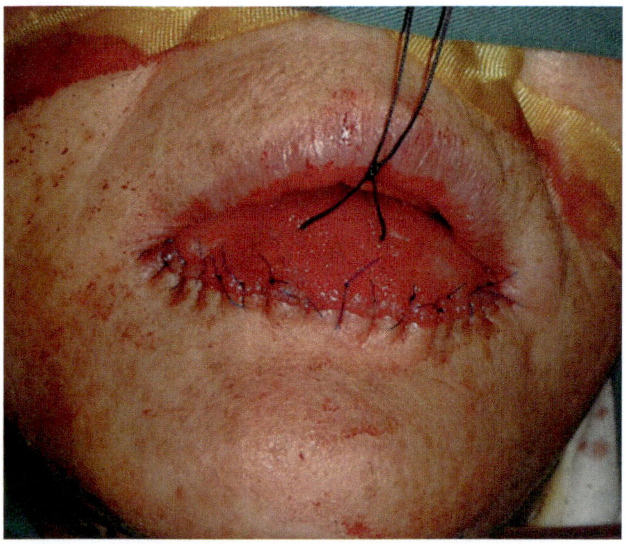

Fig. 18.25 Tongue flap secured to the lower lip defect

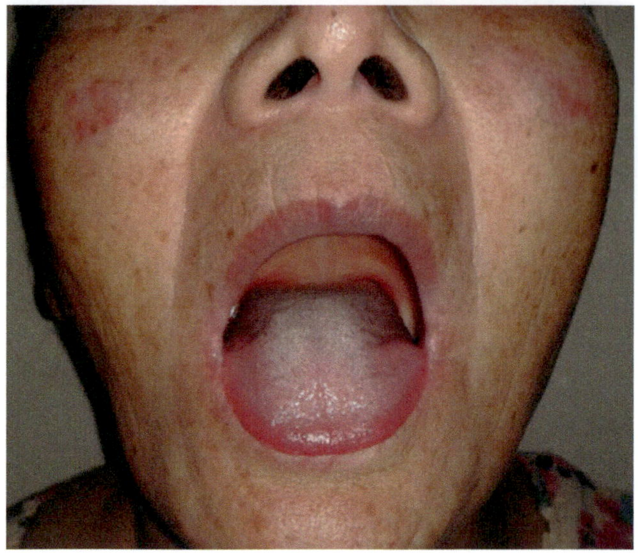

Fig. 18.26 Before dividing the pedicle

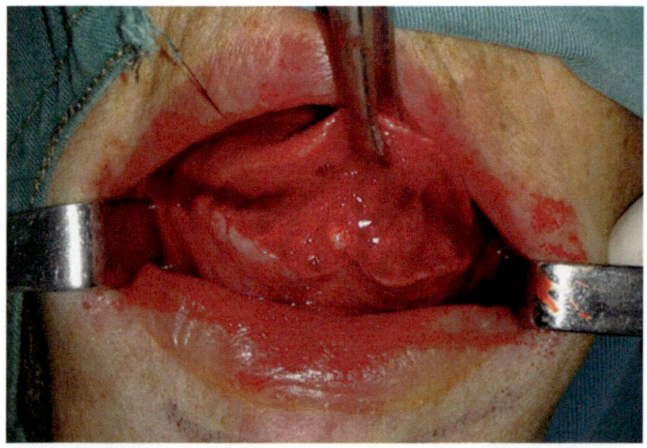

Fig. 18.27 The flap is divided from its pedicle

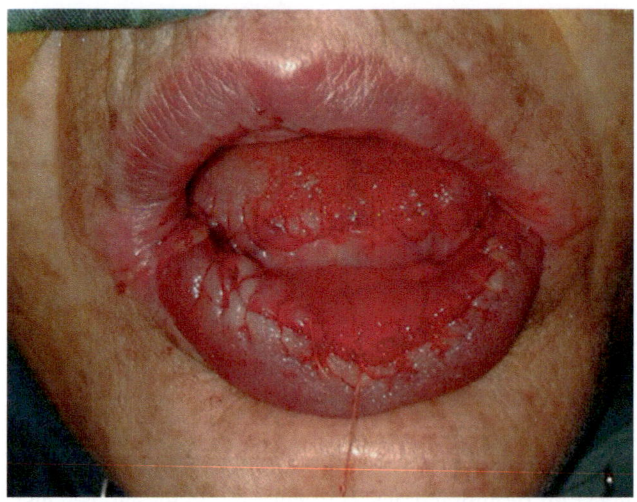

Fig. 18.28 Tongue flap divided and closed primarily

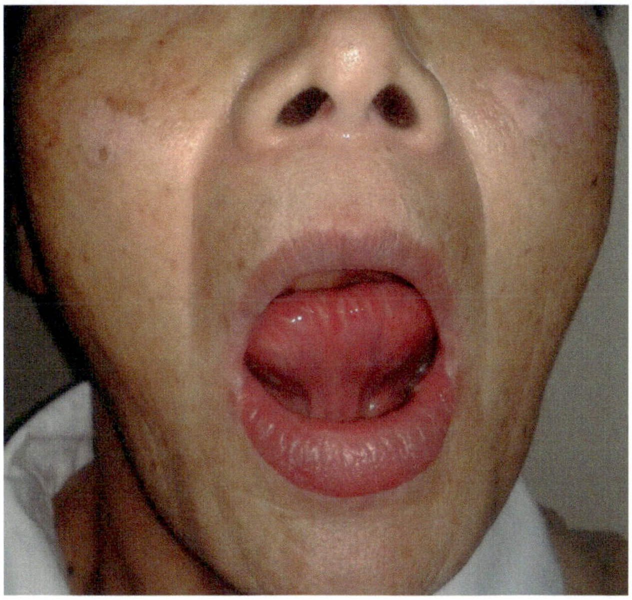

Fig. 18.29 At post-op review

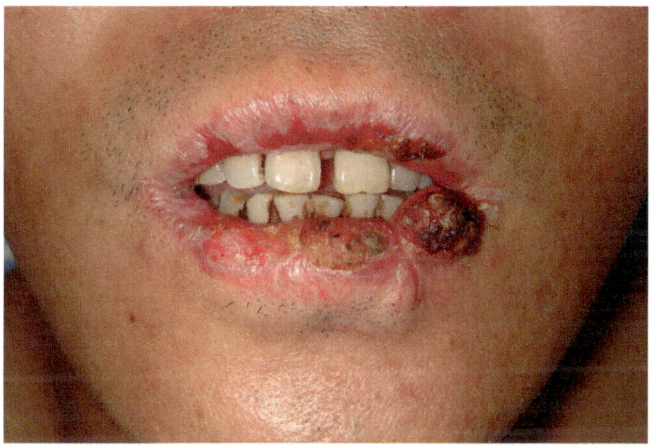

Fig. 18.30 Well-differentiated lower lip SCC

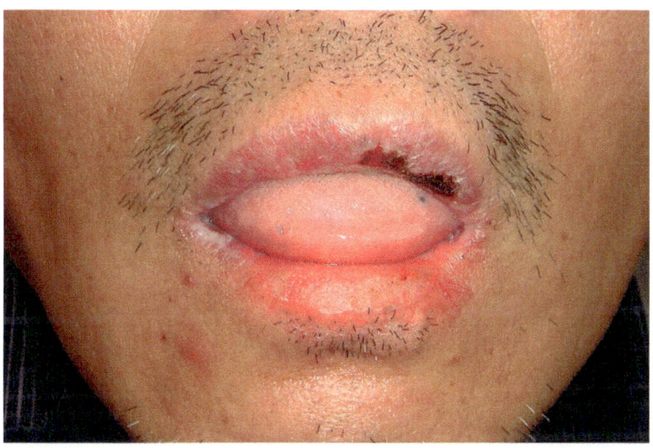

Fig. 18.31 At post-op review

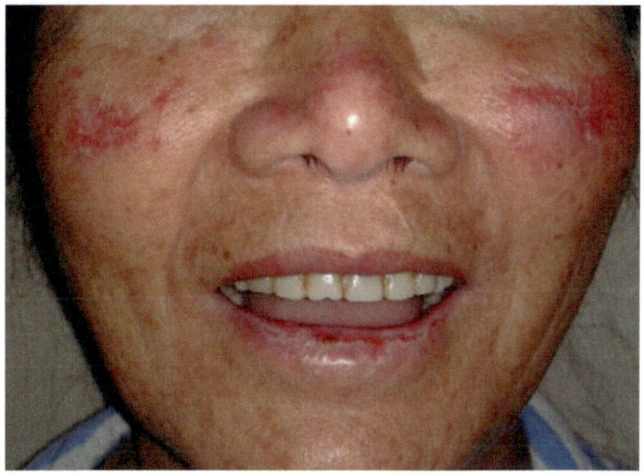

Fig. 18.32 Pre-operative picture of lower lip lesion

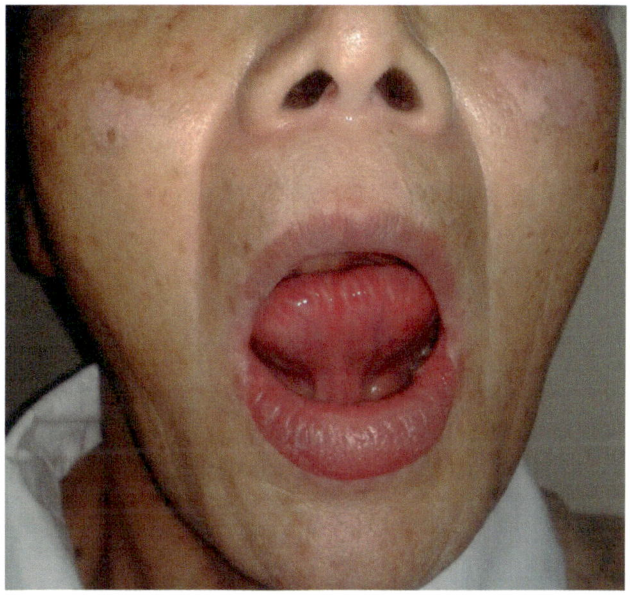

Fig. 18.33 At 1-month post-op

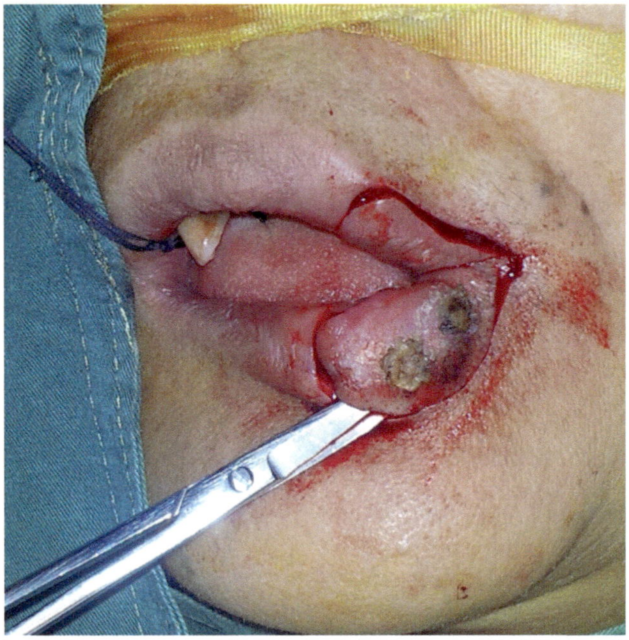

Fig. 18.34 Surgical incisions—frontal view

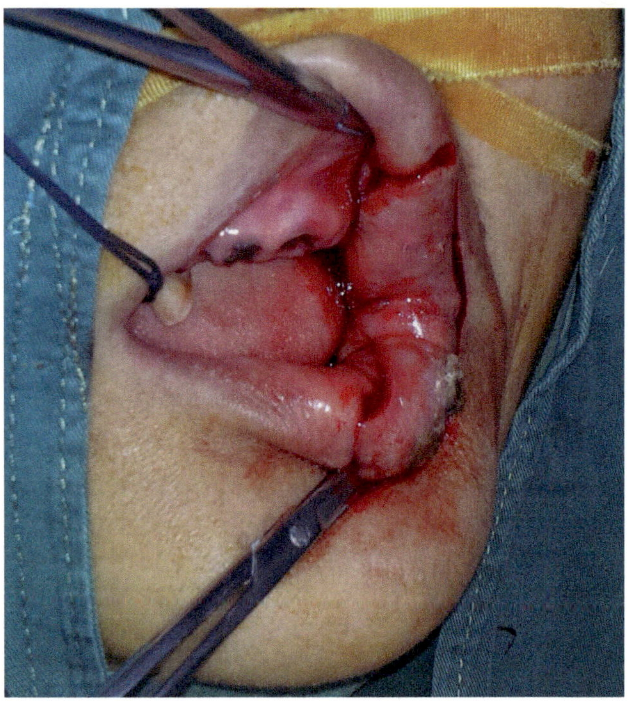

Fig. 18.35 Surgical incisions—side view

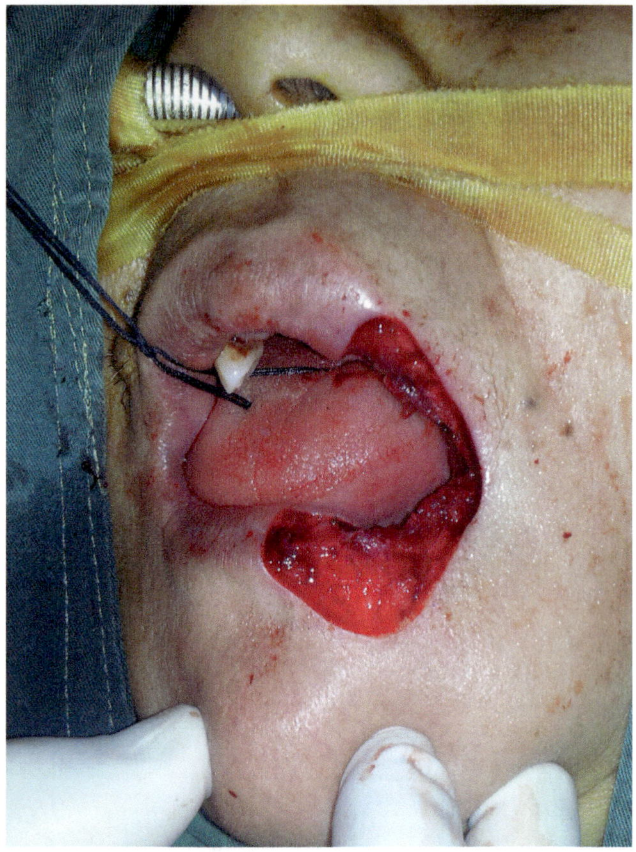

Fig. 18.36 After tumor resection

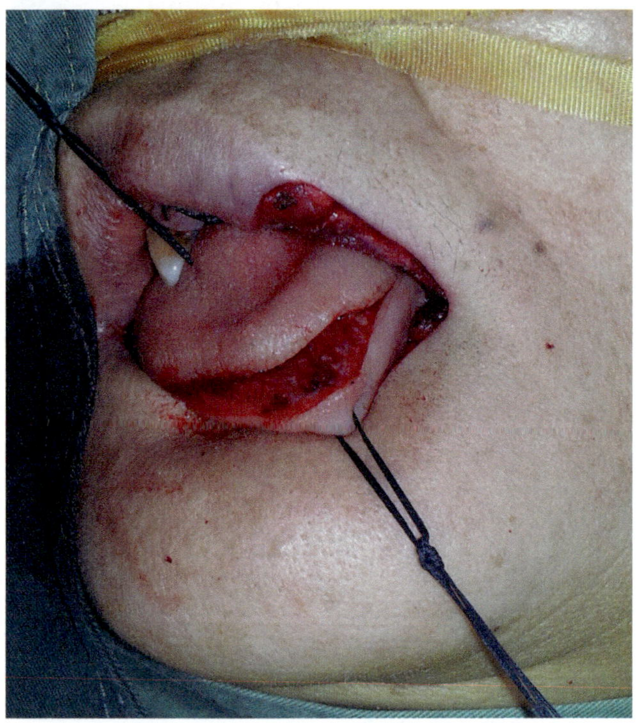

Fig. 18.37 Tongue flap design

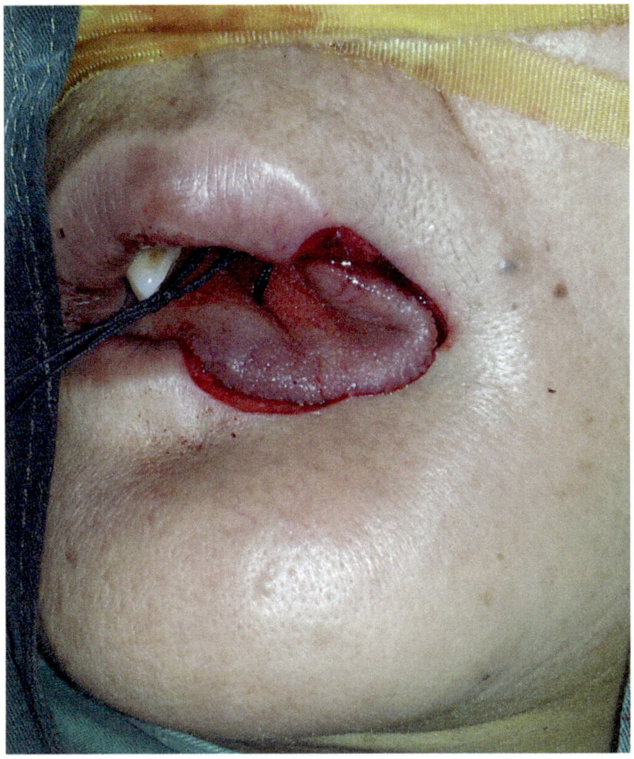

Fig. 18.38 Tongue flap in the desired position for reconstruction

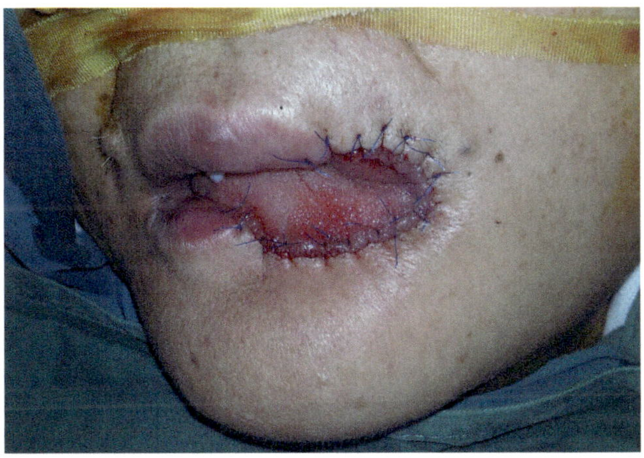

Fig. 18.39 Skin closure

(iii) The inherent difference in color between dorsal mucosa of tongue and native lower lip vermilion must be recognized.

(iv) After flap preparation, match the base of the tongue flap to the inferior border of the lower lip defect first and secure with sutures. The external edges should be closed last to form the future lower lip vermilion.

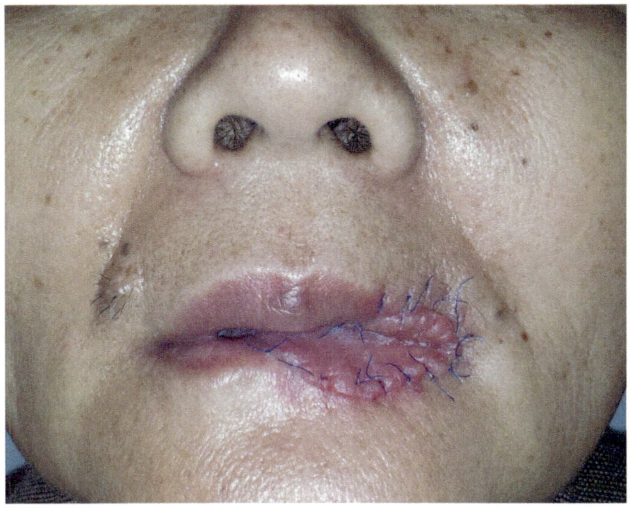

Fig. 18.40 Before flap division

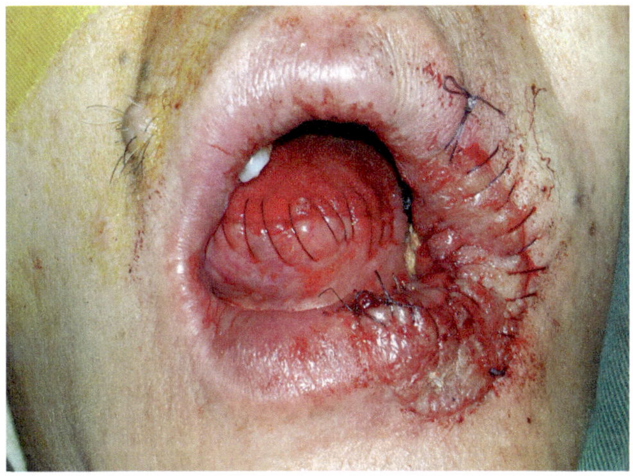

Fig. 18.41 Wound closure after flap division

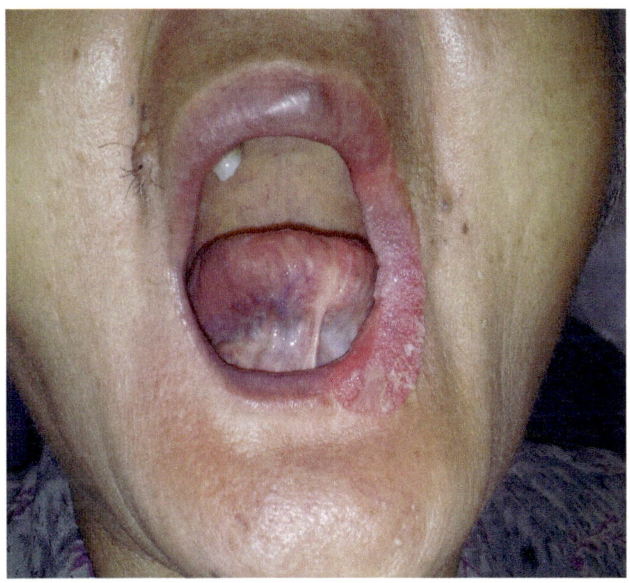

Fig. 18.42 Surgical incisions

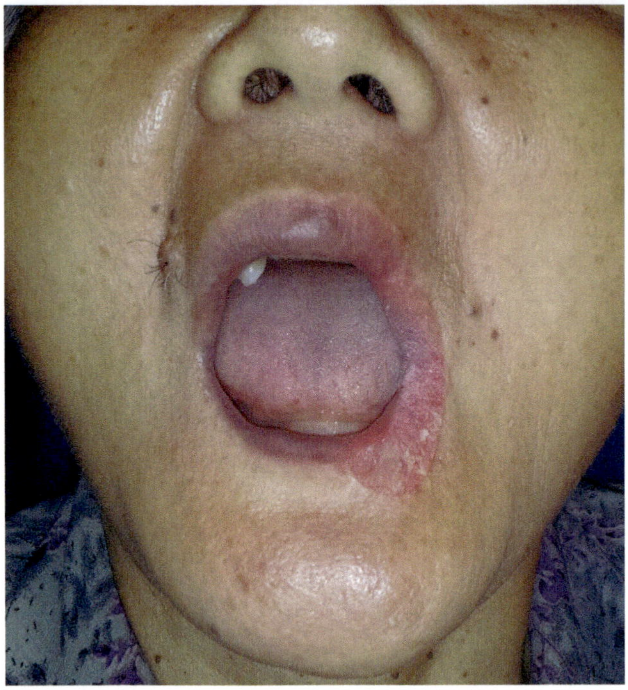

Fig. 18.43 Post-op review

References

1. Shu-Xia Z. Collected works of surgery: oral and maxillofacial surgery (in Chinese). 1st ed. Beijing: Military Science Publishing House; 1994. p. 225–36.
2. Jian-Fang T, Jian-Hua L. Lower lip pedicled composite tissue flap repairing half upper lip defects (in Chinese). J Stomatol. 2008;28(8):446–7.
3. Rui-Wu L, Chang-Fu S, Xing-Jun Q, Chun-Fu D. Functional repair of lower lip defect (in Chinese). J Oral Maxillofac Surg. 2001;11:40.

Reconstruction of Lip Defects with Composite Tissue Flap

19

Jianhua Liu

19.1 Unilateral Sliding Flap Combined with Transposition Flap for Larger Lip Defect

1. Indication
   (i) Defects of the upper or lower lip due to trauma or tumor resection, with the width about one and half – two-third of the entire lip.
   (ii) Full thickness defects involving skin, muscle, and mucosa.
   (iii) For first stage reconstruction after resection of malignant lip tumor, all frozen section margins must be negative.
2. Surgical Steps

   Although simple transposition flaps such as Abbe or Estlander flaps are well suited to reconstruct smaller defects about one and half of the whole lip, their application to larger lip defects is less satisfactory. In cases where the defects involve close to two-three of the entire lip, a combination of sliding flaps and transposition flaps can be considered. Even if such defects can be reconstructed with Abbe flap combined with a unilateral sliding flap, however, a second surgery is required for pedicle division. For defects involving the corner of the mouth, an Estlander flap combined with a unilateral sliding flap is recommended to reconstruct the commissure without the need for a second surgery to divide the flap [1, 2] (Fig. 19.1).

Illustration showing a unilateral lower lip defect after tumor resection. Design the Estlander flap on the left side of upper lip of one and half the width of the defect. Design the sliding flap with a triangular incision inferior to the defect as shown (Fig. 19.2).

After tumor resection, tissue within the triangular incision is removed. Both the sliding and Estlander flaps are formed (Fig. 19.3).

The right side of the lower lip is mobilized towards the left, while the Estlander on the left upper lip is rotated clockwise into the lower lip defect. The resultant defect on the upper lip is closed primarily.

19.1.1 Case Presentation

The lower lip tumor is resected with a safety margin. Both the Estlander flap and the lower lip sliding flap are designed one and half the width of the defect (Figs. 19.4 and 19.5).

The mucosal layer of the Estlander flap is sutured to the matching mucosal layer of the lower lip sliding flap (Fig. 19.6).

Completed reconstruction. The cervical incision was for neck dissection.

3. Special Considerations
   (i) A minimum safety margin of 5 mm is advisable during tumor resection. If the oral commissure is involved, complete resection is imperative before considering reconstructions. Intra-operative frozen sections of safe margins are mandatory.
   (ii) During the preparation of the Estlander flap, the vertical incision must stop short of the upper lip vermilion. It is essential to preserve blood vessels at the tissue pedicle to ensure flap survival. Intra-operatively and during the closure, care must be taken to prevent over-compression of the pedicle tissue from excessive rotations or surgical manipulations.

J. Liu (✉)
Department of Oral and Maxillo-facial Surgery, First Affiliated Hospital, Zhejiang University School of Medicine, Hangzhou, China

J. Liu, B. Shi (eds.), *Atlas of Lip and Nose Plastic and Cosmetic Surgery*, https://doi.org/10.1007/978-981-16-1911-3_19

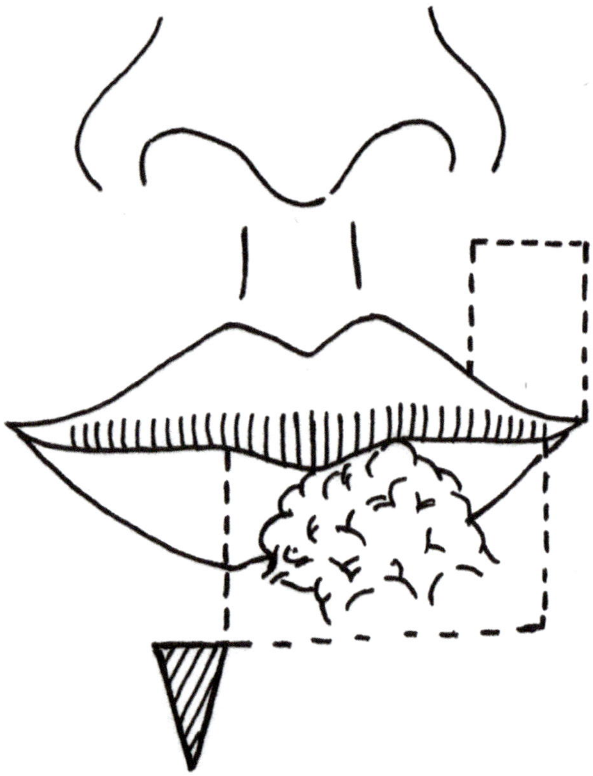

Fig. 19.1 Illustration of planned incision

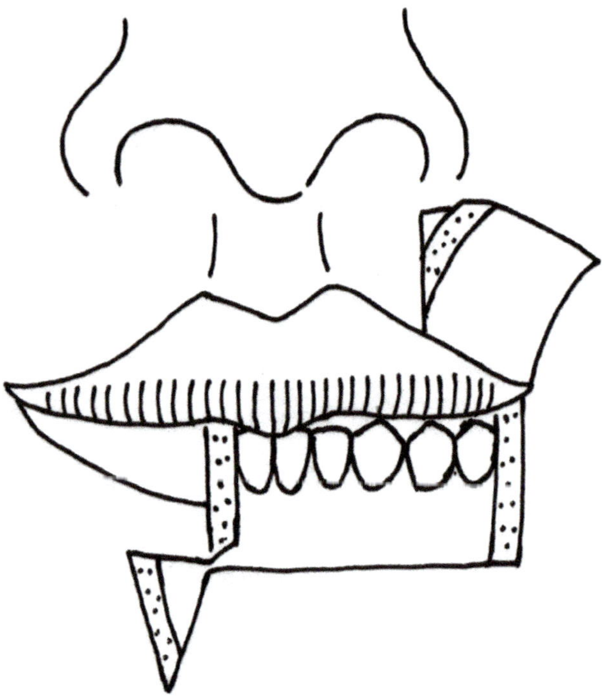

Fig. 19.2 After tumor resection

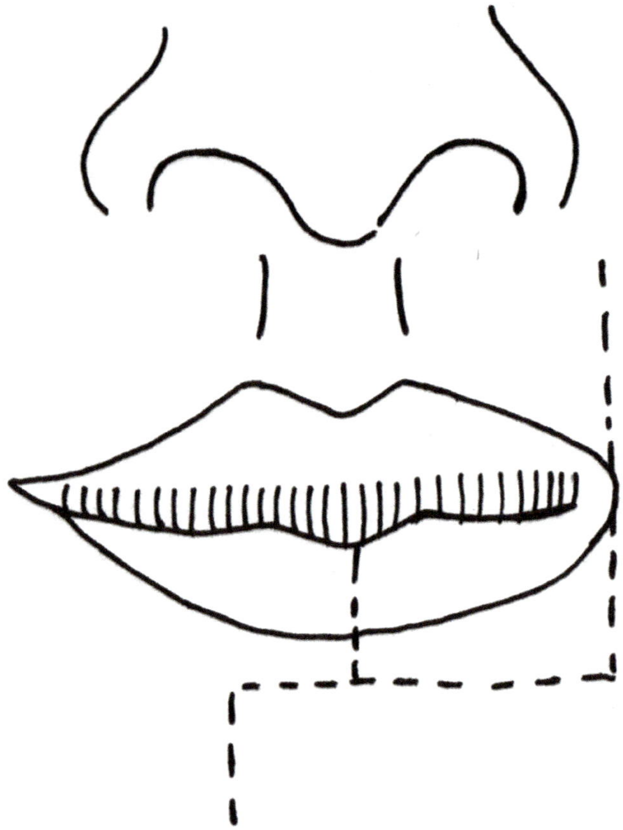

Fig. 19.3 After closure

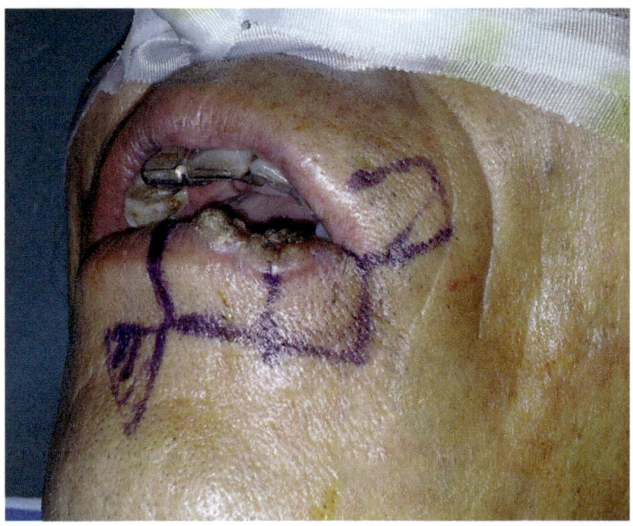

Fig. 19.4 Lower lip tumor and planned incisions

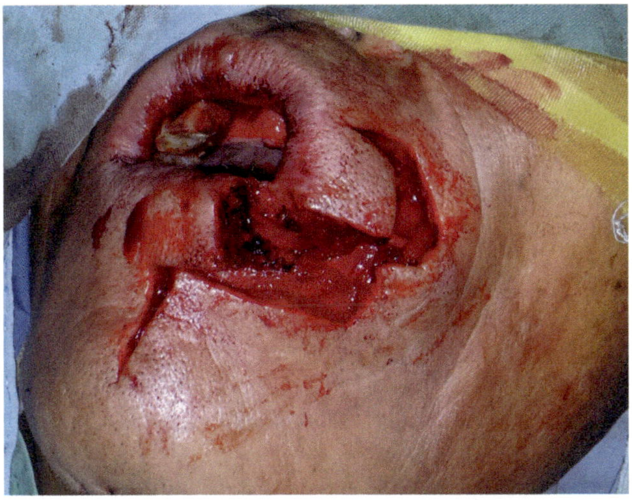

Fig. 19.5 After tumor resection, the transposition flap is prepared

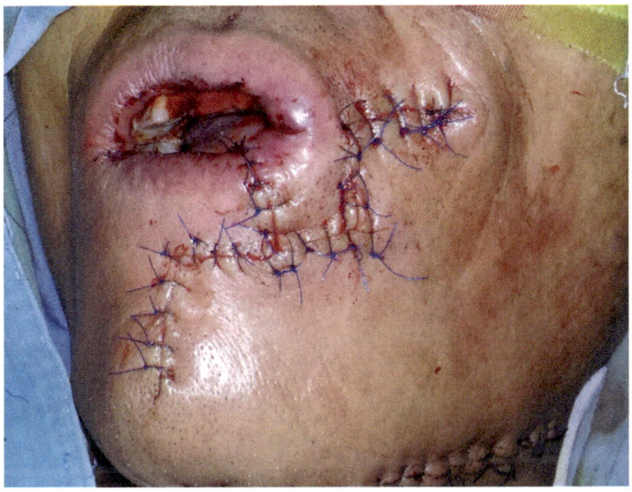

Fig. 19.6 After the closure

(iii) Full thickness surgical incisions must be closed in layers. Oral mucosa is usually closed first. Cut ends of labial muscles should be matched and sutured carefully.

(iv) Microstome and rounded commissures are commonly observed after reconstruction. A second stage commissurotomy is usually performed 3–4 weeks after the initial reconstruction.

19.2 Bilateral Sliding Flaps Combined with Transposition Flap for Larger Lip Defect

1. Indication
   (i) Defects of the upper or lower lip due to trauma or tumor resection, with the width exceeding two-third of the entire lip.
   (ii) Full thickness defects involving skin, muscle, and mucosa.
   (iii) For first stage reconstruction after resection of malignant lip tumor, all frozen section margins must be negative.
2. Surgical Steps

The Abbe flap traditionally refers to the reconstruction of the upper lip defect using a rotational lower lip flap. However, lower lip defects can similarly be repaired with an upper lip flap. Most of the larger lip defects can be reconstructed with Abbe flap combined with bilateral sliding flaps, although a second surgery is required for flap division. For defects involving the corner of the mouth, an Estlander flap combined with a bilateral sliding flap is recommended to reconstruct the commissure without the need for a second surgery to divide the flap [3, 4].

19.2.1 Surgical Illustrations

The Estlander flap is designed at the left side of the upper lip, close to the oral commissure (Figs. 19.7 and 19.8).

After tumor resection, tissue within the triangular incision is removed. Both the sliding and Estlander flaps are formed (Fig. 19.9).

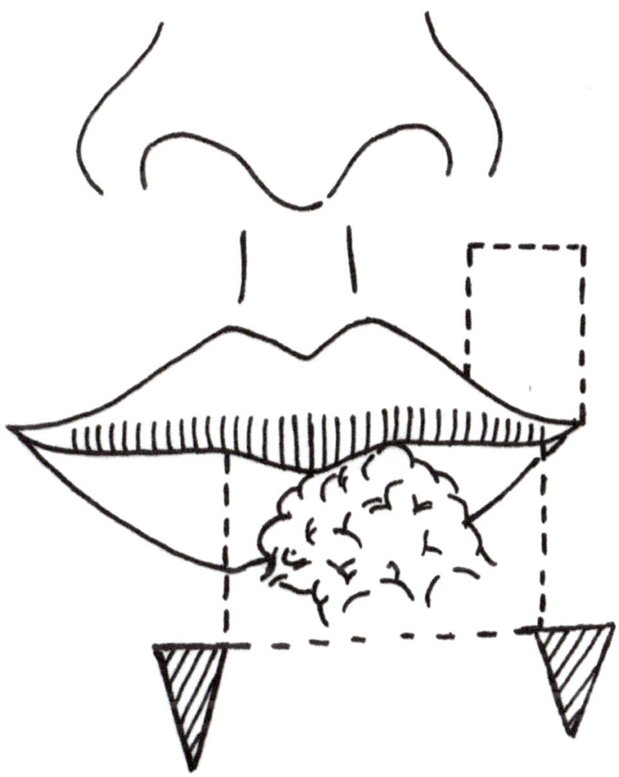

Fig. 19.7 Illustration of the planned incision

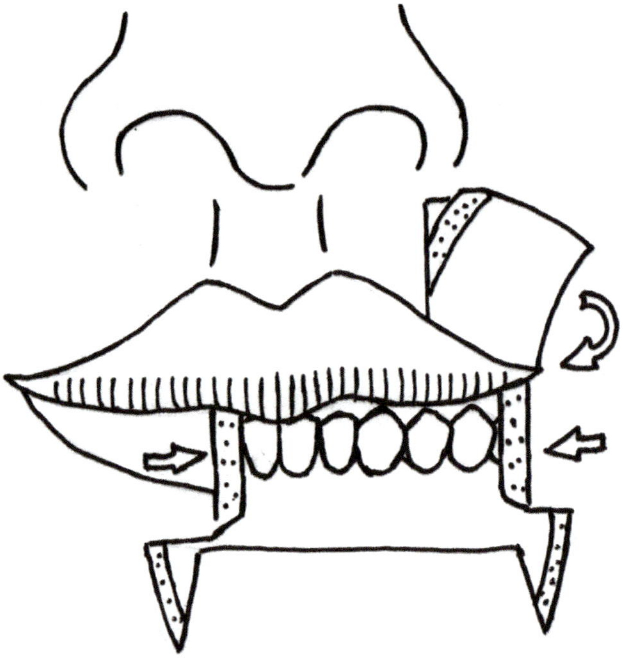

Fig. 19.8 Prepared transposition and sliding flaps

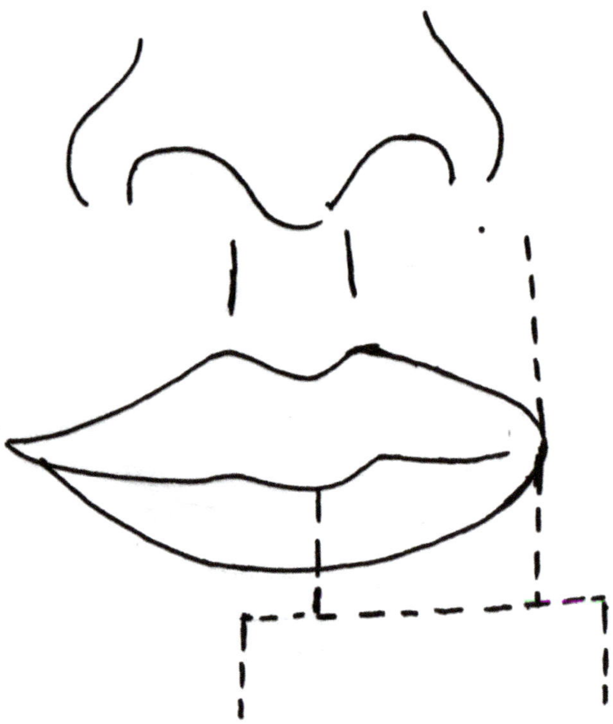

Fig. 19.9 After closure

Bilateral lower lip sliding flaps are pulled centrally and opposed accordingly. The upper lip Estlander flap is rotated clockwise into the defect and secured with sutures.

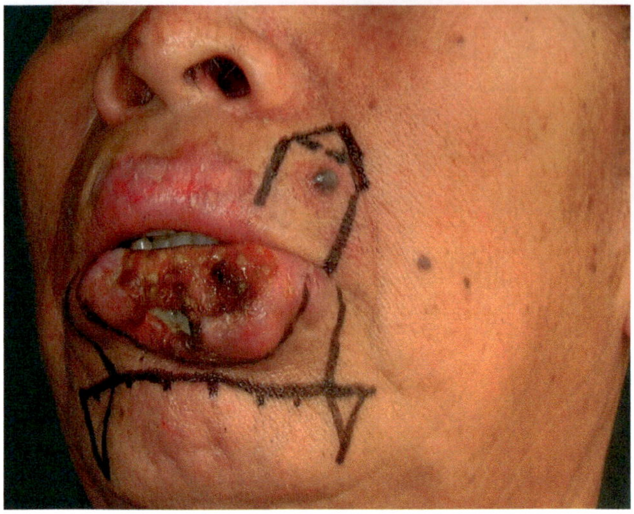

Fig. 19.10 Planned incision

19.2.2 Case Presentation

Ensure a minimum safety margin of 5 mm during tumor resection. The width of transposition flap does not exceed ½ of that of the defect. Additional triangle on the contralateral side of the lower lip is designed slightly larger to allow for greater advancement. Ipsilateral triangle can be slightly smaller as most parts of the defect will be repaired by the Estlander flap. In this case, the Estlander flap has been modified to assume a rectangular form instead of the classical triangular design (Fig. 19.10).

Full thickness resection of lower lip tumor. Arterial supply for the Estlander flap is preserved (Fig. 19.11).

Transposition flap is rotated down clockwise while bilateral sliding flaps are mobilized centrally into the defect. Incisions are then closed primarily (Fig. 19.12).

First stage surgery completed. The newly reconstructed left oral commissure deviated medially. A second stage commissurotomy was planned (Fig. 19.13).

Oral commissurotomy can be performed 1 month after initial reconstruction. The desired position of the commissure should mirror the contralateral normal side (Fig. 19.14).

19.2.3 Classic Case

A case of lower lip SCC where the tumor involves more than four-fifth of the entire lower lip (Fig. 19.15).

Wide resection with neck dissection is performed. Four additional triangles are planned for removal to facilitate the preparation of bilateral labial and buccal advancement flaps. A modified Abbe flap is designed on the right side of the upper lip to repair the lower lip defect after rotation. The flap

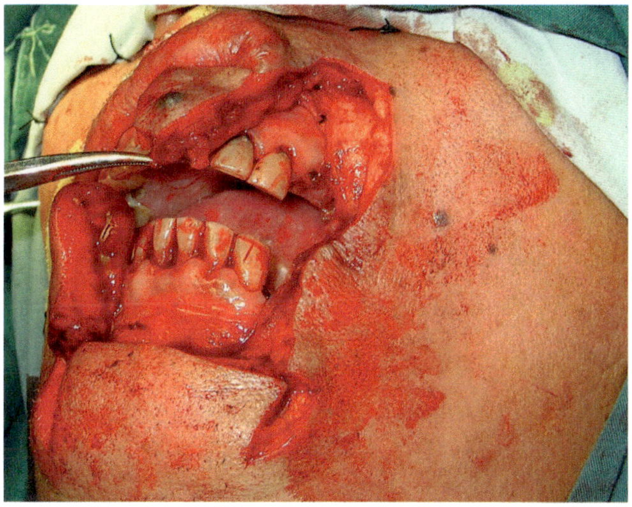

Fig. 19.11 After tumor resection

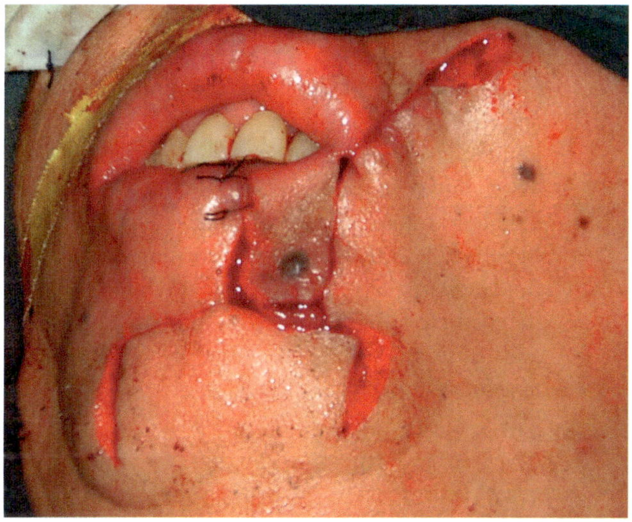

Fig. 19.12 Flaps repositioned and sutured

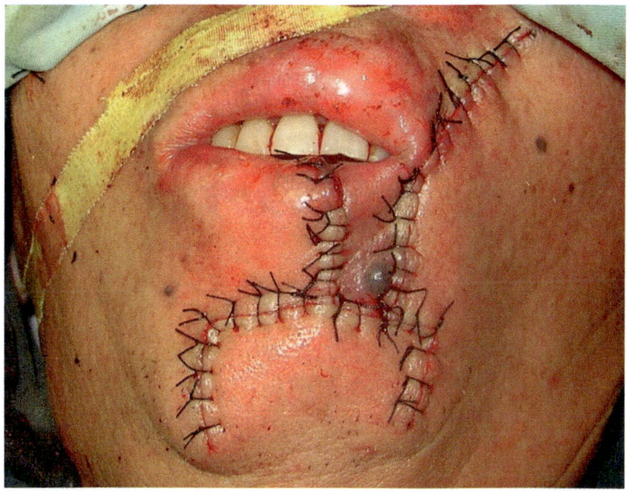

Fig. 19.13 After closure

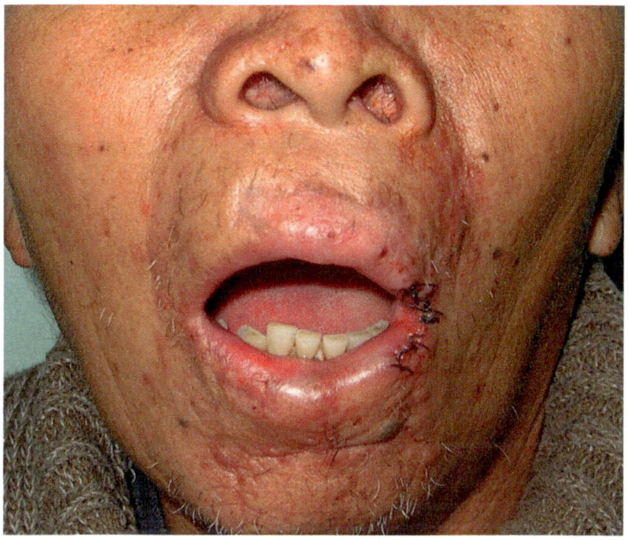

Fig. 19.14 After second stage commissurotomy

pedicle is located on the right side, while the left vermilion is to be incised completely (Fig. 19.16).

Neck dissection is completed, and all flaps are secured in respective positions. Note the pedicle is now located in the center. Alternate suture removal can be performed from 7 days post-op and complete removal on post-op day 14. Division of the pedicle should be delayed until at least 21 days post-op (Fig. 19.17).

At 4-month review, the patient presented with good facial aesthetics and function. No additional corrective or cosmetic procedures were necessary (Fig. 19.18).

3. Special Considerations.
   (i) A minimum safety margin of 5 mm is advisable during tumor resection. If the oral commissure is involved, complete resection is imperative before

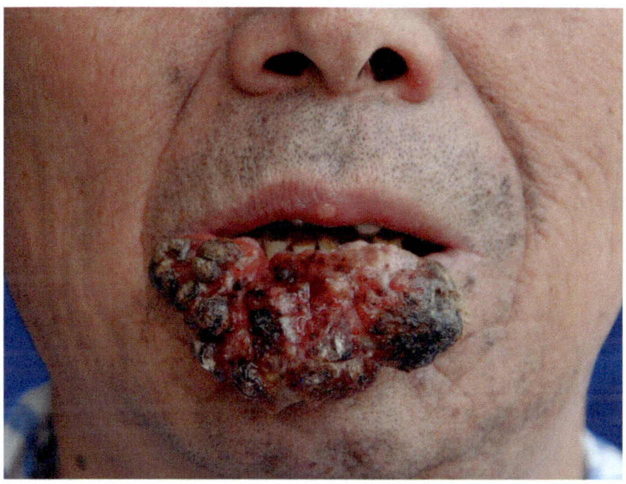

Fig. 19.15 Malignancy involving almost the entire lower lip

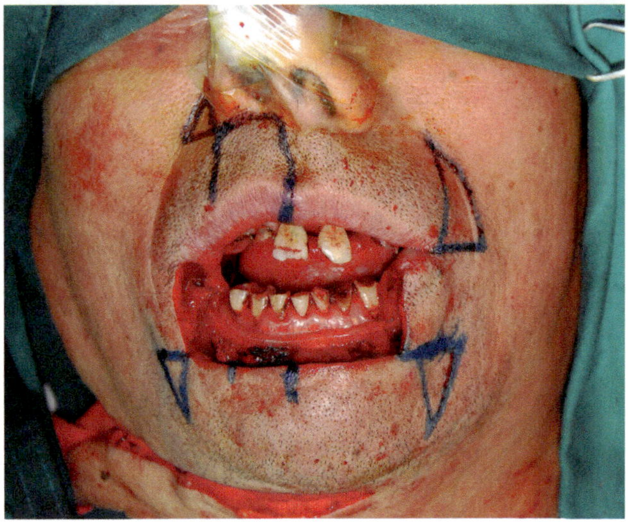

Fig. 19.16 After tumor resection

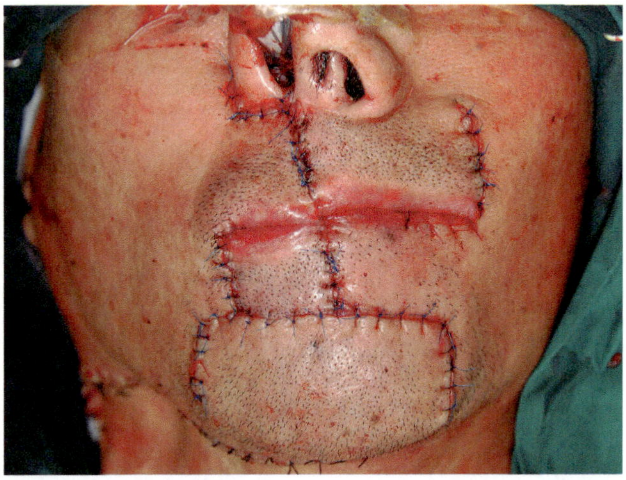

Fig. 19.17 After the closure

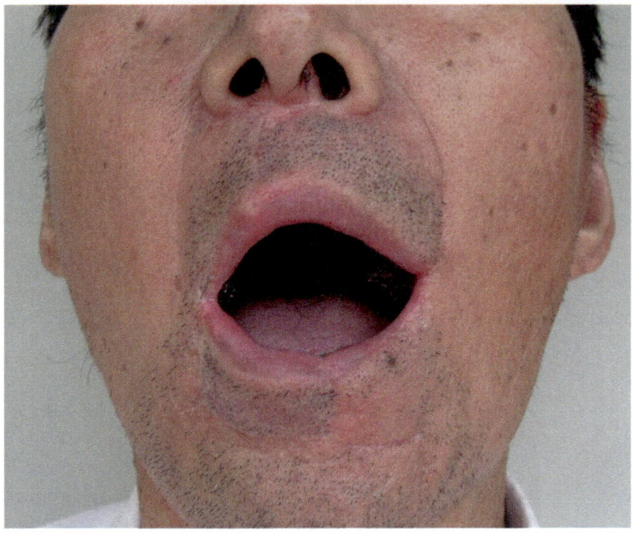

Fig. 19.18 Four months post-op

considering reconstructions. Intra-operative frozen sections of the safety margins are mandatory.

(ii) The width of transposition flap should not exceed one and half of that of the defect. For large defects where pure transposition flap proves inadequate, additional bilateral sliding flaps can be considered.

(iii) Proper design and preparation of the transposition are crucial to the success of reconstruction. Every effort should be taken to preserve the vascular pedicle. Capillary refill should be monitored frequently and regularly after flap surgery.

(iv) Pedicle is usually divided no earlier than 21 days after initial reconstruction. Patients who are unable to tolerate limited mouth opening, such as those with COPD are therefore not suitable for this method. Prior to pedicle division, restrict the pedicle blood flow with rubber bands first and observe for newly established collateral anastomosis.

References

1. Ru-Yao S, Zhang-Lin F. Cosmetic and plastic surgery (in Chinese). 2nd ed. Beijing: Beijing Publish House; 1992. p. 132–9.
2. Campbell JP. Surgical management of lip carcinoma. J Oral Maxillofac Surg. 1998;56:955–61.
3. Zilinsky I, Winkler E, Weiss G, et al. Total lower lip reconstruction with innervated muscle bearing flaps. A modification of the Webster flap. Dermatol Surg. 2001;27(7):687–91.
4. Jian-Fang T, Jian-Hua L. Lower lip pedicled composite tissue flap repairing half upper lip defects (in Chinese). J Stomatol. 2008;28(8):446–7.

20 Reconstruction of Total Nasal Defect

Kai Liu and Choi Jong-Woo

20.1 Principle of Aesthetic Subunit: Nose and Face Subunit

Traditionally, reconstructions of total nasal defect emphasize the overall aesthetic of the nasal structures. The principle of aesthetic subunit refers to the following: when the defect exceeds half of the nasal subunit, a complete reconstruction of the nose can achieve the better aesthetic result. The nasal subunits include nasal bridge, both lateral surfaces, bilateral alar and nares, nasal tip, and columella. Surgeons, for instance, tend to refrain from removing additional healthy tissues even when the nasal defect exceeds half of the entire nose. However, based on the aesthetic subunit principle, the use of a total nasal reconstruction for a partial defect provides superior aesthetics. As perceptions of aesthetics are largely subjective, it tends to depend heavily on how the face and its subunits are being observed. Russian scientist A. L. Yarbus reported that when participants were asked to focus on the central features of a face, such as facial contour, highlights, and shadows, they tend to ignore the peripheral features. As the nose is an important facial subunit, during total or subtotal nasal reconstruction the Principles of aesthetic subunits should be considered for a satisfactory result [1, 2] (Figs. 20.1 and 20.2).

K. Liu (✉)
Department of Plastic Surgery, The 9th People's Hospital, Shanghai Jiao Tong University, Shanghai, China

C. Jong-Woo
Department of Plastic Surgery, ASAN Medical Center, University of Ulsan College of Medicine, Seoul, Republic of Korea

20.2 Total Nose Reconstruction with Radial Forearm Free Flap and Frontal Flap

Choi Jong-Woo

Complete nasal reconstruction presents with several challenges including repair of internal structures, recreation of bony support and reconstruction of soft tissue exterior. Appropriate flaps should be considered according to surgical goals. The preferred sequencing of reconstruction is demonstrated in the following case study (Fig. 20.3).

1. Repair of internal nasal structures

Repair of the internal nasal structures varies from each individual case. In general, a relatively thin flap is preferred. If the septum is preserved and healthy, the septal periosteal flap is an ideal option. For patients with missing nasal septum, a free flap is preferred, ideally a thin fascial flap to reduce obstruction of the nasal passages. For this patient, the first step of reconstruction was the repair of internal nasal walls. In view of the missing septum, a radial forearm flap was selected. The flap was a combination of Dr. Menick's and Dr. Walton's designs and draped in such a way as to minimize obstruction to the nasal passages (Figs. 20.4 and 20.5).

2. Recreation of Nasal Structural Support

Proper hard tissue support is crucial to maintain a normal nasal shape. The exterior of a nose had to be simulated and recreated for this patient.

After repair of internal structures, the dorsal support is usually achieved with a rib cartilage graft. The Asian nasal structures defer from the Caucasian counterparts in that the support from the nasal septum is weaker, with relatively small and soft upper and lower lateral cartilages. The recreated nasal hard-tissue structures should simulate the natural nasal features of the Asian population (Fig. 20.6).

J. Liu, B. Shi (eds.), *Atlas of Lip and Nose Plastic and Cosmetic Surgery*, https://doi.org/10.1007/978-981-16-1911-3_20

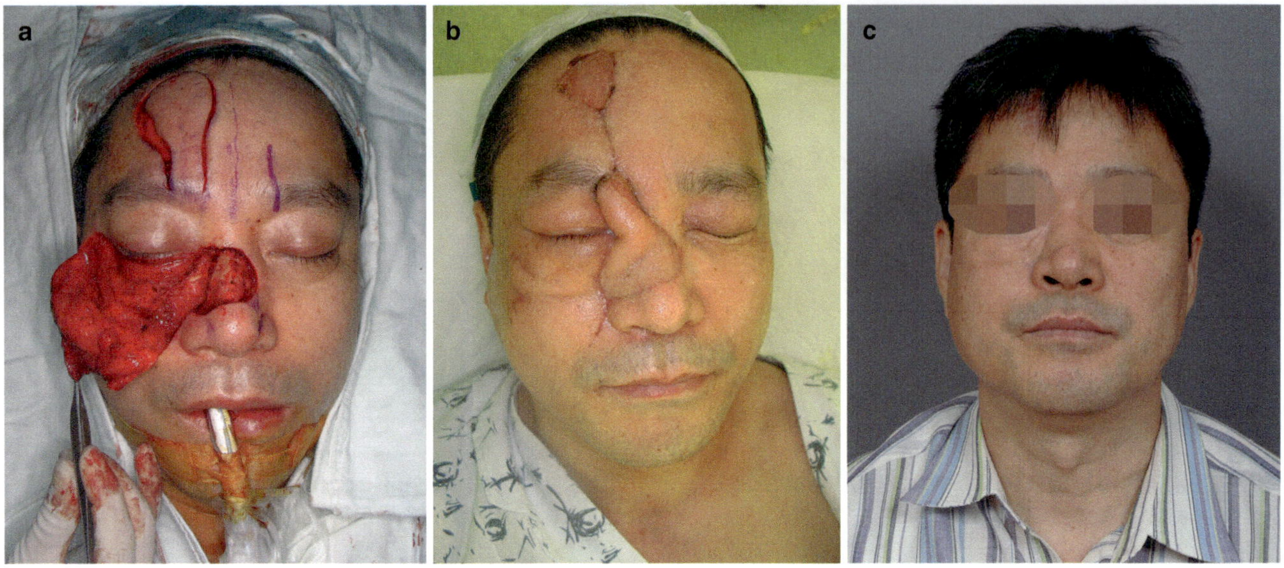

Fig. 20.1 (**a**, **b**, **c**) The nose and cheek are repaired as two separate subunits. Pictures showing a Korean patient with naso-buccal tumor. (**a**) Demonstrated the importance of separating aesthetic subunits. As defect involves the nose and cheek, spanning across multiple subunits, reconstruction with a single flap would be inadequate. (**b**) Demonstrates the satisfactory immediate aesthetic outcome after reconstructing the two subunits separately. (**c**) Shows the final healed result

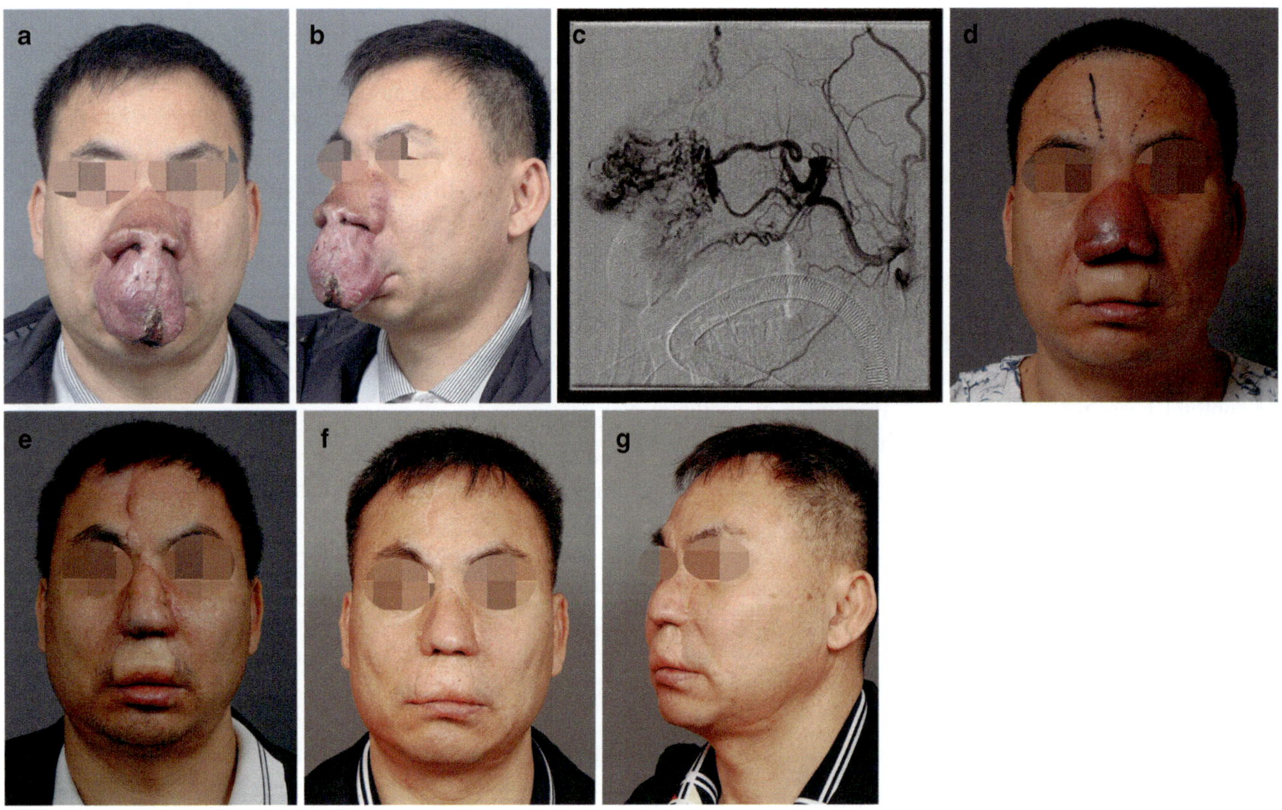

Fig. 20.2 (**a**–**g**) The nose and upper lip are repaired as two separate subunits. Pictures showing a Korean patient with nasolabial soft tissue venous malformation. (**a**) Frontal view of the venous malformation; (**b**) oblique view; (**c**) angiogram and selective embolization; (**d**) after upper lip tumor resection and reconstruction with radial forearm flap; (**e**) after nasal tumor resection and reconstruction with frontal flap and vermilion tattoo; (**f**) 3 years post-op (frontal); (**g**) 3 years post-op (oblique)

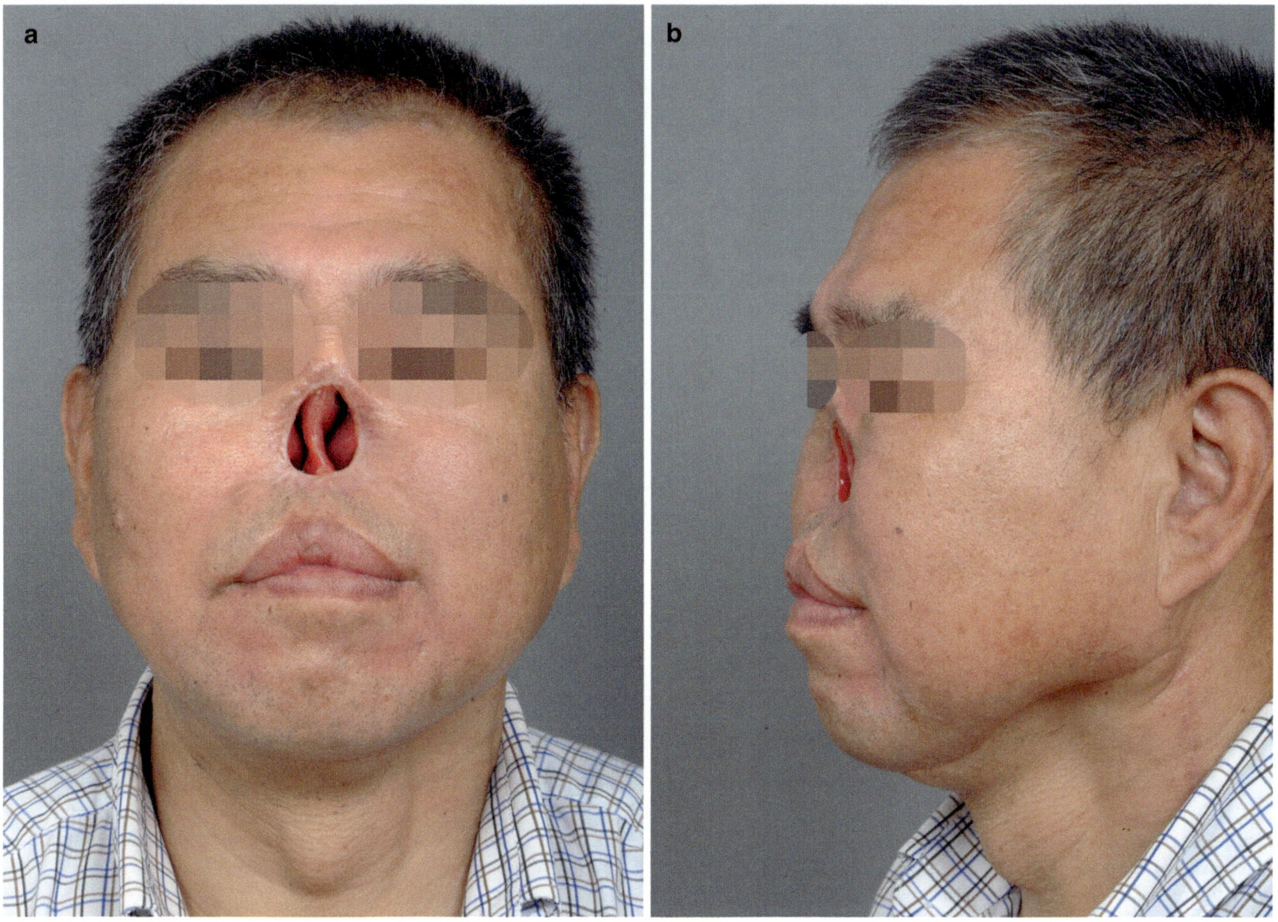

Fig. 20.3 (**a**, **b**) Total nasal defect prior to reconstruction. This patient underwent three surgeries for a nasal tumor. The resultant total nasal defect requires complex reconstruction of the internal structures, bony support, and soft tissue exterior. (**a**) Frontal view; (**b**) oblique view

3. Reconstruction of Soft Tissue Exterior

Among all the currently available flaps, such as free flaps, local flaps, and regional flaps, the frontal flap is the most suited for reconstruction of the nose with the excellent matching of skin color and texture.

In this case, a median frontal flap was used pedicled from the ipsilateral supra-trochlear artery. Usually, the complete reconstruction is divided into two or three stages. Similar to the method described by Dr. Menick, after the first stage rotation of the frontal flap, it is subsequently raised again and thinned down to improve nasal contour while maintaining the bony support. Dr. Walton however recommends a separate third surgery to readjust the soft tissue. There is no consensus on which method is better, and selection is largely based on surgeon preference (Fig. 20.7).

20.3 Total Nose Reconstruction with Expanded Forehead Flap

1. Indications
   (i) Large nasal defects (due to trauma or burns) centered on the nasal tip and exceeding four aesthetic subunits.
   (ii) Dispersed nasal defects (due to trauma or burns) exceeding three aesthetics subunits.
   (iii) Benign tumors of the nose of similar extent.

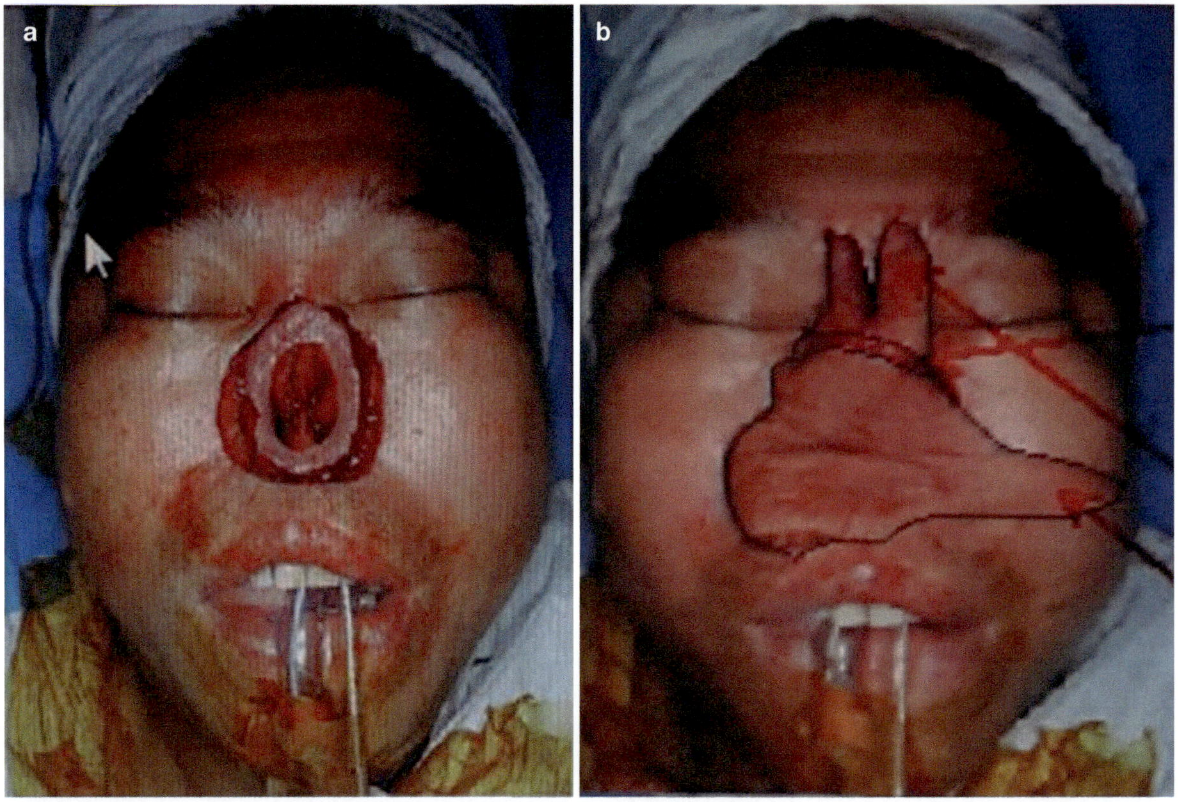

Fig. 20.4 (**a**, **b**) Reconstruction of internal nasal structures. (**a**) Nasal incisions; (**b**) draping of radial forearm flap: the superior extensions used for reconstruction of the internal nasal structures. And the left extension formed the new nare. The flap pedicles were anastomosed with facial vessels

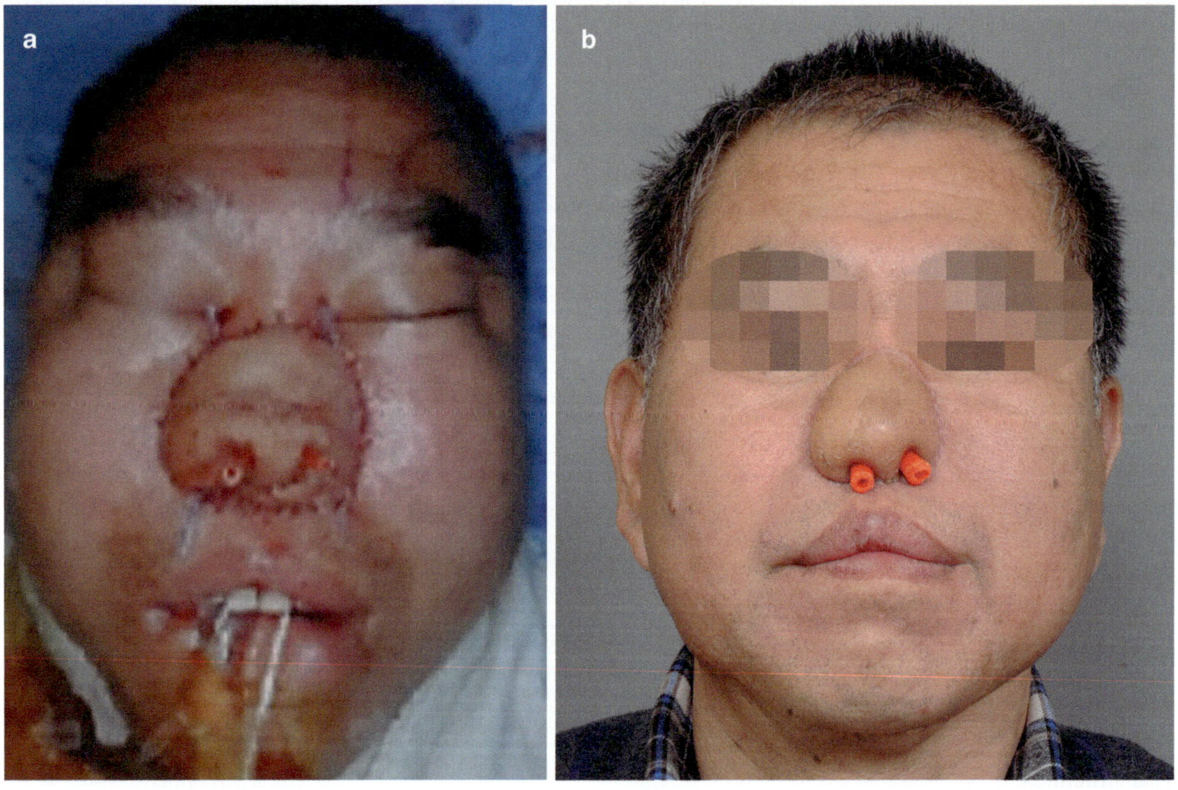

Fig. 20.5 (**a**, **b**) Completed reconstruction of internal nasal structures. (**a**) Completed reconstruction of internal nasal structures, bilateral nares supported by rubber tubing; (**b**) 3 months post-op

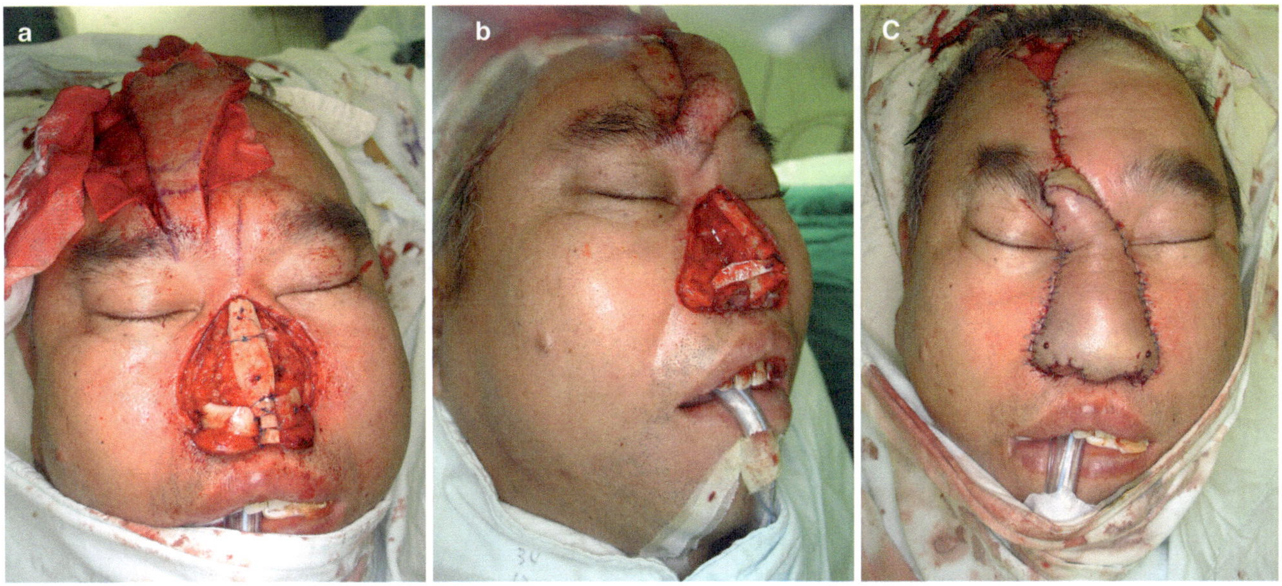

Fig. 20.6 (**a**, **b**, **c**) Recreated nasal hard tissue support. (**a**) Part of the forearm flap at the dorsum of the nose was removed. Rib cartilage was shaped to restore nasal bridge, columella, and lateral crura; (**b**) oblique view; (**c**) frontal flap was rotated to cover the nasal defect and restore exterior appearance

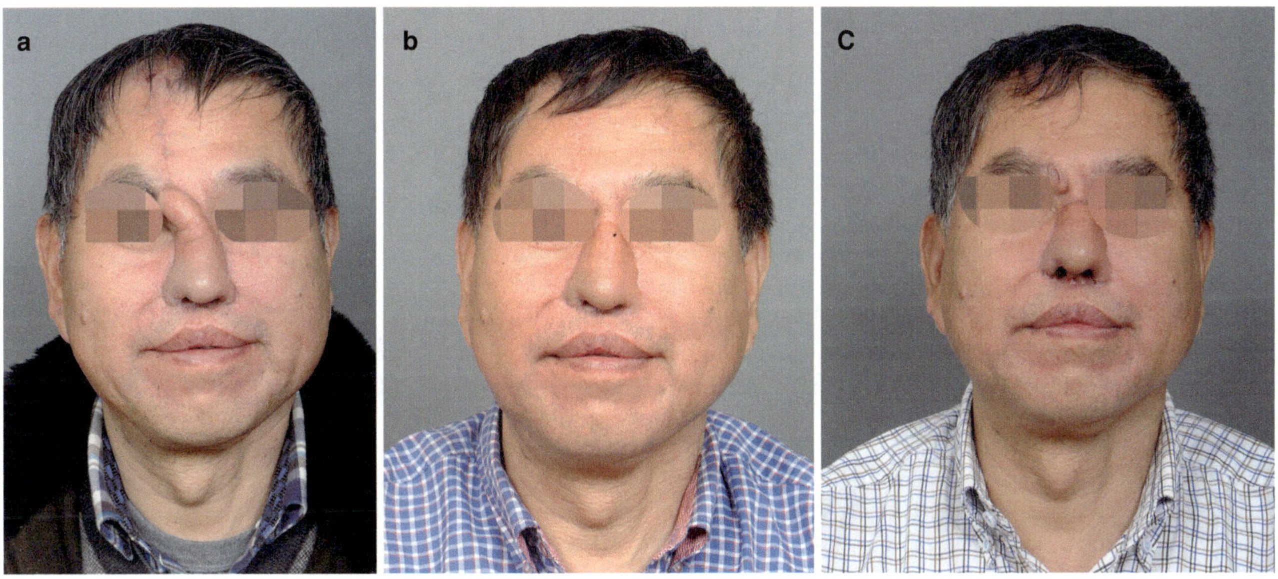

Fig. 20.7 (**a**, **b**, **c**) Reconstruction of nasal soft tissue exterior. (**a**) Frontal flap prior to division; (**b**) Frontal flap after division; (**c**) 6 months post-op

(iv) Severe malignant tumors of the nose requiring wide resection.
(v) Multiple basal cell carcinoma of the nose.
(vi) The above defects with corresponding bony, cartilaginous and mucosal defects.

2. Surgical Steps

Complete nasal reconstruction involves (1) repair of internal nasal structures; (2) recreation of bony and cartilaginous support; (3) reconstruction of soft tissue exterior.

For the repair of internal nasal structures, local rotational flaps, unilateral or bilateral island rotational flaps pedicled with external nasal arteries are most commonly used. The rib cartilage is an ideal autogenous source for the recreation of the bony and cartilaginous support of the nose. The donar cartilage is most commonly harvested from the seventh or the eighth rib and carved into the desired shape. The skin of the frontal flap is the most similar in texture and color to that of the nose, and therefore is the most preferred donor site for reconstruction of the nasal exterior. In cases where the frontal flaps are not available,

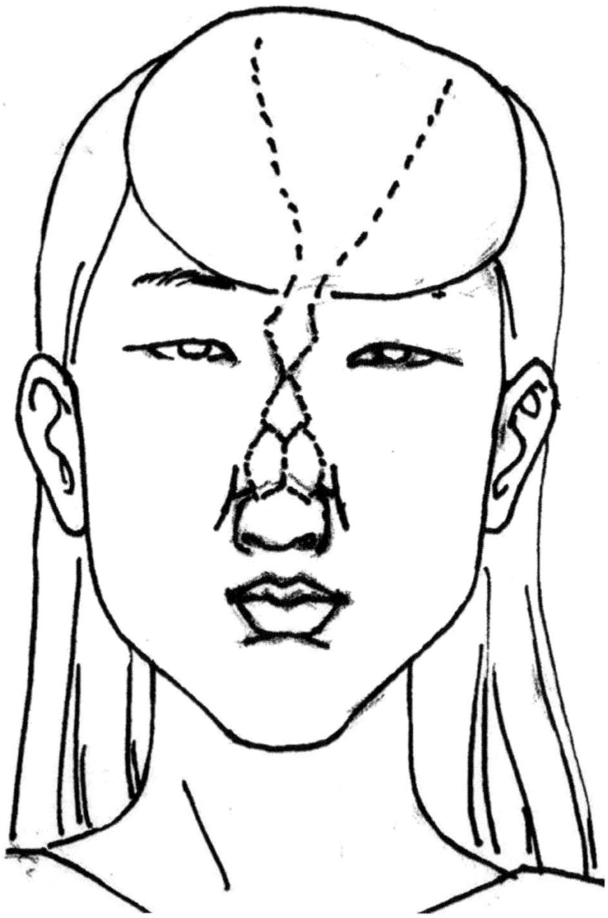

Fig. 20.8 Planned incisions

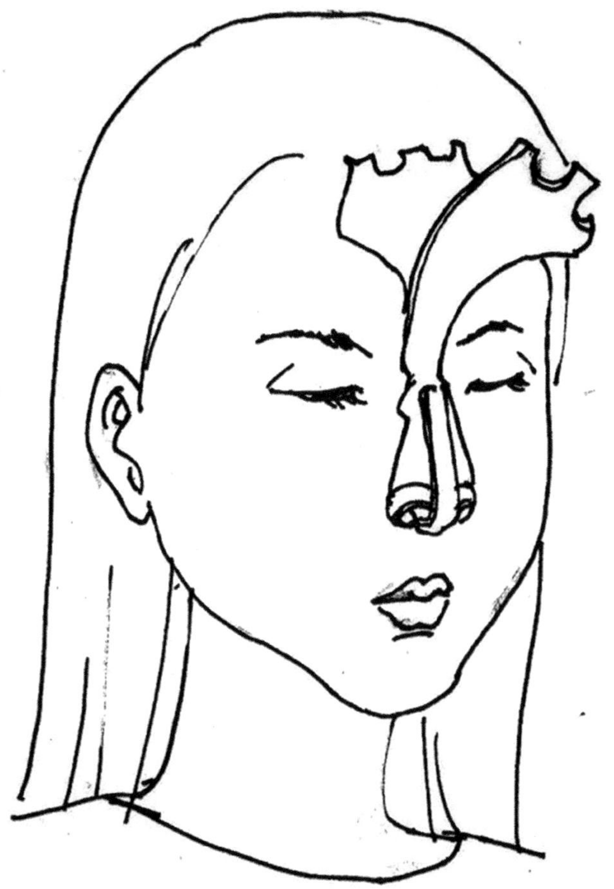

Fig. 20.9 Nasal strut with rib cartilage and formation of the frontal flap

tubular flaps of the upper arms or preconstructed flaps of the chest can be considered (Fig. 20.8).

Picture showing the planned incision of a nasal reconstruction: internal structures are to be restored with a rotational island flap with external nasal artery as pedicle; the exterior tissues are to be restored with expanded frontal flap (Fig. 20.9).

Harvest the cartilage from the seventh or the eighth rib. Shape the cartilage according to the degree of support required at the new nasal complex; raise the expanded frontal flap based on the unilateral supra-trochlear artery (Fig. 20.10).

The frontal flap is rotated 180 degrees anticlockwise to cover the cartilage strut. The donor site defect is closed primarily, and the pedicled flap divided 1 month after (Figs. 20.11, 20.12).

3. Special Considerations
   (i) Design the frontal flap 20% larger than the actual defect.
   (ii) Care must be taken to preserve the external nasal arteries when preparing the bilateral island rotational flap and ensure adequate tissue laxity when rotated to drape the defect.
   (iii) Estimate the size of the reconstructed nose with reference to that of the family members and the patient's own desire.

20.4 Preconstructed Chest Flap for Combined Total Nasal and Total Upper Lip Defect

Kai Liu and Qing-feng Li

1. Indications
   (i) Complete loss of external nose and some of upper lip or other neighboring structures due to trauma or burns.
   (ii) Patients with complete loss of external nose whose frontal skin and subcutaneous tissues are damaged as well.

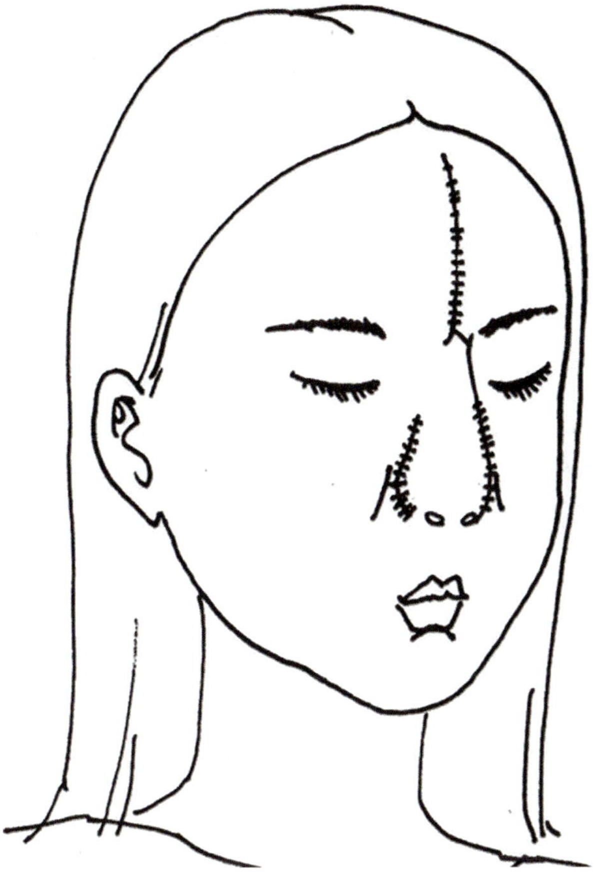

Fig. 20.10 Frontal flap rotated and secured

(iii) Severe, extensive malignant tumors of the nose requiring wide resection involving neighboring tissues.
(iv) Multiple basal cell carcinoma of the face or other malignancies requiring extensive resection and reconstruction of facial organs.
(v) The above defects with corresponding bony, cartilaginous and mucosal defects.

2. Surgical Steps

There are two donor sites available for preconstructed flaps for total nasal reconstructions: (1) Anterior neck and chest area; (2) Forearm. As the skin texture and color of the neck matches the face best, it is the preferred donor site for extensive reconstructions of missing facial organs. Raise a fascial flap based on descending rami of lateral circumflex femoral vessels from the anterior lateral thigh and re-anastomose the pedicle with facial artery and vein accordingly. Secure the flap between the skin and the subcutaneous expander placed at the chest in position. Depending on the actual extent of the defect, expansion generally takes 3–5 months to achieve a flap of adequate size.

(ii) Remove the expander after an appropriate time (generally takes 3–5 months to achieve a flap of adequate size). Harvest autologous rib cartilage to form the future nasal and upper lip structures and embed in the expanded flap. In one month, harvest the pedicled chest flap with the preconstructed nasal and lip tissues and rotate into the facial defect. Donor site defect is then closed primarily (Fig. 20.14).

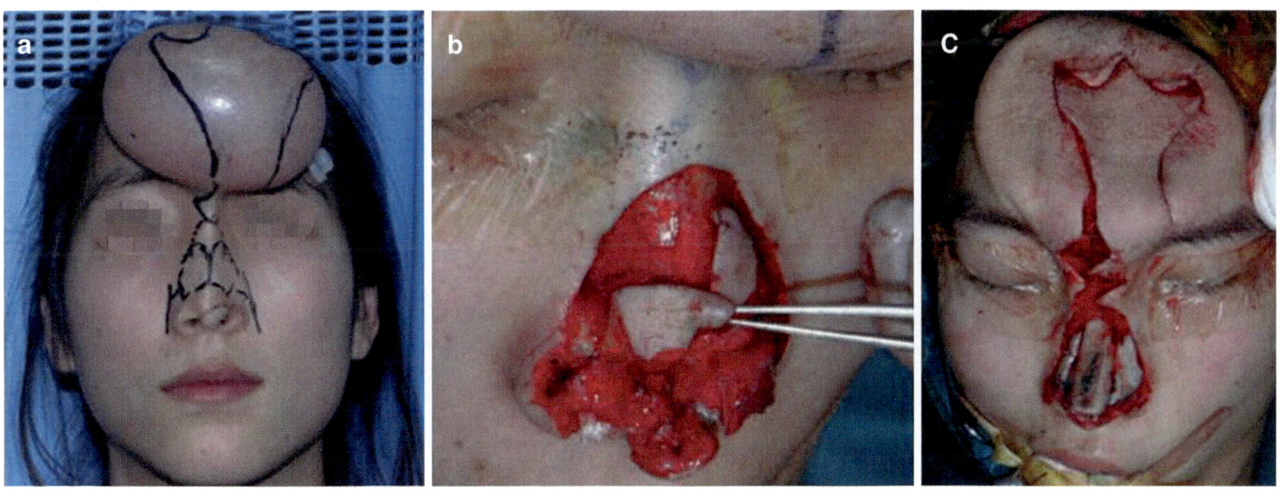

Fig. 20.11 (**a**, **b**, **c**) Pre-op design and intra-op procedures for expanded frontal flap reconstruction. (**a**) Design the frontal flap after 2 months of expansion; (**b**) bilateral island flap based on external nasal arteries rotated inwards to form the internal lining; (**c**) rib cartilage shaped and secured, the expander is removed, and frontal flap raised preserving its pedicle. The flap is then rotated down to drape the cartilage strut and secured in place. The pedicle is divided 1 month later, and incisions readjusted

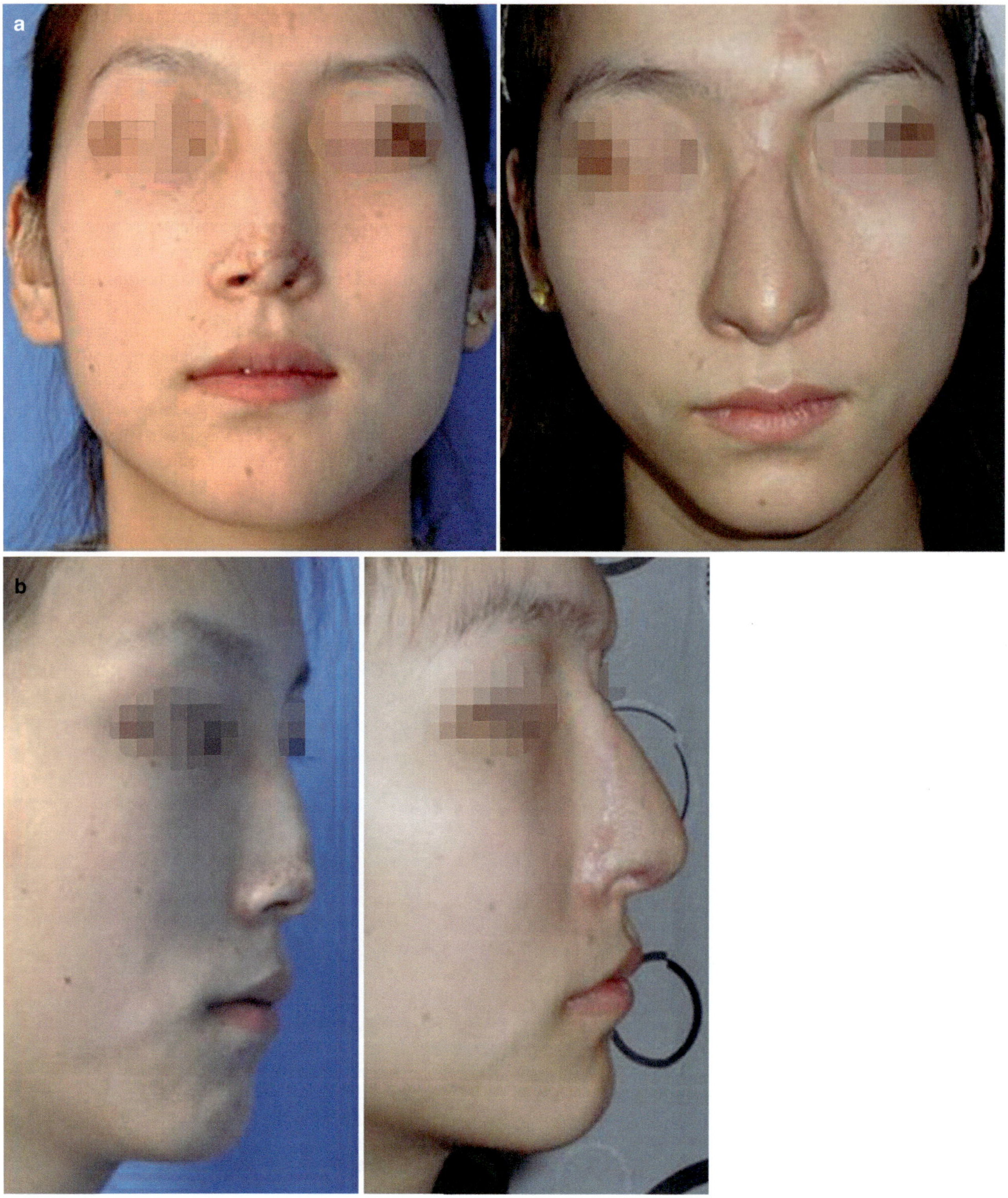

Fig. 20.12 (**a**, **b**) Total nasal reconstruction with expanded frontal flap. (**a**, upper) Same patient pre-op and 1 year post-op- frontal view; (**b**, lower) Same patient pre-op and 1 year post-op-profile view

A fascial flap based on descending rami of lateral circumflex femoral vessels from the anterior lateral thigh is prepared and re-anastomose the pedicle with facial artery and vein accordingly, as shown in Fig. 20.13. Place the fascial flap on the subcutaneous expander at the anterior chest. The skin is allowed to expand for 3 months before the expander is removed. Autologous rib is then harvested and shaped into the desired future nasal and upper lip structures and embedded into the expanded flap, as shown in Fig. 20.14. In one month, harvest the pedicled chest flap with the preconstructed nasal and lip tissues and rotate into the facial defect (Fig. 20.15).

Typical Case (Fig. 20.16):

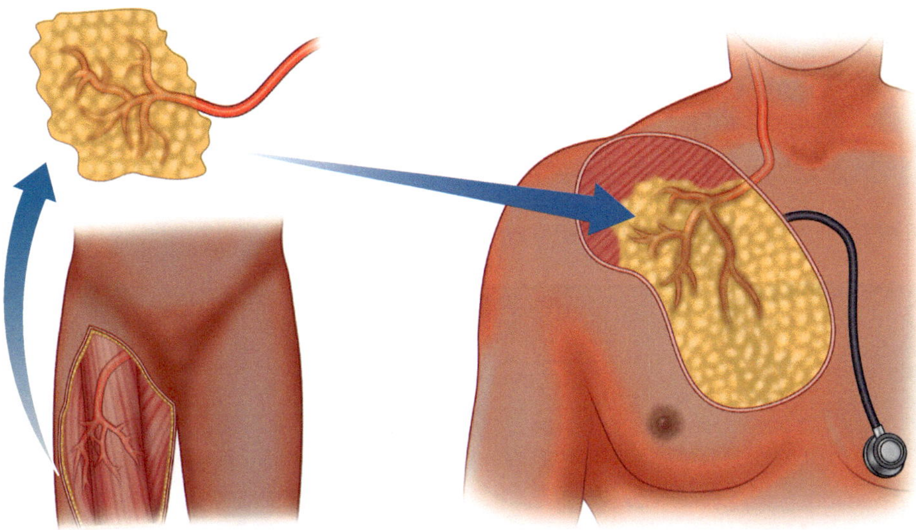

Fig. 20.13 Preconstruction of flap at the anterior chest for future reconstruction of complete nasal and lip defect

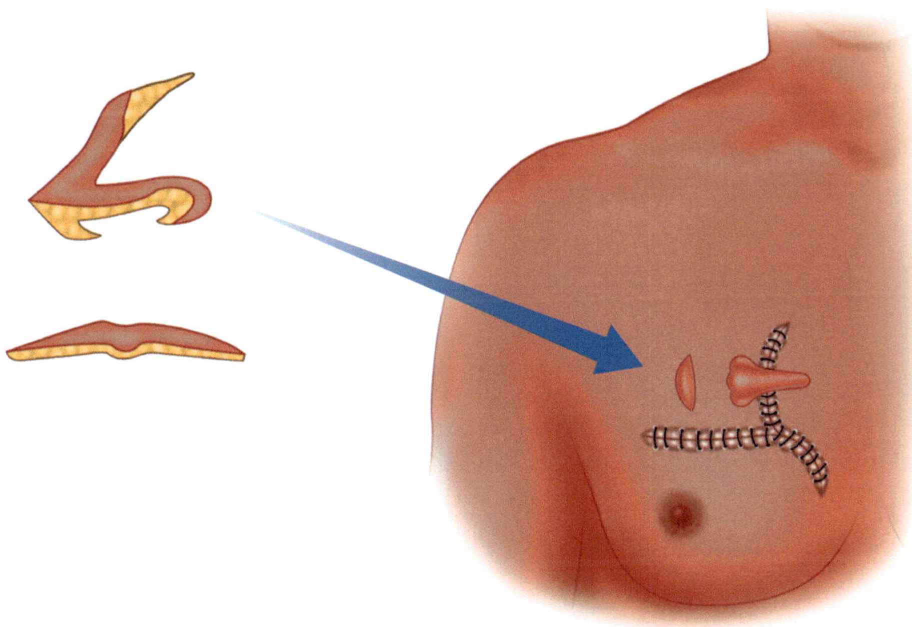

Fig. 20.14 Preconstructed anterior chest flap for reconstruction of total nasal and upper lip defect: implantation of nasal and upper lip struts

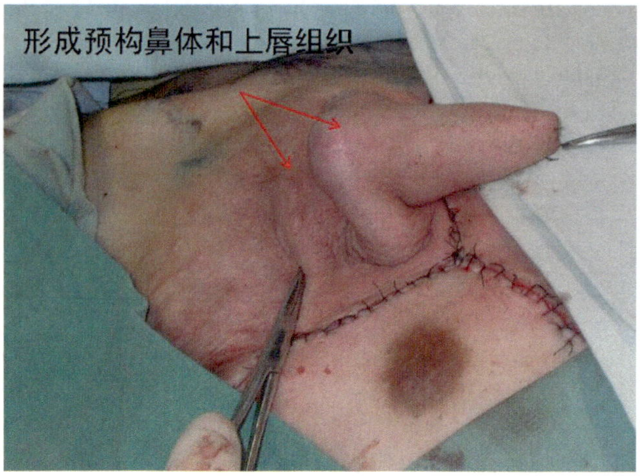

Fig. 20.15 Preconstructed nasal and lip structures at the chest flap

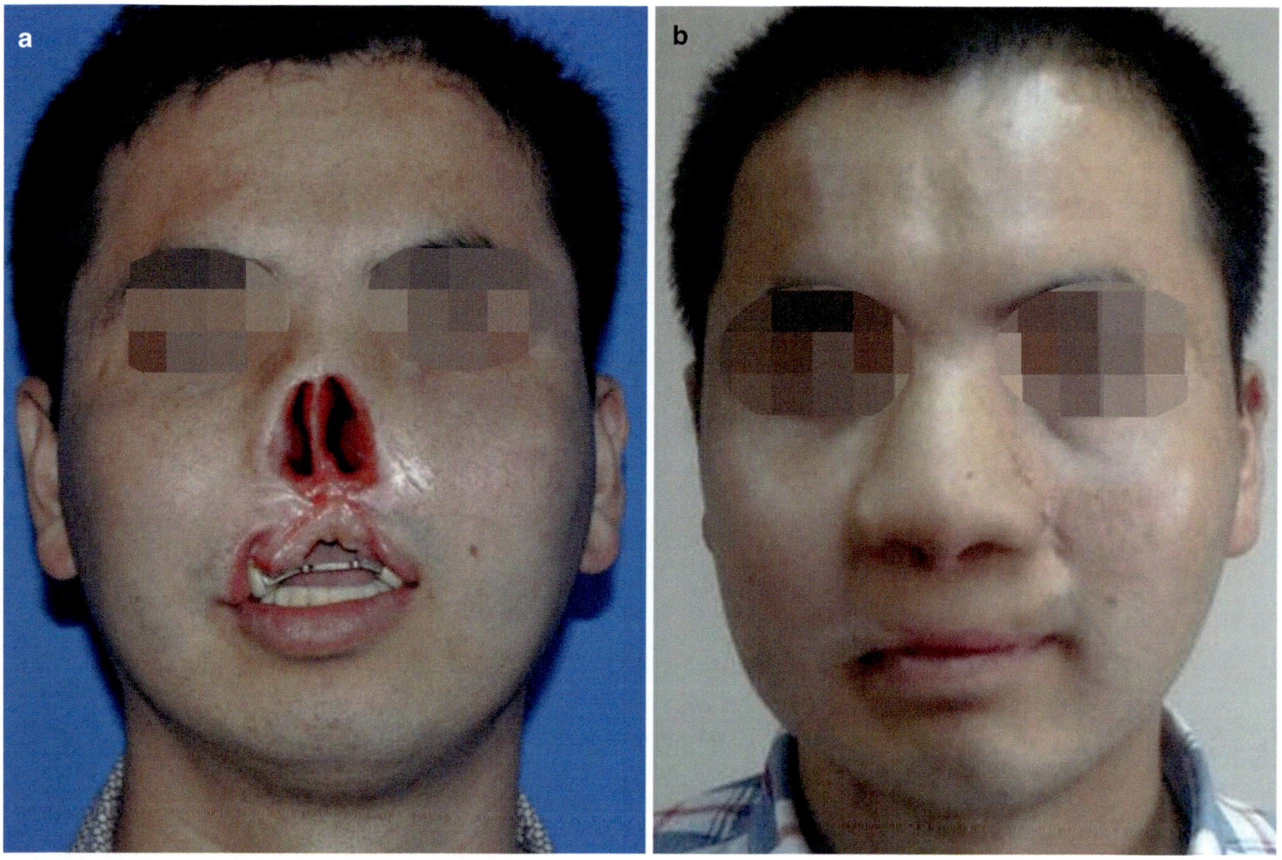

Fig. 20.16 (**a**, **b**) Typical case. (**a**) Patient with complete loss of external nose and most of the upper lip due to trauma 3 years ago. (**b**) One year after total nose and lip reconstruction using preconstructed anterior chest flap

References

1. Jang YJ, Alfanta EM. Rhinoplasty in the Asian nose. Facial Plast Surg Clin North Am. 2014;22(3):357–77.
2. Shu-Xia Z. Collected works of surgery: oral and maxillofacial surgery (in Chinese). 1st ed. Beijing: Military Science Publishing House; 1994. p. 225–36.

GPSR Compliance

The European Union's (EU) General Product Safety Regulation (GPSR) is a set of rules that requires consumer products to be safe and our obligations to ensure this.

If you have any concerns about our products, you can contact us on ProductSafety@springernature.com

In case Publisher is established outside the EU, the EU authorized representative is:

Springer Nature Customer Service Center GmbH
Europaplatz 3
69115 Heidelberg, Germany

Batch number: 09231230

Printed by Printforce, the Netherlands